The Complete Guide to
Food Allergies and Environmental Illness

By the same author:

The Allergy Handbook
The Food Allergy Plan
Allergies: What Everyone Should Know

The Complete Guide to

Food Allergies and Environmental Illness

Dr Keith Mumby

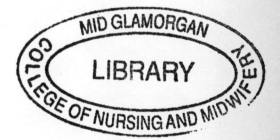

Thorsons
An Imprint of HarperCollins*Publishers*

Thorsons
An Imprint of HarperCollins*Publishers*
77–85 Fulham Palace Road,
Hammersmith, London W6 8JB

Published by Thorsons 1993
10 9 8 7 6 5 4 3 2 1

Keith Mumby asserts the moral right to
be identified as the author of this work

A catalogue record for this book
is available from the British Library

ISBN 0 7225 2504 4

Typeset by Harper Phototypesetters Limited,
Northampton, England
Printed in Great Britain by
Mackays of Chatham, Kent

To Pauline, who for a quarter of a century has been my loyal companion

Contents

Introduction 9

1. Air Purification 15
2. Alcohol 17
3. Algae 19
4. Alkali Salts Therapy 19
5. Allergy: A Definition 20
6. Anaphylaxis 22
7. Antinutrients 23
8. Anti-oxidants 24
9. Applied Kinesiology: A Way of Testing for Allergies 26
10. Atmospheric Pollution 27
11. Body Load 29
12. Brain Allergy 31
13. Bread 34
14. Brucellosis 35
15. Caffeine 35
16. Candida 36
17. Carbon Monoxide 40
18. Challenge Testing 41
19. Chemical Cleanup 42
20. Chronic Viral Infections 46
21. Co-enzyme Q10 48
22. Conventional Allergy Tests 49
23. Cyclical and Fixed Allergies 51
24. Cytotoxic Tests 51
25. Dermatitis 53
26. Detoxification 54
27. Diets 57
28. Diseases Caused by Allergies 63
29. Dowsing 65
30. Drugs for Allergies 65
31. The Dynamics of Food 66
32. Electrical Fields and Allergies 67
33. Endorphins 70
34. Environmental Allergies 71
35. Environmental Control Units 76
36. Enzyme Potentiated Desensitization 78
37. Enzyme Supplementation 81
38. Essential Fatty Acids 82
39. Flatulence 83
40. Fluoride 84
41. Food Additives 84

42. Formaldehyde 86
43. Garlic 87
44. General Adaptation Syndrome 88
45. Geopathic Stress 90
46. Gut Flora 94
47. Hair Analysis for Minerals 95
48. The Hay System 97
49. Hidden Allergy 98
50. Histamine and Mast Cells 99
51. Hormones and Allergy 100
52. Hyperactivity and Minimal Brain Dysfunction 102
53. Hypersensitivity 104
54. Hyperventilation 106
55. Hypoglycaemia 108
56. The Immune System 112
57. Inborn Errors of Metabolism/ Enzyme Deficiency 118
58. Insect Stings 119
59. Intestinal Fermentation 120
60. Ionizers 122
61. Irradiation of Foods 122
62. Lactose Intolerance 123
63. Lead 124
64. Leaky Gut Syndrome 125
65. Lectins 126
66. Magnesium 126
67. Malabsorption 127
68. Mental Retardation 129
69. Mercury Toxicity 129
70. Metal Allergies 133
71. Microwaves and the Electromagnetic Spectrum 134
72. Migraine and Headaches 136
73. Milk 137
74. Miller's Method 138
75. Moulds 141
76. Mycotoxins 143
77. Natural Gas 144
78. Nitrates 144
79. Nitrous Oxide 145
80. Noise 146
81. Nutrition and Allergies 147
82. Osteoporosis 153

83. Parasites 155
84. Peroxidation 158
85. Pesticides and Health 159
86. Phenolic Testing 162
87. Plant Toxins 164
88. Post Viral Fatigue Syndrome 167
89. Preconceptual Health Care 169
90. Premenstrual Tension (PMT) 172
91. Probiotics 173
92. Prostaglandins 174
93. Pulse Testing 175
94. Radon 178
95. Rotation Diets 178
96. Salicylates 182
97. Seasonal Affective Disorder 183
98. Sexual Hypersensitivities 185
99. Sick Building Syndrome 188
100. Stress 191
101. Sudden Infant Death Syndrome (SIDS) 193
102. Sugar 194

103. Symptoms Table 195
104. Target Organs 198
105. Terpenes 199
106. Thermal Chamber Depuration 200
107. Universal Reactors 202
108. Urine Therapy 203
109. Vega Machine 205
110. Water 207
111. Weather and Health 208
112. Zinc 209

Appendix A: Food Families 211
Appendix B: Food Contacts List 213
Appendix C: Chemical Pollutants in the Home 216
Appendix D: Top Ten Allergens 218
Appendix E: Seven-day Stone Age Diet Menu Plan 219
Recommended Reading 224
Bibliography 226
Useful Addresses 228

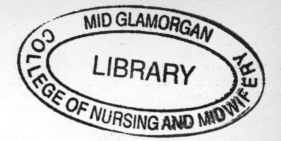
Introduction

It gave me a great deal of pleasure when Thorsons approached me about writing this book. There was something stirring about the idea of a *complete* guide. Alas, the more we worked on the planning the more it became clear that such a work would take up several volumes and that writing it would be almost impossible. This is a rapidly advancing field of knowledge: the facts are highly volatile and evolve continually. What may be a comprehensive statement could be incomplete and misleading within a matter of months. My aim, therefore, has really been to provide more of a comprehensive overview than meticulous detail.

THE BEGINNINGS

Allergy and environmental medicine began merely as an 'alternative' branch of science, as all new discoveries do; then moved into the van of medical research and progress; now it is becoming an independent corps of data, with its own unique philosophy and ethic. We share a lot of ground with conventional therapeutics but as practitioners our centre is a little way beyond the perimeter of orthodox medicine. The subject has really surpassed the confines of merely holistic healing and overlapped onto the social, political and economic agenda.

We call our modern medical interest in how the environment can make us ill *clinical ecology*. Practitioners would be called *clinical ecologists*, though I should stress that when consulting a clinical ecologist you should ensure the practitioner is medically qualified before undertaking to follow treatment. There *are* those who have moved into this field without proper medical qualifications. There is no possibility of such individuals being competent or safe without adequate medical training. The fact that most doctors are ignorant of this branch

of medicine does not excuse commercial opportunism by unqualified imitators.

Some doctors avoid the term clinical ecologist, since they want to dissociate themselves from this group. They also feel uncomfortable with the similarity to what they see as activist groups using the ecological banner. I prefer the term allergy and environmental medicine, since it is manifestly a much greater issue than just allergies and food intolerance. Clinical ecology remains a commonly used term, however, and so has been retained throughout this book.

The issues have been around a long time, but it could be said that clinical ecology began as a movement in the 1950s, with fears about radiation pollution, particularly the health risks of strontium-90. This dangerous substance was a product of fall-out from atmospheric testing of nuclear weapons. It passes from grass to cow's milk and is then taken up into bones in place of calcium, which it resembles. Its *half-life* (the time taken for half the initial dose to fade and disappear) is about 30 years. During that time, and of course for many years afterwards, it continues to irradiate bone marrow, which is where leukaemia strikes. We began to worry about the health hazards of drinking milk.

Then came fears of cancer-causing chemicals. How safe were we? A major milestone came with the proven link between lung cancer and smoking. People often forget that this is an 'environmental' illness, caused by a pollutant. Suddenly, there was no question that long-term exposure to foreign (*xenobiotic*) chemicals could be dangerous. Naturally, those responsible for the pollution denied there was any real risk. And gradually, individuals began to suspect advice and reassurances given by official government bodies. It was clear that scientists were being corrupted by vested interests and this realization itself was something of a betrayal and shock to the populace at large.

Attention soon switched to the fact that many of these potentially hazardous substances were appearing in our food. Anxiety about this issue was not helped by revelations such as the IBT scandal, in which it was found that safety tests on toxic agents were being 'fixed' to keep customers (the chemical companies) happy. Nor did it end there: during the time I have been preparing this manuscript, directors of a company marketing a sugar substitute were indicted for conducting so-called safety tests which included snipping off tumours from mice that developed cancers and reporting the results as satisfactory. Surprisingly – unbelievably, some might say – this food substance is still on the market and being sold to the public.

Add to this acid rain and atmospheric pollution, which is powerful enough to strip down the fabric of buildings, never mind our sensitive biological tissues, and we have the beginnings of a ghastly ecological nightmare for which doctors like myself were simply not prepared by our cosy medical school training. It has been a shock awakening. In Europe alone, 25 million tons of sulphur dioxide land annually on our environment in rainfall. There is understandable anxiety about what it is doing to the real estate and works of art, and even concern about what is happening to the ecosystem, but not nearly enough interest in what it is doing to ourselves.

CONTROVERSY

It has been joked that there are several stages in the development of a new medical idea:

1. 'You are mad.'
2. 'There might be something in it.'
3. 'There might be something in it, but where is the proof?'
4. 'Of course, we knew all along.'

If this is the case, we are somewhere in stage 3 at present, in respect of clinical ecology. There are already signs of stage 4. The debate hotted up recently when the Allergy and Immunology section of the Royal College of Physicians (who are still in stage 1) tried to force everyone else to accept their point of view with the publication in April 1992 of a report entitled, 'Allergy: Conventional and Alternative Concepts'. Newer methods, they stated, were fraudulent or, at best, unproven. They refused even to make mention of many published, good scientific papers that appeared to contradict their entrenched stance. Patients who claimed they had been helped were merely deluded and/or benefiting from the placebo effect. Any practitioners who claimed scientific validity for their findings about food allergies were branded fools or rogues. It was, as the late Lawrence Dickey, clinical ecologist and author used to say, 'an effective blow for ignorance'.

It is probably a cause of considerable dismay to the public at large to realize that the medical profession would stoop to this sort of political manoeuvring. The important point to remember is that it is only a few doctors who are so virulently opposed to environmental medicine; their views are not representative of the medical profession as a whole.

It seems there are those who cannot accept that anything new and important can be discovered in their lifetime. Human progress is something, evidently, from the past. Yet these are exciting times to live in and be part of. It is true, we are in the throes of a medical revolution. But I can make that seem less of a cliché by pointing out that we are, in many senses, going *backwards* towards the Earth wisdom of our ancestors. Really, it is the 'drug revolution' that is coming to an end, at the same time that new discoveries in the realm of ecology make it very opportune that this should be so.

When the drug companies are attempting to tighten their grip, using government-backed legislation to protect their monopoly, people are opting out altogether. Many are rightly concerned about drugs; some are outright afraid and not without reason.

The truth is the drug boom is over. After 30 years of hegemony, it has been exposed for what it is – a sham. The dream of universal health and magical cures for a vast array of ills, simply by popping a few pills, just hasn't happened. Instead, patients have become increasingly frightened of drug treatment, with its frequent unpleasant side-effects and manifest dangers.

This isn't to say that drugs have no place in medicine. They can and do save lives; penicillin is one of the greatest gifts Nature has given humanity, second only to fire as an aid to our survival. But those kinds of drugs are in a tiny minority. The vast bulk of substances pushed by the profit-hungry chemical cartels are useless or worse. The problem comes with long-term medication. Even conscientious and caring doctors seem oblivious to the irony that, by definition, chronic drug treatment *doesn't work*. If it cured, there would be no need to go on taking it!

At best these kinds of drugs can only suppress symptoms. But at a price. If the underlying destructive process of the disease isn't altered or stopped, then the body continues to deteriorate and the patient is given a false sense of security. There is the *apparency* that the treatment is helping, when in fact it is doing no good whatsoever. By disguising the damage, the patient may be ill served.

Also, there is the vexed question of side-effects. No drug is free of this problem, though some are worse than others. It may be very hard for a patient to live with constant symptoms he or she knows are being caused by medication. This is made even more disconcerting when the doctor under-rates the unpleasantness of these symptoms, or refuses to believe in their existence, but considers the treatment approach an unqualified success.

THE SOIL AND SEED

One of the inevitable results of the overuse of drugs and their fundamental ineffect-uality, is that the search for real causes is obscured.

Take a disease like tuberculosis. Anti-biotics now exist that can treat this condition and save lives, by killing the microbe that causes it (*Mycobacterium tuberculosis*). This puts firmly into the doctor's mind that TB is 'caused' by a bacterium. This was the sensation of medicine in the last century, the so-called 'germ theory of disease', pro-pounded by Louis Pasteur who became (quite rightly) famous as his ideas gained credence.

But it isn't at all that simple. These microbes abound everywhere, but we do not all fall prey to their pathogenic potential. Why is this? Well, the reason probably varies from case to case but it is certain that there is some weakening factor at work in those who get TB. Isn't this the *real* cause of the disease and the microbe just an opportunist?

TB is a good example because, although often cited as one of the greatest successes of modern medicine, it isn't really. The actual reason for the drop in incidence of TB isn't science or drugs at all, but improved economic factors. Poverty as it once existed is not virtually unknown in the Western world. As a result, individuals are better nourished today than ever before and have more resistance to disease. The long-term figures for mortality in TB (see Figure I.1) show a declining trend that began long before the era of modern drugs and vaccinations.

We call this a question of susceptibility, as opposed to consideration solely of the effect of pathogens (disease-causing organisms), the 'soil and seed' theory. The germs are the seeds; but whether they grow successfully and flourish, to produce a disease, depends on the character of the soil – that is, the resistance of the patient.

This brings us to the idea of the individual in medicine, which is really what charac-terizes the allergy and environmental approach. In fact, it is one of the major differences in 'philosophy' between the new and the old. Dr Theron Randolph, one of the founding figures of the clinical ecology movement, coined the expressions *exogenous* and *endogenous* medicine, to describe the two opposite ends of the spectrum. According to this view, exogeny is disease caused from without, i.e., environmentally. Endogeny is a failure from within. The second type of medicine conceives of patients only as sick people, something decrepit and malfunctioning, rather like broken-down machinery. Exogeny would see everyone as inherently

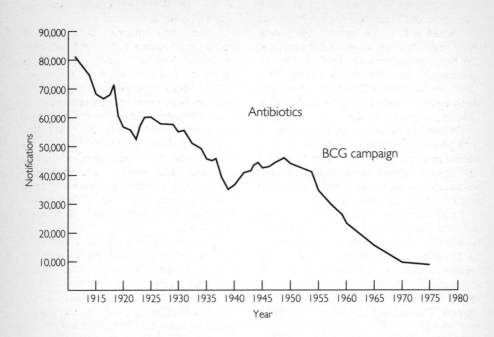

Figure 1.1: Respiratory tuberculosis notifications in England and Wales, 1912–1975. (Note the interruption of the downward trend due to the Second World War.)
Abstracted from CMO report for 1976 (London: HMSO, 1977)

healthy but for some exterior factor making them sick.

Modern medicine is endogenously orientated and its laboratory-based, reductionist, analytic, bodily-centred approach has come to dominate medicine almost entirely. Its techniques are expensive and applications complex. Without the support of Big Business and profit-making organizations it probably couldn't function at all. The clinical ecology alternative, on the other hand, is simplistic, deductive and environmentally-orientated. Patients can apply it and get well easily and inexpensively.

Unfortunately, as Randolph points out, the split between these two views and the shift in emphasis entirely to endogenous therapeutics occurred before the field of allergy and environmental medicine had developed fully. If this had not been so, it is quite possible, he argues, that the endogenous approach would not have become so firmly entrenched, though this is to ignore, somewhat naively, the influence of vested interest.

Instead, today, we have what Randolph calls a diagnostico-therapeutic gap, that is a great indifference to the actual nature and causation of disease and, instead, an almost rigid fixation on studying how to treat its end-result (symptoms). The body and its counter-role in illness is heavily subordinated to the characteristics and properties of the supposed 'pathogens'.

INTERNAL ECOLOGY

I'd like to add my own contribution to the debate by introducing the term 'internal ecology'. The concept is very simple. We live in an age that is increasingly conscious of environmental issues. It must now be obvious to all, except those who live in unimaginable isolation, that if we go on as we are doing – polluting our world, wrecking the balance of Nature, plundering its non-renewable resources and generally making a mess of things – that life on this planet will shortly become totally untenable.

Yet we seem to be doing just as much damage to our inner world of the body and its tissues and, so far, not enough people have really become aware of the problem. We have been poisoning and pillaging just as profligately but stealing something even more precious: the ability of our remarkable body defence systems to cope with the rising tide of *personal* pollution.

I'm not just talking about food additives and pesticides, which is about the limit of media awareness. We have radically altered the internal balance in our bodies, through constant exposure to a number of new hostile aspects of our environment.

Chief among these would be modern food sources, many of which we haven't had time to adapt to. Many are very poor nutritionally and we have undoubtedly added to the problems our immune systems face by distorted or inadequate nourishment. This is a problem that goes deeper than mere food allergy. The question of food quality affects everybody.

It is also true that we live under a virtual pall of chemical poisons, rained down on us from the atmosphere, polluting our water supplies and loaded onto our food. It is all in the bizarre belief that it is somehow beneficial for the human race; we are supposed to need these substances for our ultimate good; we are told repeatedly that none of it is harmful to health.

The fact is, nobody knows what the full long-term effect of this chemical onslaught will be, but you can be certain that our immune systems are among the first to suffer. Some individuals are already experiencing difficulties; hence the idea of 'human canaries'. Soon we will all follow. The warning bells have never sounded more clearly than in these closing few years of the millenium.

We live in an environment bombarded by electromagnetic radiation which simply didn't exist a century ago. The term 'electric smog' has been coined. Radio waves, radar and microwaves permeate our planet so completely that it is not possible to find anywhere on Earth to escape exposure to this unseen and little understood 'pollution'. We cannot measure what effect it has on our tissues, long or short term, except that there is new and disturbing evidence that this 'electric smog' is far from safe.

If that isn't enough, then we have destroyed or altered the normal pattern of our bowel flora by constant use and some would say abuse of broad-spectrum antibiotics. Very few people in this day and age have not been given at least one course of these ubiquitous drugs; many have had staggering quantities over the years. The result has been a virtual epidemic of opportunistic infections of the Candida sort, including other moulds. The intestine – with its dark moisture and warmth – is an ideal environment for many of these microorganisms and they flourish there quite successfully.

We are seeing so many cases that it has become almost the norm and this makes it difficult for some doctors to grasp what is really happening. There is the additional problem of malabsorption caused by so much unfamiliar growth in the gastrointestinal tract. The invaders interfere with the proper selection and processing of carbohydrates, proteins, fats, vitamins and minerals, which in turn leads back to the nutritional deficit I referred to above. Moulds also suppress the immune system, so it becomes a very convoluted, multilayered problem.

Perhaps the real question isn't 'Why are more and more people becoming ill?' but rather, 'How is it that some of us are able to remain well, despite the steadily increasing pall of toxins to which we are subjecting ourselves?' This at least would put the emphasis in the right place. We need to study the body's resources and learn how to strengthen them, before digging ever deeper into the complex detailed mechanisms of disease.

TAKE ACTION YOURSELF

I am not suggesting we go back to a medieval ecology. We all enjoy the benefits of science and technology. I would simply suggest that we begin to spend some of our vast industrial budgets on the development of safety precautions and better methods of production and disposal. This will mean exposing those who currently claim there is no problem, along with the politicians who will insist on putting the interests of big business above the common good of the people whom they are supposed to represent.

It seems there is little point in waiting for governments to act or scientific integrity to come back into fashion. Instead, clinical ecology has become very much a 'people's medicine'. For many years public awareness and personal action in health issues of this sort have been far ahead of medical competence or willingness to act. There is good and bad in this. It means no one need wait for help; the principles can be applied by anyone. But unfortunately, it has resulted in a lot of what I regard as unscientific nonsense gaining common coinage, which further compounds the problem, because unsympathetic doctors can scoff. This makes it harder for practitioners like myself, who would like to build bridges with the medical establishment.

The final answer to the myths and ignorance is knowledge and I have written this work with that in mind. Here, for the first time, are the key facts about allergy and environmental medicine, from a doctor who practises it every day and has done for 15 years. It is the 'state of the art' at present but I have tried to indicate where it is evolving rapidly. With intelligence and persistence, you should be able to use it to attain relief from illnesses of the type described and for which, previously, you have had little help.

Richard Mackarness, a consultant psychiatrist and writer who virtually brought the clinical ecology revolution to medicine in the UK, once wrote to me, 'Every idea has its time. The time of clinical ecology is now!' This heartfelt statement has only become truer with the passage of years.

Finally . . .

A word about references. It could be considered usual with a book of this genre to provide a comprehensive list of source references. Although putting across the facts is an end in itself, it is looked upon as good practice to give the origin of one's information.

After some consideration, I decided not to do this. My own personal preference is the avoidance of footnotes, which look unattractive in a text. On the other hand, confining all the notes to the end of the book, indexed to numbers in the relevant pages, is both distracting and time-consuming for the reader.

I realize that I will incur some criticism from professional colleagues for this omission. The fact is, however, that this volume has been conceived from the first as a layman's guide. It is the *only* fully comprehensive text in this field and, as such, I hope it will prove invaluable for doctors as well as laymen, but the style and approach are intended for the general reader.

This book is filled with my opinions, some of them forceful. I hold it to be a good fortune in life rather than a handicap to see things vividly, uncluttered by compromises. I do not share the thirst for obliquity and moderation that seems to be the fashion these days. You are free to disagree with any views you wish.

KEITH MUMBY
Manchester 1993

1. Air Purification

It isn't realistic to expect to achieve an environment that is 100-per-cent controlled, except in an **environmental control unit (35)**. Nevertheless there is a lot of good sense in trying to *reduce* indoor air pollution in order to lessen **body load (11)**. Some people will find the equipment below very useful, enabling restful nights and symptom-free days, perhaps for the first time; others will benefit only little and find trying to tackle inhalant particles and gases not worth the trouble. People vary and there are no hard-and-fast rules. A little experimentation is recommended. Good manufacturers and suppliers will often lend you equipment on an approval basis, so you have a chance to try it first.

FACE MASKS

There are situations where a multiply-sensitive person may want to wear a protective mask, for example when cleaning in a dusty enclosed space. However it is not a good idea to get into the habit of using artificial aids on a semi-permanent basis. Often this means little more than psychological dependence that may not have any relation to scientific removal of impurities.

There are different types of mask. Lightweight, cotton surgical masks strain out particles such as pollen, dust and smoke. People sensitive to wheat and flours who work in the catering industry may need one of these. They are *not* completely effective against particles.

For chemical vapours you may need an activated-charcoal filter mask. There are many simple versions of this design which, in its full form, is the gas-mask worn by troops in combat. Suppliers claim these are effective against benzene, ozone, diesel fumes, **lead (63)**, hydrocarbons, **nitrous oxide (79)** and sulphur dioxide. Most people would probably benefit from one of these masks when encountering smog.

AIR FILTERS

If you can't face the expense of major household air-conditioning, consider a small, mobile system. These can be used to create a clean local environment. Standards are variable and if possible you should try out a model before buying. Especially to be avoided are those with the deplorable addition of scents and 'fresh air' perfumes. There are portable models for the car that plug into the car's cigarette lighter socket.

ACTIVATED CARBON FILTERS

These are fairly effective at absorbing cooking and food smells, cigarette and tobacco odours, perfumes, diesel and petrol fumes, smog, ozone and animal smells. They are less effective against pollen, smoke, mildew, chlorine, fish odour and some noxious gases. They seem to be poor at combating **carbon monoxide (17)** and **formaldehyde (42)**.

ELECTROSTATIC AIR CLEANERS

A fan draws in particles and these are then given an electric charge that causes them to stick onto a screen or plate. Manufacturers claim they remove 90 per cent of particles. In fact performance falls off very rapidly and within days the unit may be less than 50 per cent effective. This type of purifier also needs constant cleaning and maintenance.

Another problem is that charged particles that 'escape' the screen or plate stick on walls and furniture and can cause a significant build up. This type of filter may also produce ozone, a highly toxic gas that causes headaches in some people.

Particle Size of Common Air Pollutants
(IN MICRONS)
1 MICRON = 1 MICROMETRE = 1 MILLIONTH OF A METRE

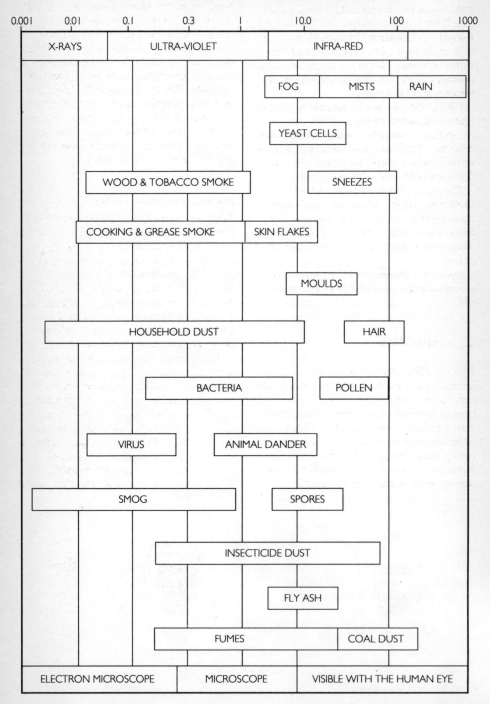

HIGH EFFICIENCY PARTICULATE AIR (HEPA) FILTERS

These are over 95 per cent efficient for particles down to about 0.1 micron in size (see Table 1.1), according to the US National Bureau of Standards. Predictably they are also quite expensive. They are sometimes called *absolute filters* and are used to maintain sterile air in hospital operating theatres and burns units.

HEPA filters work particularly well against important sensitizing allergens such as pollens, moulds, yeasts, fungi and bacteria. They are also effective against viruses, which means they may help to cut down on colds and other infections.

The only licensed company I know producing HEPA filtration units for the home and light commercial units is National Safety Associates (see Useful Addresses). They also operate a 'try before you buy' policy.

Also see **atmospheric pollution (10)**, **environmental allergies (34)** and **ionizers (60)**

2. Alcohol

Ethyl alcohol (ethanol) is consumed in vast quantities all over the world, indicating just how pleasurable most people find mild degrees of intoxication. There is little doubt that a meal without wine doesn't have the same warm glow that is so important to easing social tensions. The problem comes when this goes too far; excessive intake impairs your health (see Figure 2.1).

Short-term side-effects of drinking, such as hangover, are said to depend on 'impurities', particularly the presence of other alcohols such as isoamyl alcohol, which are known as *congeners*. Brandy contains the highest percentage of congeners and this gives it its rich aromatic smell – enhanced by gentle warming, which increases vaporization of these secondary alcohols. Clinical ecologists believe, however, that allergic reactions to foodstuffs contained in intoxicating drinks such as yeast, wheat, corn, sugar and other ingredients are also a major cause of the negative after-effects of drinking.

FOOD ALLERGY AND ALCOHOL

The great doyen of clinical ecology, Theron Randolph, likens alcoholic beverages to 'jet propelled food allergy'. Food allergics seem to suffer far worse reactions to drink than the rest of the population; indeed, for years I have regarded this as a fast rule-of-thumb criterion for food allergy. Wheat, for example, may be tolerated in some forms by a wheat-allergic, but when part of a small tot of whisky can put the patient in bed!

All alcoholic beverages contain yeast by definition. Also, there are many potential 'additives', including sulphites and other antiseptics, letting down agents in wine such as ethylene glycol (anti-freeze), asbestos, clay, seaweed, polyvinylpyrrolidine, citric acid, tannic acid, fumaric acid, sorbates, arsenic and monosodium glutamate. This doesn't mean all drinks include these substances, of course; simply that they may.

 I Unit =

single measure of spirit (¹/₆ gill)   I glass of wine   ¹/₂ pint of beer   I glass of sherry

Figure 2.1: Alcohol equivalents of I unit (8 gm)

	Corn	Wheat, barley, rye	Oats	Rice	Potatoes	Grapes	Plum	Citrus	Cherry	Apples	Hops	Juniper	Cinnamon	Mint	Miscellaneous herbs	Cactus	Beet sugar	Cane sugar
Always present = ● **Sometimes present = ○**																		
Blended Scotch Whisky	●	●															○	○
Malt Scotch Whisky	○	●															○	○
Canadian Blended Whisky	●	●				●	●	○									○	●
Irish Whisky		●	●															○
Blended Irish Whisky	●	●	●		●	●	○									○	○	
Gin (Grain)	●	●	○	○				●				●	○	○	●		○	○
Gin (Cane) High & Dry												●	●	●	●			●
Vodka					○												●	●
Jamaican Rum																		●
Tequila																●		●
Beer	●	●	○	●							●							
Grape Brandy	○					●											○	○
Cordials & Liqueurs	●	●	○	○	○	●	●	●	●	●			●	●	●		●	●
Grape Wine	○					●											●	●
Sherry	●					●											●	●
Champagne					●											●		
Cider	●									●							●	●
Vermouth	○	○	○			●											●	●
Cognac						●											○	○
Cherry Brandy	○								●								○	○

Please note that yeast occurs in all alcoholic beverages

Figure 2.2: Food contents of some alcoholic beverages
(Acknowledgements to Dr Theron Randolph)

The real trouble seems to comes from the foodstuffs themselves. For that reason I have reproduced Theron Randolph's important table of ingredients for most common alcoholic beverages (Figure 2.2). Remember, this is only a guide; individual products vary greatly. This is meant to help you to know what to look for.

Certain general observations will also help you make the right choice. Beers and stouts are the worst tolerated of all. Dry cider and dry white wine (including champagne), without contaminants, are the best tolerated. Red wine is usually disastrous since it may contain a hundred times the amount of histamine found in similar white wines. Spirits are surprisingly well taken, but people vary.

Experiment for yourself and be honest about what you find and the limitations this imposes on you.

Also see **detoxification (26)** and **phenolic testing (86)**

3. Algae

In the summer of 1989 a new ecological threat came literally to the surface in the UK when dogs and sheep died after drinking water polluted by toxic blue-green algae. Since then other incidents have been reported and this algae appears to be a growing menace to human populations.

Input of nutrients to our drinking water supplies, especially phosphates from sewage treatment works and **nitrates (78)** from agriculture run-off (called *eutrophication*), seems to favour the establishment of these tiny single-celled organisms. Warm weather is needed to enhance their multiplication. Slow-moving or stagnant water masses are particularly at risk, for example reservoirs. The result is an algal 'bloom'.

Of themselves these blooms would probably cause no more trouble than cloudy water, but certain algae produce toxins. The chief offender is *Microcystis aeruginosa*. It manufactures a highly poisonous chemical known as *Microcystin*, which is released into the water when the cells die. This is what killed dogs and livestock in the 1989 scare, though not all blooms of Microcystis

produce the toxin.

There are other possible culprits. At least five other species of blue-green algae capable of producing toxins have been identified in British waters. The extent of the problem worldwide is not known.

Microcystin is a potent liver toxin. Death can occur within hours or even minutes of drinking contaminated water. No human fatalities have been reported to date, but there was an outbreak of liver damage in 1983 in one Australian locality caused by a Microcystis bloom. Different strains of algae may also be responsible for outbreaks of gastro-intestinal upsets, rashes, vomiting, diarrhoea, fever and eye inflammations. This is a new area and research is continuing.

Note: granular activated carbon filters (see **air purification (1)**) should be competent against mycrocystin, provided they are changed regularly.

Also see **gut flora (46)**, **mycotoxins (76)**, **sudden infant death syndrome (101)** and **water (110)**

4. Alkali Salts Therapy

In 1949, Detroit surgeon Harry G. Clark formulated a hypothesis concerning allergic reactions. He reasoned that since the end-products of digestion were acids and since the allergic inflammation process accelerated intracellular breakdown, it must be bringing about an acidic state.

Theoretically then, therapy with bicarbonate salts of sodium and potassium might be helpful in treating an acute allergic reaction. On this basis they were tried and found to be extremely beneficial. The earlier they are administered the better – after the first 24 hours they may tend to make things worse.

A mixture of two parts sodium bicarbonate to one part potassium bicarbonate is normally recommended. These can be mixed in advance and, indeed, a number of proprietary products are now available with these two salts. Malic acid may be added, merely as a flavour enhancer (otherwise the taste is rather bitter).

The usual dose is a heaped teaspoon in

half a tumbler of water. This can be repeated two or three times a day but should not be used excessively, as this can be dangerous.

Also, don't forget that it makes good sense to take Epsom Salts or some other simple vegetable purge (such as Senokot) if you have swallowed something that has caused a severe reaction. The faster it is cleared from the body, the better.

Also see **anti-oxidants (8)**, **drugs for allergies (30)** and **dynamics of food (31)**

5. Allergy: A Definition

Undoubtedly, a major part of the controversy surrounding the new allergy movement, also known as clinical ecology, has been argument about the definition of the term 'allergy'.

The word was first coined by an Austrian paediatrician, Clemens von Pirquet, in 1906. He defined an allergy as an acquired, specific, altered capacity to react to a physical substance on the part of the tissues of the body. This description is worth considering in more detail:

Acquired means that it is not in-born or constitutional, though there is no doubt that the *tendency* to allergies runs in families. In what is now the 'classic' allergic reaction, an individual must meet the substance (at least once) and the allergy results from this initial sensitizing encounter.

Babies that appear to be born with an allergy do not really conflict with this theory. It's just that they made their first contact while in the womb (with, for example, a food in the mother's diet).

Specific means that it is not a generalized reaction but relates to one exact substance or, in reality, often a small part of a molecule of that substance. An individual may react to many things at once but each reaction is unique. Even if several *allergens* (allergy-causing substances) provoke the same effect, it is simply that the final end-organ stimulated is the same in each case (see **target organs (104)**).

Altered means the reaction is not 'normal'. In other words, not everyone shares the same experience. The majority of our species would probably *not* react in the way an allergic patient does. For example, most of us eat tomatoes safely, yet some people cannot do so without risking a severe asthma attack or some other unpleasant consequence.

However, there are difficulties in this last interpretation. Once you start to move outside the immunological guidelines for an allergy, phenomena such as an allergy to wheat become very common. Probably half the population or more don't tolerate it anything like as well as they suppose, once you start asking the right questions. We may retain the adjective 'altered' perhaps, but such reactions may be anything but rare or unusual.

Furthermore, when it comes to a matter such as low-grade poisoning (see below), then substances that induce symptoms are toxic for everyone. 'Allergy' then becomes only a matter of degree. Sensitive people react to levels of the toxin that would be tolerated by the average individual.

In the 1920s the sort of reaction von Pirquet was talking about was commonly found to have an immunological basis, i.e. it was an antigen-antibody phenomenon (see **immune system (56)**). Apparently, the body was responding to foreign protein (and even food is considered 'foreign' by the body since it is 'non-self' protein, namely complex polysaccharides and fats) by mounting an antibody attack. The spin-off from this interaction, rather like fall-out from a chemical battle, was what gave rise to the unwanted and inappropriate symptoms experienced by the patient.

There is something radically wrong, however, with this simplistic and narrow definition, though immunologists cling to it like a raft at sea. The great paradox – as pointed out by Professor John Soothill – is that if this explanation were true, we all ought to get allergic reactions to food every time we eat. Obviously this doesn't happen. Somehow the body knows *not* to react against food protein.

Notwithstanding this inconsistency, since the 1920s the definition of allergies has been entirely an immunological one. Any reaction outside this perimeter has been considered conveniently to be 'not an allergy'. The fact that such reactions do seem to exist, and have been reported often, has been ignored. The patients' symptoms are apparently 'all in the mind'.

Unfortunately for those who stand by this rhetoric, even as early as 1920 Dr Albert Rowe and others were able to demonstrate that there were clear reactions to ingested substances and that these could be established to exist beyond any doubt, regardless of the lack of adequate explanation. Since these reactions also accord with von Pirquet's original definition, there seemed nothing wrong with calling them allergy – in this case, food allergy.

There was no real controversy at the time, since Rowe was not an internationally-known figure. He continued his seminal researches, wrote his book *Food Allergy: Its Manifestations, Diagnosis and Treatment* (Lea and Febiger, Philadelphia, 1931) and departed the world stage. However, his successors, notably Randolph, Rinkel and Zeller, authors of *Food Allergy* (Charles C. Thomas, Springfield, Illinois, 1951), carried on Rowe's work and, particularly since the 1950s, the proof that dietary allergies could exist without there being any demonstrable antibodies became steadily more and more compelling – to the embarrassment of immunologists. If these immunologists admitted the existence of food allergy at all, they'd say it was 'very rare' and applied only to a very tiny minority of the population. Randolph, Rinkel and Zeller were finding far too many cases.

As the debate hotted up in the 1970s and 1980s the two groups polarized and antagonism grew more unpleasant. The term 'food intolerance' was introduced in a booklet published jointly in 1984 by the Royal College of Physicians and the British Nutrition Foundation. This was an attempt to try and accommodate the fact that unpleasant reactions to food clearly *did* exist, but nonetheless the die-hard immunologists wouldn't give in and allow the term 'allergy' to be applied. In many ways this was a poor compromise, especially since proponents of the term cannot provide any explanation of how 'intolerance' comes about.

Clinical ecologists continued their investigations, which were not confined to food reactions or classic dust, pollen and dander allergies. It became obvious that some individuals were sensitive to environmental chemicals. It is hard to describe this as an allergy; probably the term 'low-grade poisoning' would be better since many of these chemicals would make anyone exposed to them in sufficient concentration feel ill. The problem is just that certain individuals react to smaller doses.

Then there is the matter of hypersensitivity to metals such as nickel and chromates. These are cell-mediated immunity reactions, without antibody involvement. These too are probably best not called allergies, but clearly there is a sensitization phenomenon that fulfils the prescription of the von Pirquet phenomenon.

Confusion can arise from the fact that there may be pharmacological effects masquerading as an 'allergy'. For example, the headache, flushing, racing pulse and giddiness that can come on after too much caffeine is really a drug reaction, not an allergic one. So too are the frightening reactions to eating rye contaminated with ergot mould. This organism manufactures lysergic acid diethylamide (LSD) and victims of poisoning may experience a full-blown hallucinogenic episode but, once again, this is not an allergy (see **moulds (75)** and **mycotoxins (76)**).

Finally, there is the phenomenon of enzyme deficiency, often called '**inborn errors of metabolism**' **(57)**. Some people are made ill by their inability to detoxify or metabolize foods, chemicals and drugs. An example is lactase deficiency, which causes people to suffer unpleasant abdominal symptoms when they drink milk. Children with phenylketonuria lack the enzyme phenylalanine hydroxylase and are unable to dispose of phenylalanine, which thus accumulates and causes mental retardation and neurological damage.

Taking all these definitions together it is possible to evolve what might be called the *empirical definition* of an allergy: if it can be shown that something causes a patient harm i.e. an avoidance of it brings about a recovery and a return to it causes a recurrence of symptoms, and there is no

21

other obvious cause of the affliction, then it could be called an 'allergy'. This is eminently sensible and is how the term is used today in popular usage. The layman does not need to know the mechanisms of allergy and intolerance but can readily grasp the concept of 'something to avoid'.

All this is summarized in Table 5.1.

Types of Allergic and Sensitivity Reactions

CLASSIC ALLERGY

Atopy. IgE mediated, immediate, skin and respiratory system, anaphylaxis.

Hypersensitivity, Types II, III and IV.

Organs: skin, joints, serum.

NEWER CONCEPTS

Any end organ, immune complexes, often slow build-up, no antibodies demonstrable.

1. Intolerance
2. Pharmacological
3. Metabolic errors (enzyme deficiency)
4. Low-grade poisoning (toxicology)

This is probably a better classification than the Coombs and Gell **hypersensitivity (53)** types.

Also see **detoxification (26)** and **general adaptation syndrome (44)**

6. Anaphylaxis

Anaphylaxis is the state of sudden shock or collapse after an acute allergic reaction. Death sometimes results. It was first witnessed by the French scientist Charles Richet in 1903. He was trying to immunize a dog against the poison of a jellyfish by giving it repeated injections (prophylaxis). It had the exact opposite effect and on the second injection the animal died in seconds. Hence his term 'anaphylaxis'.

Anaphylaxis usually takes place in response to a widespread attack of an allergen throughout the body. Large quantities of **histamine (50)** and other mediator substances (by which the reaction is initiated) are released and the severity of the reaction is such that fluid loss into the tissues, together with accompanying lack of muscle tone in the blood vessels, causes circulatory collapse. Among other effects the lungs rapidly fill with fluid and breathing becomes difficult.

Death can be extremely rapid and there are many tragic cases of victims dropping down dead as they rush to get their emergency aid drugs. It is one of the most acute of all medical emergencies and there is very little time in which to act. The only treatment, once anaphylaxis is established, is an injection of adrenalin which restores the blood circulation. Any other medication is too slow.

Anaphylaxis can occur in response to a wide variety of allergens. Most common are foods such as nuts, egg and fish, or **insect stings (58)**, where the patient has become sensitized to these substances. These are always the Type I immediate **hypersensitivity (53)** reactions.

Fortunately, this kind of severe reaction is rare. Also, anaphylaxis never arises without progressing in severity over a number of exposures. In other words, the patient has warning that it is developing. The worst possible case is that it happens on the second exposure, as with the dog. This is likely to be a disaster. But more often than not, the patient has a series of reactions, each one getting more severe, until it is obvious that the next one could be fatal. Thus there is a chance to be prepared.

Patients at risk must always carry an emergency treatment kit. This consists of a syringe with a drug drawn up in readiness, for self-injection if necessary. The drug may be an injectable anti-histamine but, once the reaction has reached truly dangerous proportions, only adrenalin is suitable.

It is sensible for individuals in this risk category to carry a Medic-Alert emblem. This charitable foundation was started in 1956 by a doctor whose daughter almost died after being injected with a serum she was allergic to. It is now registered in many countries (see Useful Addresses for the Medic-Alert Foundation address). The patient wears a stainless steel bracelet or necklace showing the warning logo. The patient also carries a card giving details of what the problem is, so that if found unconscious or unable to explain the difficulty he or she will not be harmed by well-meaning attendants.

7. Antinutrients

Numerous plants such as legumes, seeds and some leaf foods (such as tea) contain anti-nutritional and toxic factors. Probably this is in part Nature's adaptation mechanism: the plant's natural enemies will learn, through experience, not to eat it. Those creatures who disregard the warnings will be de-selected for evolutionary purposes (i.e. tend to die before reproducing). As part of the ecological chain, we ignore such knowledge at our peril. However, the fact that we can cook our food has a neutralizing effect on its toxicity (raw food fanatics beware!).

WHAT ARE ANTINUTRIENTS?

The important point to make is that antinutrients are *natural* substances in food. They serve some as-yet-unknown purpose to the plant; the fact that they are bad for the likes of you and me may be incidental. They are widespread and most plants have some of these substances present.

1. Phytic Acid

Phytic acid is found in large amounts in whole grains. It impairs protein digestion by interacting with digestive enzymes and forming insoluble complexes. Also it chelates zinc, iron, calcium, copper, magnesium and manganese, which means the body cannot make use of them.

2. Enzyme Inhibitors

Enzyme inhibitors are found throughout the plant world, chiefly in the legumes, and then mostly in the seeds. This is probably to prevent digestion and ensure passage of the seed intact, ready to germinate in the animal faeces.

Several types may exist in one plant. They may interfere with a variety of enzymes, such as amylase (starch-splitters) in saliva and proteases (protein-splitters) from the pancreas. Amylase inhibitors are found in wheat, rye and taro root. Protein inhibitors are widely distributed among the cereal grains, including corn and rice, also buckwheat and beans of all kinds.

Amylase inhibitors are significant in human nutritional terms as they decrease starch availability measurably. Some of the starch may then be fermented by intestinal microflora, and absorption of fermentation products, such as acetic and butyric acids, would then follow (see **intestinal fermentation (59)**).

A special kind of toxin in this class are cholinesterase inhibitors. Solanin is a poison found in the tubers of the *Solanaceae* species (nightshades: potato, tobacco, tomato, etc.). It is also found in carrots, turnips, radishes, beets, oranges, apples and greens (celery, asparagus, broccoli). It is most highly concentrated in the skin of green potatoes, where it can be over ten times as high as that in mature potatoes.

Cholinesterase inhibition is the basis of the toxic nerve gases used in warfare.

3. Tannin

Tannin is capable of inactivating a series of enzymes, including salivary and pancreatic amylase and trypsin. It can also inhibit iron absorption – this effect can be countered by the casein of milk products, or made worse by ascorbic acid.

Examples of foods with a high tannin content are tea, beans, peas, lentils, sunflower seeds, carob, yellow peas, spinach, wheat germ and aubergine; those with a low tannin content include carrots, potatoes and tomatoes.

4. Ascorbic Acid

Vitamin C is known to lower the absorbability of iron from the gut and as such is an antinutrient as well as being vital in its own right.

5. Citral

Citral is a constituent of orange oil that can prevent absorption of fat-soluble vitamins and possibly, if taken in excess, cause damage to blood vessels and contribute to cardiovascular disease. It is present in orange skin and therefore found in orange juices flavoured with orange oil and in marmalade or orange drinks made from compressed whole fruit.

6. Pectins

Pectins are potent chelating substances found in apples and particularly in lemons. Environmental medical practitioners sometimes use these substances in a nutritional programme to help remove heavy toxic metals from patients' systems. But it must be remembered that as well as removing toxic metals like mercury the pectins are quite capable of doing the same thing to zinc.

7. Other Antinutrient Factors

It should not be overlooked that drugs also interact with nutrients and reduce their efficacy. For example, antibiotics reduce the availability of B vitamins, anticonvulsants remove vitamin D and oral contraceptives interfere with a wide number of vitamins: C, E, B_1, B_2, B_6 and B_{12}.

Note also that rancid fats and oils remove vitamin E and mineral oil (liquid paraffin) depletes the fat-soluble vitamins A, D and K.

Also see **endorphins (33)**, **lectins (65)**, **nutrition and allergies (81)** and **plant toxins (87)**

8. Anti-oxidants

Oxygen is essential for the basic functioning of all life-forms. Without it we would die in a matter of minutes. However, it has long been known that oxygen is toxic to cells. Hydrogen peroxide, which vigorously gives off 'live' oxygen, is used as an antiseptic to kill microbes. This 'excited' oxygen strips off the lipid (fatty) envelope surrounding the cell walls, making them collapse. It is equally inimical to bacteria, viruses and yeasts.

In fact white blood cells in our immune system have a **peroxidation (84)** mechanism for producing this 'live' oxygen on the spot,

precisely for the purpose of attacking foreign organisms. Fortunately Nature also sees fit to supply an enzyme – peroxidase – to get rid of it as fast as it is formed, otherwise it would harm the body's own cells.

Even so, this highly active oxygen produced in the tissues is likely to react with other molecules nearby, energizing them and making them in turn super-reactive and hungry to grab onto something – any nearby chemical. We call these fiery groups of atoms 'free radicals'. They can damage the body inappropriately and we now believe that certain degenerative diseases such as cardiovascular disease, rheumatoid and other arthritis conditions, loss of immunity and allergies, cancer and possibly the process of ageing itself are all in some way bound up with this unwanted oxidation process.

However, the mere existence of these radicals does not pose a threat. It wouldn't make sense for Nature to *ensure* harm. Instead, it seems the damaging effect of oxidation is only made manifest by existing weaknesses in the tissues. We know that nutritional deficits, for example, can make normal healthy cells vulnerable. Lack of selenium, copper, manganese and zinc can each result in increased susceptibility to free-radical damage of the fat part of cell membranes.

Nutrients that we now believe are provided by Nature as a means of combating free radicals we call anti-oxidants. These include beta-carotene, vitamin A, vitamin E, vitamin C, selenium-containing amino acids (such as cystine) and enzymes such as glutathione reductase, peroxidase (catalase) and superoxide dismutase.

Trace elements are vital for integrity of this anti-oxidant system of enzyme defences. Thus, for example, glutathione and superoxide dismutase require copper, manganese and zinc. However, excessive copper (or iron) can actually increase free-radical production.

EXTRANEOUS FACTORS

Our environment provides us with what might be termed 'oxidative stress': atmospheric pollution, especially petrochemical smog, produces potent oxidants such as ozone, nitrogen dioxide, peroxyacetyl nitrates and other hydrocarbon-derived free radical substances (see **atmospheric pollution (10)**).

Ionizing radiation (radioactivity) is damaging precisely because it produces free radicals by destabilizing existing molecules (ions are free radicals). We are all subject to a certain degree of 'natural' radiation of this sort, with or without additional man-made sources.

Smoking (active and passive) subjects the lungs and other organs to chronic oxidative stress. Xenobiotic chemicals – including medical and street drugs – can also be sources of oxidative stress.

Poisons can do it. The pesticide paraquat's toxicity, for example, is believed to result from its free radical form. It is made a free radical by the action of an enzyme on the paraquat molecule in the presence of NADPH (nicotinamide dinucleotide phosphate with an added hydrogen atom, a detoxifying co-enzyme). The transformation results in the removal of one electron (reduction).

In the presence of oxygen this paraquat free radical generates a superoxide radical, which attacks lipid membranes. This step takes away the excess electron, returning the paraquat to its original form, ready to start all over again. This can go on indefinitely, each time using up the body's precious stores of co-enzymes. It means that paraquat cannot be adequately metabolized and removed from the body. The victim dies slowly and painfully.

These reactions are probably easier to see diagrammatically and are shown in Figure 8.1.

TESTS

Oxidation stress can be measured by looking at the degree to which the patient's red and white blood cells break up when subjected to a particular dilution of hydrogen peroxide. The more they break up, the less anti-oxidant potential of the individual.

Enzymes such as red cell glutathione peroxidase can also be measured, and if levels are low we know that oxidative stress is high. It makes sense also to measure

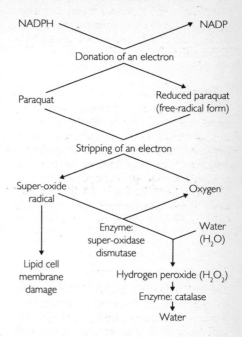

Figure 8.1: Metabolism of paraquat

selenium, manganese, copper, and zinc levels, as well as those of vitamin C, vitamin A, vitamin E, and beta-carotene, to get a complete picture of the patient's anti-oxidant status before embarking on treatment.

WHAT TO DO

The reader will see that increasing anti-oxidant potential is vital in an increasingly xenobiotic world. Fortunately, this isn't difficult to do. Ensuring that you eat a healthy diet is part of it and also making sure that you have adequate supplements of selenium, vitamins E, A and C and beta-carotene.

Note: the recommendations of this section are in direct conflict to the claims of the **Peroxidation (84)** lobby. I do not recommend the peroxide approach, but at least one clinical ecology doctor in the UK uses it extensively.

Also see **nutrition and allergies (81)**

9. Applied Kinesiology: A Way of Testing for Allergies

This method of testing for allergies usually raises a few medical eyebrows. It has its origins partly in chiropractice and partly in acupuncture and was first described and developed by George Goodheart in the USA. As its name suggests it is primarily concerned with the dynamics of posture and movement. Although it has no proven scientific basis it does seem to be founded on a certain body wisdom. A simpler version for the layman, called Touch for Health, was developed by California practitioner John F. Thie.

Allergy testing is only a small aspect of this discipline. Applied kinesiology is based on the discovery that if the body is subjected to adverse influences, certain muscles go weak. This can be demonstrated with a high degree of consistency, even if performed double blind – that is with neither the practitioner nor the patient being aware of what is being tested. No one pretends to know the physiological basis of this effect, simply that it can be shown to exist.

TECHNIQUE

The practitioner gauges the strength of a group of muscles (techniques exist to improve the tone of weak muscles and generally 'balance' the body's dynamic status before starting). Then, by putting a sample of food under the tongue and retesting, he or she is able to tell whether that substance is 'hostile' to the patient's body. If the muscles weaken significantly, the food is deemed to be an allergen. Actually, those who practise this method say it is only necessary for the patient to hold a bottle or a sample of the substance being tested – the muscles will still go weak, which means non-food substances can be tested also.

AK, as it is expediently known, probably isn't as accurate as the more 'scientific' methods, but that doesn't mean it isn't successful most of the time. Remember it isn't necessary to identify absolutely every allergy to make someone well. Even if it was only 60 to 70 per cent accurate (and it is probably much better than that when carried out by a skilled practitioner) it is still the most cost-effective testing method of all.

THE AURICULO-CARDIAC-REFLEX METHOD (ACR)

Even stranger than applied kinesiology is the auriculo-cardiac-reflex method, developed and taught by Dr Julian Kenyon of the Centre for the Study of Complementary Medicine in Southampton. Quite a few GPs have studied with him and you may therefore encounter this testing technique.

It is based on the fact that stimulation of the sympathetic nervous system causes the rate of maximum pulse amplitude to shift along the artery. *Note:* this has nothing to do with pulse rate, which does not necessarily alter.

The test is calibrated as follows: the practitioner rests his or her thumb over the radial artery at the wrist so that the impulse is just out of reach beyond the tip of his or her thumb. A bright light is then shone onto a sympathetically enervated portion of skin, either the earlobe or the back of the hand. This causes the point of maximum amplitude of the pulse to move till it comes directly under the practitioner's thumb (see Figure 9.1).

Done properly, it is like feeling nothing until the light shines, at which point the pulse suddenly starts to bump under the counting thumb. This response to light is called a *positive reflex*.

Testing foods and other allergens is then simply a matter of holding a filter containing each substance over the skin of the forearm. A positive auriculo-cardiac reflex lasting a dozen or more pulse-beats is a sign of an allergy. If it lasts 20 or more beats, that is a severe allergy.

With a set of filters covering common foods and other allergens, it is possible to test quickly a wide range of substances. Once again, the patient must simply avoid the food but, since only the most pronounced allergens show up, it doesn't

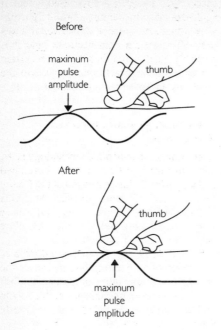

Before

maximum
pulse
amplitude

thumb

After

thumb

maximum
pulse
amplitude

Figure 9

usually lead to a long list of banned substances.

As with the applied kinesiology method, the ACR technique is a fast and cost-effective means of allergy testing, sacrificing high accuracy for expediency but a very useful method, nonetheless, particularly with children.

Also see **cytotoxic tests (24)**, **dowsing (29)** and **Miller's method (74)**

10. Atmospheric Pollution

The air we breathe today, especially in cities, could hardly be awarded the term 'fresh'. It is so corrosive that it damages the fabric of our buildings. St Paul's Cathedral, London, the Parthenon in Athens, the Roman Colosseum, Chartres Cathedral and the Taj Mahal are all disappearing gradually under this onslaught of chemicals. It would be a foolish individual who claimed these substances had no effect on the humans who breathe them continuously.

Table 10.1 lists some of the main components of the pollution of urban air.

Factors in Atmospheric Pollution-

CHEMICAL SOURCE
Hydrocarbons from fuel combustion
Carbon monoxide
Oxides of nitrogen
Sulphur dioxide
Ozone
Formaldehyde
Pesticides
Chlorine
Mercury
Lead
Nickel
Manganese
Cadmium

Most of these substances come from the burning of fossil fuels, especially within a petrol combustion engine. Other sources of pollution include smelting, agricultural spraying and waste incineration. Some highly toxic substances such as peroxyacetyl nitrate and **nitrous oxide (79)** are caused by the effect of sunlight on existing atmospheric pollutants.

We are used to thinking of ozone as valuable and healthy, because of fears for its loss in the upper atmosphere. It is important to remember, however, that it is toxic to life and that levels reached in modern cities on a summer's day can be dangerously high.

Many people experience a dramatic improvement in their tolerance of food and other items when they get away from city life. This may be true for you. Holidays abroad sometimes offer the clue: if you can eat and drink widely without ill-effects when you are in, say, Greece or Spain, atmospheric pollution may be the reason.

The comprehensive **environmental control unit (35)** is the only definitive way to diagnose these problems, but until these are more widely available there are one or two things you can do to help yourself. Firstly, if you suspect atmospheric pollution and your diet is reasonably under control, go away for a few days in the country or, even better, abroad. If you improve markedly, you have pin-pointed something about your home environment.

The trouble may be either within your home or outside of it. To establish which with a fair degree of certainty, on the day you return home stay outside your house for several hours. Walk around, expose yourself to traffic and other fumes before entering your home. If you feel ill *before* going indoors, then clearly the problem is outdoor atmospheric pollution.

Ascorbic acid (vitamin C, 4 to 20 g daily, depending on tolerance) may enable you to combat the worst effects of atmospheric pollution. Taking Miller's neutralizing drops to combat exhaust fumes, **formaldehyde (42)**, synthetic alcohol and other chemicals may also help.

Best of all, if you can manage it, is to move to a less polluted area. This might seem drastic, but most people who have done it reckon that it was preferable to a lifetime battle with ill-health.

INDOOR POLLUTION

A major aspect of atmospheric pollution, often forgotten, is indoor air in the home or office (see also **sick building syndrome (99)**). The atmosphere indoors is loaded with formaldehyde from fabrics and furnishings, with cigarette smoke, products of combustion from stoves and heaters (such as nitrous oxide and carbon monoxide), sometimes asbestos, biological elements (such as dust mite, moulds and bacteria) and numerous trace toxins from modern plastics and resins, such as xylene from paints and toluene di-isocyanate from varnishes.

A good clue to the fact that you may be suffering from indoor air pollution is that you feel worse in winter. Hay-fever sufferers, as you know, experience an allergic peak in the warm months. A number of allergy conditions have no seasonal element. But those who become worse in winter generally do so because of the build-up of indoor pollution at that time.

The reason is simple. When the weather turns cold we retreat indoors, closing all the windows and doors. Draughts are discouraged and often sealed against. Then we turn up the heating systems, such as gas fires and stoves, which themselves are the principal causes of the pollution. Some tests suggest that carbon monoxide levels in the home may rise by as much as 200 per cent at this time. Yet quite small amounts of this poison, breathed over a period, have serious effects.

The inference is quite clear. Get plenty of fresh air, even in the middle of winter. Open doors and windows as much as you (and those you live with) can stand. Don't huddle over stoves and fires. Change your heating system, if practicable, to less polluting types such as electric oil-filled radiators. Avoid tobacco smoke.

CIGARETTE SMOKE

This is a potent pollutant. Some patients are made very ill by it quite apart from the risk of cancer from the side-stream elements.

Freedom from this peril may not only include changing your own personal habits but those of your immediate family. It may be very difficult to get them to give up smoking when they are not the ones who are ill. In the meantime, avoid crowded, smoky bars and other obvious places of contact; for most this will hardly be a major deprivation.

CROP SPRAYS

Each year there are some 1,000 million gallons of pesticide spray dispensed on to farming land. Droplets under 10 microns in diameter mist and do not settle. In other words, they remain permanently airborne. This is the reason pesticides travel widely in our atmosphere, forming a major contribution to atmospheric pollution. One study showed that tagged chemicals released in the Paris area were picked up as far away as Scandinavia *within 24 hours*.

Talk of limited applications is essentially meaningless. Remember, the effects are cumulative; last year's residue is not suddenly eradicated but must be added to this year's total.

MOTOR CARS AS POLLUTANTS

The internal combustion engine is a major – if not *the* major – source of environmental chemical pollution, emitting hydrocarbons, oxides of nitrogen, formaldehyde and other toxic fumes, not to mention **lead (63)**. Some of the worst air you will ever breathe comes from behind a smoky lorry, and at least one company produces an in-car air filter designed to remove chemical fumes in the vehicle. Some countries have vigorous laws to control emissions, but in the UK to date we have none.

If you must own and use a car there are certain things you need to know. Firstly, the inside of the car itself is a source of many chemicals. Most of the fittings are plastic and give off fumes. This is quite apart from any seepage of petrol odour into the cabin space. It takes several years for these odours to die away to a 'safe' level (for some patients, of course, there is no safe level), but in practical terms a new car becomes usable by all but the most sensitive people after about three months.

Don't choose a car that is too old, otherwise leaks and general deterioration will cause a recurrence of the chemical problem. Always keep the boot closed and do not travel with the hatchback open (as when carrying large items); this sucks in exhaust fumes, enough to cause carbon monoxide poisoning, never mind a sensitivity reaction.

Also see **chemical cleanup (19)**, **environmental allergies (34)** and **weather and health (111)**

11. Body Load

One of the most important of all healing principles, if not *the* most important, is that of *total body load*. It is the key to all recoveries and overcoming all disease processes. No doctor really cures anything; Nature does that. All the successful physician can do is to reduce body load to allow this process to take place. Unfortunately, modern medicine and its drugs often *adds* to the biological burden instead of relieving it.

Along with all living creatures we are endowed with a number of key regulatory mechanisms. One can only be amazed that they rarely seem to break down, rather than being surprised and disconcerted when they do. The skin protects us from temperature variation and dehydration, the immune system wards off micro-organisms, the kidneys eliminate poison waste, the liver detoxifies an ever-increasing amount of xenobiotic (alien) chemicals and other factors regulate the acid-base balance within the body.

Every day, every minute, trouble is nipped in the bud before it gets started and we remain unaware of what is taking place; we feel OK. It is only when the defences are overworked that we actually experience any health problems at all. By the time we are aware of a symptom, any symptom, the defences have already broken down and matters are really quite serious.

OVERLOAD

Overloading the system is thus asking for trouble. There are many ways to overload – Table 11.1 summarizes most of these. A mere glance will tell you that this list is also a summary of clinical ecology to date.

Conditions Contributing to Overload

    Stress
    Allergies
    Chemical pollution
    Drugs
    Geopathic stress
    Mercury toxicity
    Hidden infections
    Endocrine disorders
    Electromagnetic fields
    Fatigue
    Nutritional deficiencies
    Radioactivity
    Alcohol
    Oxidative stress

Overload can lead to an almost infinite variety of disease symptoms. Mental breakdown, heart disease, ulcers and cancer are just some of the possibilities. Which symptoms arise from which stressor comes under the consideration of so-called **target** (or 'shock') **organs (104)**. Something will break down and usually it is the inherent weak link that snaps first. If the overload is prolonged or severe, more and more end-organs will fail and symptoms and complications will multiply.

REDUCING THE LOAD

The opposite side of the equation works just as effectively and can be turned to good use by a physician with the requisite skills. Any legitimate means of reducing body load helps, directly or indirectly, with any illness: better nutrition will aid the fight against cancer; eating fewer stress foods can help hay-fever (stress foods include those you are allergic to, refined carbohydrates – which can cause adrenal stress – or food additives (chemical toxins), etc.); clearing up hidden infections such as Candida will reduce PMT; eliminating hairsprays and perfumes may improve catarrh (even though dust is the main cause); stopping smoking aids fertility and moving away from geopathic stress will help alleviate almost any disease process. Even a divorce might lead to a recovery!

Now you may understand why you can eat a food you are normally allergic to while on holiday (where your mental stress and, probably, the amount of chemical pollution are far less) with not ill effects.

If you understand overload and work to avoid it, this very important principle will serve you well.

THRESHOLD VALUES

It is implicit that you will be able to tolerate a definite level of each stressor and only by exceeding that do you move into overload. These limits may shift under different circumstances but there is always a line, drawn somewhere, which you must not cross if you want to remain well.

Bad allergens, then, are the ones of which even a tiny quantity puts you over the limit. Mild allergies are those which need a big dose of an allergen to come into effect. Probably mild allergies would not arise at all if the allergens were encountered in normal quantities, but several together can add up to trouble. It is even possible to imagine a scale and assign arbitrary numerical values. If your threshold limit is, say 10 points, a 12 allergy would put you straight into symptoms. But one or two 3s taken together would still have no effect; two 4s and a 3 might, and so on. This can be represented diagramatically (see Figure 11.1).

The 'values' scale may be a bit artificial but if you get the idea of allergies being cumulative, you will avoid unpleasant consequences more often. You will also begin to understand why sometimes you can eat a food without any effect and at other times be ill.

Incidental life events can play havoc with these threshold levels. Virus infections often shift the values markedly, usually to the patient's disadvantage; so does emotional stress.

Also see **anti-oxidants (8)**, **cyclical and fixed allergies (23)** and **universal reactors (107)**

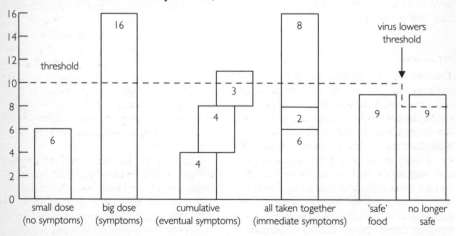

Figure 11.1: Threshold values

12. Brain Allergy

GENERAL

One of the most fascinating **target organs (104)** for allergy is the brain. The effects can be subtle, amusing, bizarre, dangerous or disastrous, in varying combinations. I have seen allergy lead to heightened sexual feelings, murderous assault, schizophrenic psychosis, woolly thinking, hallucination, hyperactivity, depression, anxiety, learning difficulties, dyslexia and autism, with many intermediate types and mixtures of symptoms.

Minimal brain dysfunction in children is probably one of the commonest allergic effects (see **hyperactivity and minimal brain dysfunction (52)**). It may lead to antisocial acts, poor concentration, learning difficulties and emotional unhappiness. Dyslexia is an interesting and unusual condition which may respond dramatically to the clinical ecology approach. Some youngsters afflicted with these problems have a very bad time in life; everyone thinks they are naughty, stupid or lazy and they get no help and may even be scolded or punished for things they have no control over.

Naturally, if undetected these difficulties may roll on into adult life. There the condition shifts emphasis often, causing more inner neurosis and unhappiness. Patients may brood and feel melancholy; life doesn't seem worth living and many patients have said they would like to end it all, if only they had the courage.

PYROLURIA

The late Carl C. Pfeiffer was noted for his work in this and related nutritional topics concerned with mental illness, especially schizophrenia. His writings are a seminal source of ideas for future researchers. He made famous the 'mauve factor', though in fact it was first identified by doctors Abram and Mahon in 1961, who discovered that when a certain reagent (known as *Erhlich's reagent*) was added to the urine of 39 schizophrenic patients, 27 patients' urine samples turned mauve. The actual substance present in their urine that caused this change

is called pyrrole and the condition is more clumsily known as 'pyroluria'. Pfeiffer even identified subjects from history who were said to manifest the symptoms of pyroluria – being withdrawn, melancholic, experiencing blinding headaches, nervous exhaustion (neurasthenia), abnormal sensitivity (one might almost say paranoia) about stressful changes and outside influences, palpitations and digestive disorders, even handwriting abnormalities – naming Charles Darwin, Charles Dickens and Emily Dickinson as possible sufferers, among others.

It is worth pointing out also that pyrroles were originally found in the urine of several patients undergoing severe LSD psychosis. This probably tells us something, but as yet we don't know what. The importance of the possible role of pyrroles in mental disease is that they reduce available zinc and B_6. Large supplements of these two essential nutrients are thus beneficial to those with schizophrenia and pyroluria. B_6 – enough for nightly dream recall (see **nutrition and allergies (81)**) but not exceeding 2,000 mg (this level is dangerous and should only be attempted under skilled medical supervision); zinc – 30 mg night and morning; and manganese gluconate 10 mg, night and morning.

HISTAMINE

Pfeiffer also stressed the possible role of **histamine (50)** in mental disorder. He hypothesized two types, according to blood levels. Fifty per cent of tested schizophrenics, he said, had *low* serum histamine (histapenia). Twenty per cent had *high* levels (histadelia). Histapenics, he said, usually have high copper levels as well. Since this may occasionally be primary, it is essential to remove any environmental source of copper pollution, such as in the water supply.

Pfeiffer gave symptoms for the histapenic patient, which included difficulty achieving orgasm, increased body hair, the absence of allergies and headaches and some of the symptoms suggesting schizophrenia itself, such as the feeling of being mind-controlled by other people, seeing or hearing things abnormally and undue suspicions – in other words, anxiety, hallucinations and paranoia. Histapenic patients are said to respond well to nutritional supplements, as given below:

● Niacin, 100 mg twice a day
● Niacinamide 250 – 500 mg twice a day
● Folic acid 1 mg daily
● B_{12} by injection
● Zinc 15 mg and manganese 5 mg daily
● A high-protein diet

The histadelic patient, on the other hand, will feel effects referable to the presence of excess histamine. It mimics allergies. Symptoms would include sneezing in bright sunlight, seasonal allergies and headaches, itching, restlessness, crying, salivation, nausea, shyness and oversensitivity as a teenager, given to tears and over-emotional reactions, backaches, stomach cramps, ease in achieving orgasm, tensions, fears and phobias, with suicidal depressions. Pfeiffer cited Marilyn Monroe and Judy Garland as likely histadelics.

He treated histadelics with a low-protein, complex carbohydrate diet (whole grains), calcium supplements (500 mg twice a day), methionine (500 mg twice a day) and possibly anti-convulsant drugs.

OTHER PSYCHONUTRIENT FACTORS

The benefits of B_6 and zinc supplementation have already been noted in certain schizophrenics. It is worth pointing out that one sub-group in this illness is made *worse* by the addition of these two nutrients and a physician would have to be alert to this possibility and discontinue treatment immediately.

Other trace element deficiencies have also been considered. In 1927 Dr Reiter in Denmark treated 30 schizophrenic patients with intravenous manganese injections and reported improvements in 23 of them. In 1929 Dr English of Brookville, Ontario, tried manganese again with 181 patients and about 50 per cent of them improved. Then Dr Hoskins of the Worcester Foundation tried it, using intramuscular injections of a different, non-absorbable form of manganese, and found no effect. Manganese was promptly forgotten.

The psychiatric profession is currently investigating abnormal metabolic pathways involving a number of neurologically active 'transmitters' such as dopamine and serotonin. There is much complex pharmacology here, enough to maintain centre stage for many decades to come at the expense of more holistic approaches.

Only in one area is 'nutrient therapy' or supplementation the fashion and that is in treating mania. It has been found that lithium calms manic patients. It will not stop hallucination and mania once developed, but it makes these symptoms less likely. This may mean that only a reduced amount of a more 'orthodox' psychotropic drug is necessary or, in some cases, no drug at all. Because of the marked Parkinsonism-like side-effects of some of these drugs, this is a welcome aspect.

It isn't possible to accord lithium the status of a trace element, but it is close. Animal studies have shown its efficacy and 'essential' status and psychiatrists are in danger of joining nutritionists and clinical ecologists in so-called *orthomolecular medicine!*

Conventional thinking says lithium therapy should only be administered where regular checks on blood levels are available. Pfeiffer claimed it is safe in dosages as low as 300 mg lithium carbonate twice daily, without any such monitoring. On no account should patients be tempted into self-dosing.

Lithium carbonate is manufactured as Liskonium, Camcolit, Priadel and Phasal.

BRAIN ALLERGY

By far the most interesting discovery in psychiatric medicine, though most psychiatrists are unaware of its existence, is in the realm of 'brain allergy', whether due to real allergy, intolerance, low-grade poisoning, etc. Theron Randolph, who began to notice unusual cerebral manifestations in his patients, went to the trouble of cataloguing these and drawing up a table (see Table 12.1, below). It was quickly apparent to him that there were varying stages of excitation and depression during allergic and hypersensitivity reactions, passing through gradually deepening levels

Stimulatory and Withdrawal Levels of Manifestations

Directions: Start at zero (0)
Read up for predominantly Stimulatory Levels
Read down for predominantly Withdrawal Levels

++++	MANIC WITH OR WITHOUT CONVULSIONS	Distraught, excited, agitated, enraged and panicky. Circuitous or one-track thought, muscle twitching and jerking of extremities, convulsive seizures, and altered consciousness may develop.
+++	HYPOMANIC, TOXIC, ANXIOUS AND EGOCENTRIC	Aggressive, loquacious, clumsy (ataxic), anxious, fearful and apprehensive; alternating chills and flushing, ravenous hunger, excessive thirst. Giggling or pathological laughter may occur.
++	HYPERACTIVE, IRRITABLE, HUNGRY, AND THIRSTY	Tense, jittery, hopped up, talkative, argumentative, sensitive, overly responsive, self-centred, hungry and thirsty, flushing, sweating and chilling may occur as well as insomnia, alcoholism, and obesity.
+	STIMULATED BUT RELATIVELY SYMPTOM FREE	Active, alert, lively, responsive and enthusiastic with unimpaired ambition, energy, initiative and wit. Considerate of the views and actions of others. This usually comes to be regarded as 'normal' behaviour.
O	BEHAVIOUR ON AN EVEN KEEL, AS IN HOMOEO-STASIS	Children expect this from their parents and teachers. Parents expect this from their children. We all expect this from our associates.
−	LOCALIZED ALLERGIC MANIFESTATIONS	Running or stuffy nose, clearing throat, coughing, wheezing, (asthma), itching, eczema and hives, gas, diarrhoea, constipation, colitis, urgency and frequency of urination, and various eye and ear syndromes.
− −	SYSTEMIC ALLERGIC REACTIONS	Tired, dopey, somnolent, mildly depressed, oedematous with painful syndromes (headache, neckache, backache, neuralgia, myalgia, myositis, arthralgia, arthritis, arteritis, chest pain), and cardiovascular effects.*
− − −	DEPRESSIONS AND DISTURBED MENTATION	Confused, indecisive, moody, sad, sullen, withdrawn, or apathetic. Emotional instability and impaired attention, concentration, comprehension, and thought processes (aphasia, mental lapse, and blackouts).
− − − −	SEVERE DEPRESSION WITH OR WITHOUT ALTERED CONSCIOUSNESS	Nonresponsive, lethargic, stuporous, disoriented, melancholic, incontinent, regressive thinking, paranoid orientations, delusions, hallucinations, sometimes amnesia, and finally comatose.

*Marked pulse changes or skipped beats may occur at any level.

as the brain became more and more over-charged or somnolent. Moreover, people would 'roller-coaster ride' between different stages. These ups and downs, he pointed out, were exactly like the manifestations of addiction.

Two points need making clear. Firstly, there are no hard-and-fast gradations: these symptoms blend subtly one into another and indeed it is possible to have 'minus' reactions present at the same instant as 'plus' reactions. Secondly, each individual, though he or she may move around on the ladder, tends to gravitate towards a permanent level appropriate to him or her. Even this 'chronic' level may move in time, usually ultimately tending towards the extreme minus end of the scale which represents a total inability of all body resources to oppose stress. So-called allergic reactions are thus, in reality, short-term departures from this chronic level.

Minus reactions are easy to equate with illness but the over-stimulatory phase is not, except in its extreme. Rather it is sometimes looked on as a good thing to be 'energetic', charging around all the time, 'getting things done'. Moreover, inappropriate laughter and enthusiasm tend to be viewed as evidence of a cheerful disposition when in fact they are merely the result of a minor degree of intoxication, corresponding to a plus 1 or 2 reaction. This only becomes clear when working daily with people being allergically challenged and using provocation techniques; the difference between genuine emotion and a pathological state then becomes easy to discern.

The speed with which people can move from one phase to another is on occasion quite astonishing. I have seen patients, challenged with a food or chemical, appear excited, giggling and intoxicated yet within minutes be slumbering soundly, difficult to rouse. It is well known that for every 'high' there tends to be a corresponding 'low'. The transition can be sharp and the effect very unpleasant indeed. So much so that patients who have never touched alcohol can suffer alarming hangover symptoms. Indeed the inebriation effect caused by foods has often been taken for drunkenness, leading on occasion to unfortunate encounters with the police, who have needed a great deal of convincing.

Incidentally, sexual excitation and destimulation follow patterns that are similar, and Randolph produced a table to this effect too (see **sexual hypersensitivities (98)**).

Not all psychiatric manifestations are organic, of course. But *all* psychiatric illness, I believe, is complicated by organic processes and these aspects of an individual's illness, even assuming there are genuine *psychogenic* (coming from the psyche, caused by the mind) components, will only respond to the ecological approach. Drugs (more chemical pollution) are the last thing that these individuals require; yet that is usually their fate.

Lastly, crime too is influenced by the above criteria. Many violent and destructive individuals in society are simply manifesting the effects of brain allergic reactions. I myself made medico-legal history here in the UK when in 1986 the Crown Court in Ballymena accepted my evidence that a youth who had tried to strangle a member of his family was made aggressive by a potato allergy. Since that time, other similar cases have appeared before the courts. As well as doctors, police should be made aware of what the Randolph brain allergy table means in terms of human behaviour.

Also see **alcohol (2)** and **endorphins (33)**

13. Bread

Long known as the staff of life, bread is actually a food that causes a great deal of ill-health due to the widespread prevalence of wheat allergy and intolerance. There is also a great deal of misleading propaganda from manufacturers. An example is their use of the term 'improvers' as an ingredient. These additives fluff up the loaf to make it lighter; that means you are sold more air and less bread.

Another deception is the redefinition of 'wholemeal'. Traditionally this sort of bread contained *only* wholemeal flour, yeast and something to texture the rough grain (usually soya oil or similar). Due to an increasing interest in healthy eating in the 1970s, more and more people began to turn to this kind of loaf and abandoned commercial white bread. What did the manufacturers do? They lobbied to have a law passed relaxing the legal definition of wholemeal so that they could sell an inferior product to the unsuspecting public under the label 'wholemeal'. Now bread only has to *contain* wholemeal flour to be called wholemeal in the UK.

Paradoxically, many allergics cannot eat the whole grain product but can tolerate white bread satisfactorily. The refined loaf has less of the characteristics of 'wheatness' and so may not provoke any allergic response. If you are one of these individuals, try to get a simply made white loaf from a small local baker. They tend to use fewer ingredients and bake a better product anyway.

Avoid loaves guaranteed 'fresh for days'. The ideal loaf for allergics is one that is uneatable next day and has to be bought daily, as the French do. A loaf that is too poisonous for mould and bacteria isn't very healthy for humans, after all. Forget what you thought; change your habits and seek out a simple unadulterated bread, without additives, and you'll soon learn to enjoy it.

Those intolerant to wheat in all degrees will have to try wheat-free bread. Unfortunately, even most rye loaves also contain wheat. Rye on its own is very leaden and unappealing, but the exception is German black rye bread or pumpernickel, which is usually wheat-free.

If you cannot eat yeast but wheat is safe your problem is different. You'll need to make soda bread. The commercial kind usually contains buttermilk which is fermented and not allowed on a yeast-free programme. Actually, after a bit of practice you will be able turn out a very palatable product.

MAKING SODA BREAD

This traditional Irish soda bread is surprisingly quick and easy to prepare. For one 8-inch loaf you will need:

1 tsp butter/dairy-free margarine/oil
1 lb/455 g flour
1 tsp bicarbonate of soda/baking soda
1 tsp salt
4–8 oz/115–225 g buttermilk/goat's milk/ soya milk (water if you are stuck)

Preheat the oven to *hot* (475°F/220°C/Gas Mark 7). Grease a large baking tray and set it aside. Sift the flour, soda and salt into a large mixing bowl. Gradually beat in the buttermilk or other liquid. The dough should be smooth but firm. If necessary add more liquid. Transfer the dough to a floured board and shape it into a flat round loaf, approximately one and a half inches thick and eight inches in diameter. Place on the baking tray and with a sharp knife make a deep cross on the top of the loaf. Place the loaf in the oven and bake for 30 to 35 minutes or until the top is golden brown. Remove from the oven and allow to cool. Best served slightly warm.

Also see **diets (27)**, **food additives (41)** and **milk (73)**

14. Brucellosis

Brucellosis (also known as Malta fever and undulant fever) is a great mimic and is usually a cryptic or masked infection. It can certainly reproduce the profound fatigue of myalgic encephalomyelitis (ME) and maladaptation syndrome and has to be considered as part of the differential diagnosis of any patient with chronic fatigue or multiple allergic-type symptoms.

Pasteurizing milk kills Brucella. Infections come from drinking raw milk from infected animals. Brucella produces a toxin which is responsible for widespread symptoms. The name undulant fever comes from the fact that the patient tends to have a relapsing illness, with a temperature that roller-coasters up and down.

Chronic brucellosis is characterized by fatigue, myalgia (muscle pain) and depression which may persist for weeks or months. This is very like ME or **post viral fatigue syndrome (88)**. The onset is often insidious, with a general feeling of being unwell, headache, weakness, night sweats and muscle pains, usually ascribed to flu. Lymph nodes are usually swollen and painful and the liver and spleen may be enlarged. Arthritis, spondylitis (spinal inflammation), bursitis, osteomyelitis, orchitis (testicular inflammation), epididymitis, meningitis and endocarditis have all been described in association with brucellosis.

The organism can be identified from blood samples, although this can be difficult. It is usually treated with tetracycline.

Research suggests that in recent years most cases of brucellosis come from occupational exposure and direct contact with animals rather than by consuming infected milk.

15. Caffeine

Many reported allergies to tea and coffee are not allergies in the true sense of the word but simply caffeine poisoning. Doses above 250 mg a day are potentially harmful. Children are more prone to caffeine's negative effects, yet cola drinks may legally contain up to 60 mg of caffeine per portion.

People have been drinking caffinaceous drinks since the dawn of time. Maté, still drunk by 20 million South Americans, was known to Paleolithic man. Tea from the bush *Camellia chinensis* has been drunk in China for 2,000 years. Coffee – taken from the *Coffeia arabica* plant – was established more recently, because without the fermentation, extraction and roasting processes, which must have taken some ingenuity to discover, its taste is unpleasant.

The distinctive aroma of coffee comes from over 500 compounds that arise during roasting. Almost none of these compounds have been properly evaluated for toxicity; they include thiopenes, thiazoles, oxazoles, furans, pyrroles (see **brain allergy (12)**), pyridines, quinolines, quinoxalines and indoles. There are others.

We drink caffeine beverages for their energizing effect and to enable more rapid, 'positive' thought. Unfortunately the effects soon wear off and the subsequent fatigue necessitates that we drink yet another cup to clear our head. Symptoms generated by excess caffeine include irritability, rest-lessness, nausea and headache. Withdrawal produces the reverse, with drowsiness, lethargy and low mood. Research shows caffeine can aggravate cystic mastitis; women with this condition should avoid it.

A typical cup of coffee contains 90 to 100 mg of caffeine. So-called de-caffeinated coffee has about 2 mg. A 5-oz cup of tea contains about 50 mg caffeine and 1 mg theophylline. Cocoa and most chocolates have significant amounts of caffeine, a fact that is often overlooked.

De-caffeinated drinks may be preferred but take care: some have the caffeine removed by chemical treatments using formaldehyde or dry-cleaning fluid! Vacuum extraction is best.

Theophylline is a similar chemical and has extra properties as a broncho-dilator (helps asthmatics breathe more easily, as it dilates the bronchi). It is found in tea and coffee. Aminophylline, a relative, is frequently used as an emergency asthma drug. Once again children are more sensitive to theophylline. Anti-asthma drugs may be a potent cause of hyperactive behaviour because of this theophylline connection.

A number of pain-relief drugs such as *Anadin*, *Hypon*, *Pardale* and *Solpadeine* contain caffeine as well as analgesics; usually around 10 to 30 mg. Migraine-specific drugs such as *Cafergot* and *Migril* contain much more: generally 100 mg of caffeine. Over-the-counter cold remedies and proprietary slimming preparations may also contain significant amounts of caffeine (around 30 mg and 200 mg respectively).

Stimulant drugs such as *Pro Plus*, designed to combat fatigue, are essentially caffeine.

Also see **phenolic testing (86)** and **plant toxins (87)**

16. Candida

Candida – that is, infection with *Candida albicans*, the thrush germ – is now big business. Probably no condition in the natural health arena is attracting more interest at present. Many magazines and newspapers feature articles on it, yet doctors' journals virtually ignore it. It recently gained notoriety in the UK when a pop star's wife was said to suffer from it and the public watched her getting sicker and sicker until it was obvious that the treatment was more deadly than the disease.

What are the real facts? So much ignorance and misinformation abounds that you may be wondering if there is anything *really* known about the topic. I will attempt to summarize just what we *do* know about Candida and also put an end to some of the nonsense and falsehoods, spread principally by unqualified medical practitioners. Many of these enthusiastic amateurs have set themselves up as 'Candida experts' and are making belligerent claims they cannot justify and treating individuals with tech-niques that are sometimes worthless or – at worst – downright dangerous.

FALSE CLAIMS

Some of the confusion about Candida comes from the fact that a number of widely circulated 'anti-candida diets' do have beneficial effects, at least at first. What isn't understood is that the mechanism at work is often that of eliminating a food allergy and not eradicating the Candida at all. I saw one diet in Sweden which asked patients to exclude dairy produce as part of an anti-Candida regime; a naturopath here in Britain says 'no grains'. There is absolutely no rationale for these omissions in the fight against Candida but these methods ensure that a great many people who are dairy or wheat allergic will 'miraculously' get better. This creates the false impression that the patients had indeed had Candida.

Another incorrect datum that has gained much currency is that once you have got Candida you are stuck with it. One hears of people who are supposed to have had it for years. Again, the amateur meddlers' fundamental lack of knowledge is to blame. Because they are not able to prescribe proper anti-fungal drugs – and indeed, to protect their own shaky position as 'experts' some even say that it is undesirable to take anti-fungals – they are not able to effect proper eradication. This means that many sufferers are denied the full treatment that they need, treatment that would enable them to overcome their condition.

WHO GETS CANDIDA?

A number of factors are known to predispose infection with Candida. Anything that compromises the immune system is likely to have this effect (AIDS patients often die of severe systemic Candida; they are simply unable to fight it off). ME cases seem to get it very consistently. *Any* long-term debilitating illness may be accompanied by what we call 'opportunistic infections' (those that get under way while the patient's resistance is low).

Steroids (including the birth control pill, which is often overlooked as a steroidal) sometimes lead to Candidiasis. However, there is little doubt that the single most widespread cause of Candidiasis is the administration of broad-spectrum antibiotics. Incidental to their main, beneficial effect, these antibiotics kill off resident bacteria in the gut. This '**gut flora**' (**46**) is needed for optimum health and proper gut performance. When the bacteria are killed off other pathogens are free to move in, and Candida is one of the most common of these. Countless patients have become chronically ill after frequent or prolonged use of antibiotics and can pinpoint the onset of their troubles to such a course of treatment.

Finally, some Candida patients have none of the above predisposing causes yet they seem to have the condition. Perhaps our modern, manufactured 'junk' diets are partly to blame.

TOXICITY

Candida is able to ferment and release alcohols from sugars in food (see **intestinal fermentation (59)**). To many people these alcohols are quite allergenic. There have been several celebrated cases in which individuals who were guilty of driving under the influence of alcohol were able to show they had not been drinking but that they did have significant infections with Candida and so escaped the law. Remember Candida is a yeast, related to moulds, and these organisms themselves are also often quite toxic and may be highly allergenic in their own right.

But the real problem is that Candida also appears able to generate food and chemical sensitivities. Increase in food intolerance has been blamed on damage to the gut wall. Like many yeasts and fungi, Candida has a vegetative form, which grows out small threads or *hyphae* into the surrounding cells. It has been hypothesized that these hyphae may provide channels through which the products of digestion escape prematurely into the bloodstream. This means that food substances have not been broken down fully and are thus still biochemically 'wheat', 'pork' etc.

If this were so we would certainly expect trouble from allergies, so the supposition fits with the observed facts. But please remember, it is only another theory. It sounds good but may be totally wrong. Clinical ecologists call it the '**leaky gut syndrome (64)**'.

I believe personally that Candida doesn't really cause allergies but that Candida and allergies share a common origin: a poor or 'flat' immune system.

THE MOULDY PATIENT

I use the concept of Candida in talking to patients since most people have heard of it and believe that is what they have got. However, I prefer the label I used in my *Allergy Handbook* (Thorsons, 1988), the so-called 'mouldy patient'. It is a term that stays in the mind, broadens out the debate and gives better insight into what we are dealing with. Whatever the nature of this illness, its manifestation is of a disease caused by encountering and being sensitized by biological products from yeasts, fungi and moulds.

Patients are made worse by anything that can be fermented, such as starch and sugars; they react to foodstuffs containing yeast or mould (bread, wine, mushrooms; etc.); they are often ill in mouldy or musty surroundings (old buildings, woodlands or animal byres); some are even sensitive to damp weather, when moulds are sporing freely; often there are accompanying infections of the fungus type including athlete's foot or other skin infections such as *Tinea* and *Epidermophyton*; finally, the patient may have been diagnosed as having Candida, either in the mouth, gut or vagina.

DIAGNOSIS

We are plagued by the lack of a suitable diagnostic test to show whether or not a patient has Candida. Some practitioners use **applied kinesiology (9)** techniques but this is hardly acceptable to the medical community. Until the time comes that we have a proper test we must rely heavily on taking a careful patient history, seeking to elicit symptoms typical of those outlined above.

Fatigue is an almost constant accompaniment of Candidiasis and mould problems; depression and disturbance of mood are also particularly prominent. However, lists of symptoms are *not* reliable guides to Candida infection or any other mould problem. Most such lists give symptoms that are typical of food allergy, ME and many other states. These simply reflect a body under stress and not some specific condition.

However, there are four symptoms that I have found very helpful in pin-pointing Candida: a craving for sweet foods, a poor tolerance of alcohol, chemical sensitivity and bloating. This is the 'awesome foursome'! All four means a certainty, any three will do. Craving for sugary foods is often outstanding among Candida victims.

One thing is certain, there is virtually no correlation between Candida in a stool sample and the existence of the 'yeast syndrome'. Indeed, Candida albicans is rarely identified in specimens, despite its known very wide occurrence.

Researchers in the UK are trying to establish a valid gut fermentation test. The idea is to take a resting blood alcohol level and then repeat the test some hours after a sugar feed. If alcohol appears in the blood this would suggest that fermentation is going on. But it doesn't tell us *what* is doing the fermenting.

A likely improvement is to look for a wider range of fermentation products. At the moment Biolab (London) are testing for short-chain fatty acids such as acetate, proprionate, succinate and butyrate, and for other alcohols such as iso-propanol, butanol and 2,3-butylene glycol. The advantage of this newer test is that it doesn't need 'before' and 'after' samples, so it is easier to do.

At the end of the day, we rely mainly on what is called a therapeutic trial. That is, we give the patient the appropriate treatment and, if it works, we infer he or she must have had the disease.

TREATMENT

A successful anti-mould programme must include efficacious restoration of bowel flora. That means removing the offenders and replacing them with 'friendly' bacteria. Several steps are necessary: killing off the moulds, avoiding sugars, minimizing further contact with mould and yeast, especially in the diet and, lastly, recolonization with suitable flora.

The most important step is medication with suitable anti-fungals. These *must* be prescribed by a competent physician. Nystatin is the most popular. Even among allergics it is well tolerated, probably because it cannot be absorbed. The usual doses are in the range of 1,000,000 units four times a day (1,000,000 units = quarter of a teaspoon).

Remember: Nystatin can act as a chelating agent (that is, it binds to metals and blocks them) and so should not be taken with nutritional supplements (it would remove zinc, magnesium etc.).

Alternatives include ketoconazole (*Nizoral*) tablets and fluconazole (*Diflucan*) capsules. The latter is expensive but easy to take. A 'one-shot' form exists, for those likely to develop reactions to medication. Except for Nystatin, lengthy treatments should not be undertaken, as side-effects are potentially serious.

Capricin, a trade brand of caprylic acid, has been frequently advocated as an antifungal. Other substances include **garlic (43)** and Taheebo tea (Pau D'Arco).

Much is disseminated about the 'burn off' reaction patients sometime get when first starting anti-fungal treatment. This is similar to the Herxeimer reaction that syphilis patients used to get when starting a course of penicillin; it was caused by a flood of circulating dead spirochetes (syphilis germs). Burn-off (a sudden exacerbation of symptoms) does exist but is much exaggerated and rarely amounts to anything serious. Discontinuance allows it to settle and, nine times out of ten, when the patient resumes the treatment there is no further trouble.

Medication needs to be supplemented by avoidance of added sugars in the diet. Extreme denials are not called for. Some writers foolishly recommend avoidance of fruit and similar natural foods. This may lead to dangerous inadequacies in nutrition and is bad advice because *it isn't necessary*. Anyone with 'Candida' made ill by eating fruit has a fruit allergy, almost certainly. Those who feel unwell after eating sugars

may really have a degree of carbohydrate intolerance due to deficient enzymes (see **inborn errors of metabolism/enzyme deficiency (57)**).

Similarly, with avoidance of yeast or mouldy foods – fanaticism is not necessary and may be counter-productive. Patients willing to experiment a little will find suitable tolerances to a number of items in this category. The full list of ferments is very extensive and your physician will probably give you more detailed information. Table 16.1 summarizes all the main yeast and fermentation products.

Fermentation and Yeast Products

1. Substances that contain yeast, moulds or ferments as basic ingredients:

- All Raised Doughs: Breads, buns, rolls, prepared frozen breads, sourdough and any leavened food.
- All Vinegars: apple, distilled, wine, grape, pear, etc. This includes all foods containing any vinegar, e.g. salad dressings, mayonnaise, pickles, sauerkraut, olives, most condiments, sauces such as barbecue, tomato, chili, green pepper and many others.
- All Fermented Beverages: Beer, lager, stout, wine, champagne, spirits, sherries, liqueurs and brandies as well as all substances that contain alcohol, e.g. extracts, tinctures, cough syrups and other medications, including homoeopathic remedies.
- All Cheeses: Including fermented dairy products, cottage cheese, natural, blended and pasteurized cheeses, buttermilk and sour cream.
- All Malted Products: Milk drinks that have been malted; cereals and sweets that have been malted.
- Ferments and Moulds: Such as soy sauce, truffles and mushrooms.
- Antibiotics: Penicillin, ampicillin and many other '-illins'; '-mycin' drugs and related compounds such as Erythromycin, Streptomycin and Chloramphenicol; tetracyclines and related derivatives; all the cephalosporin derivatives and all others derived from moulds and mould cultures.
- Vitamins: B, B complex and multiple vitamins containing B complex. All products containing B_6, B_{12}, irradiated ergosterol (Vitamin D). All health products containing brewer's yeast or derivatives.

2. Substances that contain yeast- or mould-derived substances:

- Flours that have been enriched (most)

- Milk enriched or fortified with vitamins
- Cereals fortified with added vitamins, i.e. thiamine, niacin, riboflavin, etc.

3. Substances that may contain moulds as allowed contaminants commercially:

- Fruit Juices: canned or frozen. (In preparation the whole fruit is used, some of which may be mouldy but not sufficiently so to be considered spoiled. Fresh, home squeezed should be yeast-free.)
- Dried Fruits: Prunes, figs, dates, raisins, apricots, etc. Again, some batches may be mould-free but others will have commercially acceptable amounts of mould on the fruit while drying.

GUT FLORA

Finally, it makes sense to try and recolonize the bowel with friendly bacteria. Most well known among these friendly bacteria is Lactobacillus acidophilus, the yoghourt-making germ. Many supplements of 'acidophilus' are currently being marketed. Some contain very few live bacteria and are of poor value if not completely fraudulent.

In fact Bifidobacteria is much more prevalent in the gut, comprising some 90 per cent of natural bowel flora. Top brand **probiotics (91)**, as these flora supplements are known, now include primarily Bifidobacteria. Look for those that provide human-strain acidophilus; logically these are more likely to establish themselves in the human colon.

17. Carbon Monoxide

Carbon monoxide poisoning is a major cause of death each year, either accidentally or through suicide. But it is the lesser effects that concern us here and these, though common, are usually overlooked. Ambient raised carbon monoxide levels in the home and at work are a major source of indoor pollution and can lead to headaches, weakness, mental confusion and dizziness. Just the kind of thing a busy primary care doctor is likely to shrug off as psychogenic (mental or emotional rather than physical) symptoms.

In 1972 a branch of the US Department of Health, Education and Welfare surveyed 25 communities where fossil-fuel burning space heaters were in use. Air sampling was done in homes and blood sampling of children was done as they arrived at their nursery schools, kindergartens, elementary schools, etc. Out of 2,229 children tested for carbon monoxide levels, 22.5 per cent had levels of 3 per cent or more. Readings were found as high as 8 per cent. Of the 1,820 homes tested, over 16 per cent had concentrations of carbon monoxide of 10 parts per million (ppm) or more.

Smoking constitutes the greatest source of exposure to carbon monoxide, since the mean level for smokers was more than four times the level for non-smokers (up to 7 per cent carboxyhaemoglobin in the blood). Sidestream smoke from cigarettes contains two and a half times more carbon monoxide than inhaled smoke.

Outdoors in a city air is not so 'fresh', as we all know, due to power station emissions and motor exhaust fumes. Typical carbon monoxide levels on the street are around 10 to 20 ppm and may reach 100 ppm in traffic queues and congested areas such as enclosed car parks. Cardiac symptoms such as raised blood-pressure and speeded pulse start at ambient levels of around 75 ppm.

PHYSIOLOGY

The primary toxic mechanism of carbon monoxide is its high affinity for haemoglobin – about 250 times that of oxygen. Since carboxyhaemoglobin which is formed is not capable of carrying oxygen to tissues, tissue hypoxia results. When exertion is high and breathing is rapid, carboxyhaemoglobin levels can increase very rapidly. One study showed that in firefighters exposed to 1 per cent carbon monoxide for two minutes, their carbon monoxide blood levels rose 30 per cent.

The brain is especially affected by hypoxia. The initial symptoms of low level intoxication are non-specific, such as headache, dizziness, weakness and difficulty thinking; these symptoms get worse as the length of exposure increases. Flu is often diagnosed, especially since family members in the same environment present similar symptoms, and if carbon monoxide poisoning results from faulty or unvented heating devices this coincides with the onset of cold weather or 'flu season.'

To protect your family, make sure any fires, stoves, boilers and furnaces in or near your home are efficient and well-ventilated. Get expert advice if there is any doubt. Remember, when carbon monoxide strikes, the first faculty you lose is the sense of danger!

Also see **atmospheric pollution (10)**, **chemical cleanup (19)** and **nitrous oxide (79)**

18. Challenge Testing

Eating a portion of food to see if it causes a reaction is called *challenge feeding*. It is vital to 'unmask' a food allergy before attempting to do this test, otherwise the results are meaningless.

As Randolph, Rinkel and Zeller state: 'Actually, the most discerning patient is rarely ever able to detect the presence of a masked food allergy. In fact, the most skilled allergist cannot do so either until he tests for it. Masking may be 100 per cent perfect, even with an individual food test, if steps have not been taken to avoid it.'

To unmask a food you are at present eating you must avoid it for at least four days and preferably five before testing – longer if you suffer from constipation.

Then proceed as follows:

1. Test only on a day when you are feeling well. If, for example, you are still undergoing a reaction to a food tested the day before, wait until this clears up before proceeding.
2. Eat only the food you are interested in for the test meal. Spring water and salt (if needed) are permitted, but nothing else. Eat a substantial portion to be sure of provoking a reaction.
3. Eat the food raw or prepared only very simply. Compound foods (mixtures) are not allowed. It is best to use organic produce, free of any chemical contamination if possible. If not, carry out the test anyway.

4. Lunchtime is the best meal. If you use the evening meal it is possible to sleep through any allergic reaction and miss it. If you test at lunch and symptoms occur in the afternoon you can be fairly certain the food was to blame. If there are no symptoms at all you then eat a normal evening meal but include more of the test food. If no symptoms are experienced by next morning you are justified in treating it as a safe food.
5. It is possible to increase the accuracy of this procedure by including a pulse count. A resting pulse is taken before and after the test meal – actually two or three times afterwards, say 30 and 60 minutes later. By 'a resting pulse' I mean that the patient sits still for two minutes before counting it (longer after exertion). A rise or fall of ten or more beats after challenging is considered highly suggestive of an allergy and it is best to avoid such food even if no overt symptoms have developed.
6. It is sensible when testing a food for the first time to *smell and taste* it before committing yourself. Animals do this all the time: you may notice a dog sniffing and licking any unknown substance before ingesting it. They follow their instincts as to whether or not a substance is safe to eat. Humans can also easily learn to develop this faculty. If when you smell it or taste a little, you get a distinct negative impression *don't* make yourself ill by eating the whole portion.

   This can be carried further. Some people get immediate symptoms around their mouth if they put their lips or tongue to a danger food. Others notice soreness or itching if handling or cutting up food. It may be possible to challenge a food by placing a fresh-cut portion of it on an exposed area of your skin – say the cheek or inner forearm. If the skin goes red, itches, blisters or reacts in some other way it should obviously not be eaten. This simple preliminary test can be very useful for children who are too young to describe their reactions.
7. If the results of a test are confusing or equivocal repeat the whole procedure but avoid other members of the same botanical or phenolic family: otherwise

there may be cross-reactions. If the outcome is still doubtful, treat the food as an allergen. Avoid it for a few months, then try again.

Note: If you experience unpleasant reactions while challenge testing foods you can clear them more rapidly by taking epsom salts and sodium and potassium bicarbonate mix (see **alkali salts therapy (4)**).

Be aware of the fact that if you stay off a food too long, even as little as a few weeks, the reaction could die down and you might miss it.

Finally, some patients report a 'build-up' effect with foods, that is, it may be safe to eat once or even for a whole day, but if eaten more often than this a reaction appears. Stay alert to this possibility. If you feel ill after introducing several new foods and can't say for sure which was the culprit, this may be the reason. You may need to eliminate all these foods and repeat the tests, taking your challenge foods over several days, just to be sure.

Foods that cause a build-up effect may be retained in your diet but you must make a point of rotating them carefully so that you don't eat any individual food more often than every four or five days (see **rotation diets (95)**).

CHEMICALS

Testing for chemicals is not very different from the procedure recommended for foods. Proceed as follows:

1. Avoid the substance strictly for four or five days. You are more likely to succeed if you eliminate as much chemical pollution as possible prior to testing.
2. Test only on a day you are feeling well. There must be few or no symptoms for the test to be valid.
3. Take your resting pulse before and afterwards, at intervals of 10, 20 and 40 minutes. Observe changes and any subjective symptoms. Note these down. As with food, a rise or fall in pulse rate of more than 10 beats is considered significant.
4. Make sure you come into fresh contact with only one substance in each test. Give

yourself a significant exposure, for example three deep breaths, repeating this *once* after a minute has elapsed.

Note: Take care, as this could be dangerous with some chemicals such as ammonia or carbon tetrachloride. For these and similar items it is sufficient to sit a few feet away from a dish or saucer holding about an ounce of the fluid or from a bottle of it with the top removed. As the substance evaporates and diffuses towards you, you will notice the smell first and then the symptom, if there is one.

5. When you have experienced symptoms, cease testing until they have cleared. This may mean no more testing for the day or even for several days.
6. As with food reactions, alkali salts may help the clearing process. Also take substantial doses of vitamin C (up to 20 g).

Warning: Always tell someone what you are doing and have him or her keep an eye on you. If you pass out during one of these tests you could be in real difficulties. Fortunately, this is rare; but it can happen.

Tell the other person if you are overcome to simply lay you horizontally, remove the offending substance and open all the doors and windows. If any amount of the substance has been spilled, you must be taken to a different room. *Discontinue all further tests if this happens.* Seek help from a clinical ecologist.

Also see **conventional allergy tests (22), cyclical and fixed allergies (23), diets (27)** and **hidden allergy (49)**

19. Chemical Cleanup

Probably the main bone of contention between allergy and environmental medicine doctors and the conventional die-hards is the recognition of 'chemical allergies'. Leaving aside the dispute over the term allergy it is an undeniable fact that many individuals are made ill by traces of the numerous toxic chemicals in our environment. Dr Theron Randolph of Chicago, doyen of the modern allergy movement, first called attention to this in his brilliant book *Human Ecology and Susceptibility to the Chemical Environment* (Charles C. Thomas, 1962).

A better term for this effect might be low-grade poisoning; it is as if sensitive people are feeling the toxic effects even when these chemicals exist at levels that do not perturb the rest of us. It has been hypothesized that such individuals probably have some deficit in their enzyme **detoxification (26)** pathways: so-called slow reactors.

THE CHEMICAL ENVIRONMENT

Human beings are exposed to tens of thousands of chemicals today that simply were not present in our environment a few decades ago. Before the Industrial Revolution there were virtually none other than the products of living organisms. These occurred naturally and our biological systems had millions of years to grow accustomed to and deal with these types of foreign substance. The trouble with our modern world, apart from the sheer amount of toxins present, is that we haven't had time to adapt physiologically and so develop the means to render these substances less harmful to us.

The very fabric of our homes is now loaded with chemicals: wallcoverings are probably vinyl (paper hangings or emulsion paint); the furniture we sit on is mostly synthetic (laminates, fabric and upholstery foam); petrochemicals are added to our food and are present in increasing amounts in our water supply; on the way to work we sit in a car that gives off traces of gas from the upholstery and the plastic panelling as well as the engine; when we arrive at work or school there is a whole host of new chemicals such as those found in photocopying fluids, cleaning aerosols, detergents and – for many workers – risky construction and manufacturing chemicals with which they must work; our hobbies, too, may bring us into contact with more substances, cosmetics certainly will; and finally, if we feel ill from all this, the doctor will want to prescribe yet more of these xenobiotic (foreign-to-life) chemicals – supposedly to make us well.

POTENTIATION

It would be unbelievable if a large number of these xenobiotics were not toxic, either singly or in combination. The potential hazards are made worse by the interaction of substances over which we have no control and pathetically little knowledge. All that we can say for certain is that such interactions are bound to occur and they will enhance the toxicity of some chemicals many times over. The extra effect of two or more substances present at the same time we call *potentiation*.

It's a case of two plus two equalling six, eight or ten. For example, most people have read in pulp detective novels about the fatal combination of quite moderate doses of barbiturates and alcohol. The trouble is that there may be many such combinations at work in our environment and it is impossible to assess their long-term effects.

Remember, official safety tests do not take account of these interactions. Each substance scrutinized is tested in isolation. Thus a clean bill for any one substance should be far from reassuring.

ENERGY EFFICIENCY

The problem of environmental hazards for chemical sensitives is made far worse by the modern craze for energy efficiency. In sealing our homes and buildings to keep heat in we also raise the levels of indoor pollution. This is an example of conflicting interests, even within the ecological field.

In fact modern buildings can be disasters. Most people have now heard of **sick building syndrome (99)**. One architect boasted he could design a home that would cause any couple to divorce – so beware! These are not trivial considerations. Many patients trace the origins of their allergic illness to a particular home. Earth radiation (**geopathic stress (45)**) could be a factor. Chemical pollution almost certainly is.

SUSPECTING CHEMICAL ALLERGIES

A number of observations should cause you to suspect you are suffering a chemical allergy. You may already be aware that certain substances such as perfumes or bleach give you a headache or some other symptom; being made ill by long car journeys is a clue, as is getting a headache from exposure to gloss paint. You may get a rash from a particular cleaning agent. Some patients find that certain chemicals give them a lift or that they 'like' the smell. This too should be taken as a sign of sensitivity (think of glue-sniffers).

You may notice you are ill in certain locations and not in others (this is true with any environmental allergy, not just a chemical allergy). If the city centre makes you tired, sick and headachy, a likely reason is petrol-fume allergy.

Table 19.1 lists factors that should cause you to suspect you are allergic to certain chemicals.

Symptoms Suggesting Chemical Sensitivity

Already know that some chemicals cause you to feel unwell

You feel particularly bad in enclosed areas (e.g. shopping malls)

You get a lift from or like certain smells

Gloss paint makes you headachy

Your sense of smell is lost or heightened

You suffer a reaction to perfume (which is ethanol-based)

You are sick on long car journeys

You feel unwell in certain locations

CHEMICALS AT WORK AND AT SCHOOL

Chemicals at work can be a problem to some individuals. What is harmless to some may be toxic to others. The classic pattern for such individuals is that they feel worst at work and generally tend to improve at weekends and on holidays. Every Monday they have an unpleasant reaction on returning to work which is, in effect, a **challenge test (18)** with chemicals. By Tuesday the symptoms have often settled down and disappear on Wednesday, Thursday and Friday.

The individual then goes home for the weekend, clears him- or herself of all the chemicals and unmasks the allergic reaction so that by Monday the process starts all over again when a new round of symptoms

occurs. 'Monday morning blues' are famous and, although there are other explanations, the one that is most often missed is the person sensitive to the work environment.

Table 19.2 summarizes the symptoms that would suggest chemical sensitivity at work.

Symptoms Suggesting Chemical Sensitivity at Work

The presence of any known hazards (e.g. toluene diisocyanate, formaldehyde

You feel better at weekends

Symptoms clear up on holidays

Co-workers also affected ('sick building syndrome')

Reaction began when you started your present employment

Worst on Monday and Tuesday

Keep in mind potential physical factors, e.g. VDUs and back or eye strain – not necessarily an allergy

In some trades there are specific hazards; since the Health and Safety at Work Act of 1974 the monitoring of these exposures has come under the control of the Environmental Safety Officer (ESO) in the Environmental Medical Advisory Service (EMAS). However, to pretend this system is working efficiently and protecting workers properly is foolish in the extreme.

Only a very small percentage of workers – those employed in larger factories and offices – effectively come under this sort of umbrella. Although the Act supposedly covers all offices, factories and places of work, in actual fact it is impossible to monitor the countless small businesses that this represents. Only if an individual worker complains is any action likely to be taken in the event of a hazard – and many workers are reluctant to report breaches of the codes for fear of losing their jobs, either in retribution or indirectly because the works are closed down.

It may be obvious to you that you are working with major chemical toxins. However, many chemical allergens at work are insidious and difficult to detect.

Problems can come from photocopier fluids, solvents, aerosols, powerful cleaning agents and detergents (common where contract cleaners are employed), air purifiers and, last but not least, the fabric of the building and its furnishings (**formaldehyde (42)** particularly). If your office has that new 'plastic' smell, this could be a problem. Air conditioning often makes matters far worse by circulating indoor pollution.

Factors Suggesting Allergies at Home

(Includes sensitizing allergens, as well as chemicals)
You feel worse in the evenings and at weekends
When you wake the symptoms are at their worst
You feel better when on holidays (as also with chemicals at work)
You feel worse in certain rooms of the house
Other family members/friends may be affected

Nose Survey

Our sense of smell can provide us with important clues. Sense of smell tends to alter or even diminish in response to a chemical sensitivity. This may be accompanied by rhinitis (catarrh) and a blocked nose, through which no positive sense of smell is possible. But most patients experience a heightened sense of smell before this stage is reached.

To pinpoint potential chemical hazards, I usually get patients to comb the whole house, room by room, cupboard by cupboard and shelf by shelf, listing all the chemicals they find. Sometimes the list itself is a shock and this is salutary.

This procedure can be made much more effective by tracking down *smells*. I call this a *nose survey*: the Mumby rule of thumb is simply that, if you can smell it, it can make you ill. That is, if there is enough to cause an odour, there is enough to cause symptoms. Obviously, those suffering a loss of their sense of smell will have to enlist someone's help in this procedure.

CREATING A SAFE OASIS

It makes good sense to clear your environment of as many unnecessary chemicals as possible. This will reduce your overall burden. The best place to start is in your home, where you have the most control. You may be able to influence changes at work, especially if you have a private office, but for many people this isn't practicable. 'Open plan' offices, in

particular, often mean allergics sharing their workspace many hours a day with those who smoke or wear perfume and with equipment, fabrics and carpets that give off fumes such as formaldehyde and other vapours. Modern offices are among the worst imaginable places to be; down a coal mine would be healthier than many of the environments people have to put up with. If you are faced with this difficulty at least try to press for an open window near where you work.

Once you have created your safe 'oasis', you can come back to it in times of overload and de-stress your chemical detoxification systems. But don't forget the value of fresh air. In almost all situations it is better than indoor air. If it isn't, you might want to consider moving!

There are now available some very good personal environmental air systems for creating a clean local environment. These are a remarkably good investment for anyone with this kind of sensitivity problem.

There follows a list of some of the modern chemical hazards and ways to go about achieving a smaller chemical load. It makes no pretense to be an exhaustive treatment, which would require a full-length book, but it will get you started. Finally, remember you will not be able to eradicate these hazards altogether, nor should you become fanatical and try to do so. It is also a Mumby maxim that you don't need zero load to get zero symptoms!

- Aerosols
  We all know about the effect aerosol propellants (CFCs) have on the environment. What is more important and often forgotten is that they have a bad effect on humans too!
  Also, beware of so-called 'ozone friendly' products. These simply contain alternative chemicals. Remember that ozone friendly doesn't mean 'bio-friendly'.
- Air fresheners
- Tap water
- Cavity wall insulation
  Urea-formaldehyde foam insulation (UFFI) is a cause of considerable health problems; so much so that it was banned

some years ago in the US – although we are still being told it is safe here in the UK.

● Cleaning materials

There are always simpler alternatives, even if they do call for a little more manual effort. Sodium bicarbonate or borax can often be made to serve where more powerful alkaline agents would be used. Avoid 'biologicals' like the plague. Especially avoid fabric 'conditioners', which seem to cause strong reactions in some.

For personal washing use *Simple*, *Castille* or *Neutragena* soaps. For household duties try soft green soap (that's its name!) obtainable from chemists.

● Cooking utensils

Allergics should avoid using non-stick pans with Teflon-type coatings. Nor is aluminium cookware recommended, due to toxicity problems. Glass and enamel are best.

● Fabrics

Most people are better off in natural fabrics, such as wool and cotton. Man-made fabrics all give off fumes long after they are new. Of course some people are allergic to natural fabrics, especially wool, and trial and error is required to find what suits you best.

● Flues

Chimney flues may present problems as they can leak and give off serious fumes. The only safe course is to have the flue lined with a modern flexible flue liner which, although expensive, can be passed up the chimney with the minimum disturbance and mess.

Better still, change to electrical radiators and eliminate gas or open fires.

● Garages, integral

Petrol fumes are a common concern, I find. It is far better (and safer!) to park the car outside and to use the garage to grow mushrooms or for a model workshop.

● Gas

All chemically-sensitive patients should get rid of gas from their homes if it is at all practicable and economically viable to do so.

Avoid open gas fires.

Do not use gas for cooking, even if you have to retain it for heating purposes.

A final word of warning: Under no circumstances whatever be tempted to use the free-standing butane gas heaters which can be wheeled from room to room. These give off very toxic fumes.

● Heating

Avoid ducted air systems, fan heaters and, to a certain extent, open bar electric fires. Best are central heating radiators or, for portable use, small oil-filled electric radiators, such as the Dimplex type.

● Make-up

Cosmetics are generally biologically unfriendly. Try to get the hypoallergenic kind but remember there is no such thing as non-allergenic.

● Paints

Paints can cause many unpleasant symptoms. There are a number of 'organic' paints coming onto the market. These are watersoluble and free of the toxic solvent fumes. If you don't want to use water-based paints, latex paint is said to be best for allergics. Stir in sodium bicarbonate until the paint stops bubbling. Richard Mackarness suggests about 100 g to 5 litres of paint.

● Toothpaste

Toothpaste may contain ammonia, ethanol, artificial colours and flavours, formaldehyde, mineral oil, saccharin, sugar and carcinogenic PVP plastic.

Weleda (Ilkeston, Derbyshire) do a simple salt gel or plant gel paste, safer than any others. For the exquisitely sensitive, try oil of cloves.

Also see **atmospheric pollution (10)**, **natural gas (77)** and Appendix C

20. Chronic Viral Infections

It has been well said on occasion that a virus is a piece of bad news wrapped up in protein. Apart from being witty, this remark makes a good point: viruses are not 'alive' in the strict sense of the word. They are protein bundles that cannot reproduce themselves. Instead, they hijack healthy cells and force them to produce more of their own kind. It is a strange existence but phenomenally successful.

Medical virology has been hitherto concerned with acute infectious illness, however it seems certain in the future that trends will be towards the damaging effects of chronic virus infections such as herpes simplex, cytomegalovirus, Epstein-Barr, varicella-zoster (chicken pox and shingles), hepatitis B and, of course, HIV.

Viruses do not always kill the host cell in which they replicate and may not provoke an immune attack, which is why the body cannot shake them off. Instead they alter the function of the cells they invade, to the detriment of the host organism. It seems increasingly likely that many familiar diseases such as diabetes, multiple sclerosis, dwarfism and even chronic hypoglycaemia are caused by viruses. Suppression of the immune system is just one likely result: this would result in allergies and intolerance.

VIRAL RECEPTORS

The effect of a viral infection depends on the organism and the host. Effects may be produced at the site of the virus or on distant organs. If specialized cells are involved, such as neurological tissue, the effects can be disastrous. By contrast, many less specialized cells such as fibrous tissue and epithelial cells can be widely infected without any life-threatening consequences. We now have the concept of *viral receptors*, that is, specific target areas to which a virus will gravitate.

Once inside a cell, a virus can cause many effects. The polio virus, for example, can block or divert enzymes necessary for cell metabolism. Other viruses may disrupt the membranes within cells and cause the release of products that will kill and digest cells. They may damage cell walls and alter their integrity. Some viruses such as the measles virus can cause cell walls to fuse and cells to group together uselessly.

This is important to those of us in the field of allergy and immunology, since chronic viral infection of many types may lead to a breakdown of tolerance and the development of allergic reactions and other immune

dysfunction. In fact we are working gradually towards the idea that probably any organism – viral, bacterial or protozoan – can have this adverse effect.

CHRONIC INFECTIOUS MONONUCLEOSIS (EPSTEIN-BARR VIRUS)

Infectious mononucleosis (or glandular fever) is caused by Epstein-Barr (EB) Virus. There is an acute phase of the illness, usually attacking the upper respiratory tract (the throat, etc.). But the virus may linger and cause a chronic condition, characterized by fatigue, low mood and other non-specific symptoms. In a proportion of cases, a relapsing illness results which is very like ME.

It would seem that some forms of Chronic EB Virus (CEBV) are normal for most adults. It may become activated only in states of immune deficiency.

Positive antibody *titres* (levels of antibodies high enough to suggest an infection) are the mainstay of diagnosis. The classic test is the Paul-Bunnell antibody test. However, many normal, healthy individuals may also have anti-EB Virus antibodies and this has sometimes led to confusion.

SLOW VIRUS INFECTIONS

This term refers to virus infections that have no acute phase but take many years, sometimes decades, before the disease assumes any outward manifestation. The concept has been around for a long time but we are being forced to confront it more urgently with the growing anxiety about the possibility that certain animal diseases may be transferred to humans, particularly bovine spongiform encephalopathy (BSE).

The causative agent for this condition, which has proved very elusive indeed, appears to be an odd-ball virus. The worry is that it is very much like the agent that causes a recognized disease in humans, namely Creutzfeldt-Jakob Syndrome. This is a pre-senile dementia that occurs in mid-adult life, caused by a spongiform degeneration of neurological tissue (a sort of 'brain rot'). It is uniformly fatal and there is no known cure.

A similar condition was once prevalent in New Guinea and was known as KURU. The victim lost control of motion and walking, began to shake inexorably and death was rapid, usually within a year. It was probably caused by the ceremonial practice of eating the brains of deceased relatives. KURU declined when cannibalism was banned.

There are a number of such diseases, including scrapie in sheep and distemper in dogs. Professor David Anderson at Salford University has drawn a connection between distemper and the human affliction known as Paget's disease. This is a curious disorder characterized by a thickening of the bones, leading to fracture and deformities. It is very prevalent in Britain, which would make sense since we are said to be a nation of dog-lovers. Paget's disease can develop up to 50 years after contact with an infected dog.

It has even been suggested that multiple sclerosis, diabetes and systemic lupus erythematosus could be slow viruses. There is no proof for this. However, multiple sclerosis has all the appearance of a viral disease, leading to the breakdown of fatty insulation tissue in nerves which then sets up an auto-immune reaction, precipitated by the breakdown products.

But the real agony of BSE (if we are to get it), and of Creutzfeldt-Jakob Syndrome, is that we will have inflicted it on ourselves through carelessness, greed and stupidity. The modern agribusiness practice of feeding cows deceased animal products may unwittingly have led to a huge build-up of afflicted animal stock. The causative agent is not inactivated by cooking, so the practice of eating very 'rare' beef is irrelevant: we may already have infected countless humans.

Also see **immune system (56)** and **post viral fatigue syndrome (88)**

21. Co-enzyme Q10

This vitamin-like substance (also known as Ubiquone-50) was discovered in 1957. Since then a deluge of scientific papers have shown it to be involved beneficially in strengthening the immune system, lowering blood-pressure, preventing heart attacks, countering obesity and slowing ageing. A pretty formidable list. Yet most doctors have never heard of this substance.

In comparison to the major impact of an awareness of the health effects of vitamin C, zinc and essential fatty acids, and other new interests in nutrition, Co-enzyme Q10 seems almost to have been underplayed to the point of being lost in the transmission 'noise'. Yet in Japan some 10 million people (10 per cent of the population) take it daily and swear by it. In fact that country offers over 200 commercial brands to choose from, marketed by 80 pharmaceutical companies.

Why haven't we heard about it? Are the claims made of it exaggerated? Or are vested interests at work again?

Co-enzyme Q10 (also known as CoQ10) is a quinone. This family of substances includes vitamins E and K1. A potent anti-cancer agent, Adriamycin, also has a quinone-like structure. There are 10 ubiquinones (the name comes from the Latin: *ubi* – 'everywhere'), numbered Q1–Q10. Numbers Q1 to Q8 are found entirely in yeasts, moulds and bacteria. Q9 and Q10 occur only in plant and animal life. In fact, with very few exceptions (rats, mice and the wall-eyed pike, which also have CoQ9), all vertebrate animals (those with backbones) have only ubiquinone Q10.

CoQ10 is found in all cells, where it is responsible for the manufacture of adenosine triphosphate, the body's basic energy molecule. Highest levels are found in the cells of the heart, the liver – our powerful detoxification factory – and the immune system. This observation alone argues it is of vital importance to health and indeed survival. Without a heart we wouldn't live minutes, without an immune system we wouldn't last hours, without a liver no more than a day or two.

It is now being said that if CoQ10 levels in the body drop by 25 per cent or more, disease and probably cancer will follow inevitably. If levels drop by 75 per cent, then life itself is no longer sustainable.

CoQ10 is also an **anti-oxidant (8)** and will prevent 'free-radicals' from attacking and ageing tissues. Significantly, animal experiments on mice showed that CoQ10 increased the life-span of mice by around 50 per cent. Equally interesting was that it seemed to be a type of 'youthful' life, not just an extended old age. Improvement in some phsyiological parameters was hard to dispute; for example, increased cardiac output and stroke volume (the amount of blood thrust out over one contraction or stroke).

It also seems to be able to lower blood-pressure, though how exactly isn't known, and to reduce weight, presumably by increasing metabolic performance. CoQ10 also seems to diminish the effect of histamine on the tissues.

Those concerned about boosting their immune system (which would include cancer and AIDS patients, as well as allergics) will be glad to know that CoQ10 increases phagocytosis and raises antibody levels. Mice with chemically-induced tumours fed on CoQ10 survived, on average, over twice as long as controls with the same tumours. What is more, the tumours actually diminished in size.

All in all then, a remarkable chemical.

Supplementation can be considered. A suitable dose would be 10 to 30 mg daily. This can rise to 100 mg in certain cases but, in our present state of knowledge, should not exceed this amount.

However, don't forget that CoQs occur in *all* living tissue. CoQ10 specifically is found plentifully in heart, muscle, kidney, eggs and milk (animal sources) and also in potato, sweet potato, spinach, alfalfa, soybean, wheat, rice bran oil, soya bean oil and cottonseed oil.

Also see **nutrition and allergies (81)**

22. Conventional Allergy Testing

PRICK TESTING AND HYPOSENSITIZATION

Conventional allergy testing has not advanced significantly since 1911, when the prick and scratch test method was first developed. For this method a small drop of the substance being tested is dropped onto the skin, which is then scratched or pricked with a needle at that spot. The amount of flare and wheal compared to that caused by a control (inert) solution gives an indication of how allergenic the substance is.

It is a very inaccurate method, with many false negatives, and subjects seldom react to food at all in this way, though a demonstrable allergy may be present on **challenge testing (18)**. An important migraine study at the Great Ormond Street Hospital for Sick Children in 1983 showed that none of the cases would have recovered by following an exclusion diet based on the results of prick testing (though 93 per cent improved on a suitable diet, showing that food allergy was the cause). Because the prick and scratch test can be misleading, many conventional allergists prefer not to use it.

The hyposensitization method aims to find out which substances the patient is allergic to and then to give injections of a mixture of these, increasing gradually in strength, until quite large amounts are being tolerated. The body is often then found to be able to cope with normal ambient concentrations. The process is not unlike that of *mithridating* – named after king Mithridates, a Persian ruler who protected himself against poisoning by taking larger and larger doses of poison daily until he could tolerate amounts that would normally kill a recipient.

There are two major drawbacks to this hyposensitization treatment: (a) it rarely works and (b) it can be extremely dangerous. Patients sometimes react severely and deaths due to **anaphylaxis (6)** used to occur regularly until by common consent its use was abandoned in the UK, except in special circumstances and where full cardio-pulmonary resuscitation equipment is at hand.

The only suitable indications for the use of this method are in cases of perennial rhinitis and asthma due to dust and dust mite allergy, seasonal rhinitis due to pollens and the danger of anaphylaxis due to insect stings. Even so, very brittle (vulnerable) cases, especially children, are better left un-desensitized, since the dangers of the method are very real. We have better, safer methods, in the form of **enzyme potentiated desensitization (36)** (EPD) and Miller's low-dose desensitization (see **Miller's method (74)**).

PATCH TESTING

Another fairly primitive technique is patch testing. Small quantities of different suspected substances are placed under individual cups which are taped to the skin for a number of hours. A reddening of the skin under the patch denotes a sensitivity to that substance. A control is used, since some people react to the pads or tape, etc.

A positive reaction is probably fairly dependable, but it rarely happens. Even substances known to have a marked effect often don't affect the skin. In other words, negative reactions do not exclude significant allergens.

This method works best for identifying causes of contact dermatitis, such as nickel, soap powders or industrial chemicals.

All other conventional allergy tests are based on immunological reactions of the IgE antibody type (see **hypersensitivity (53)**). Naturally, classic antigen-antibody reactions are the only results to be expected, which precludes a large number of allergic and intolerant reactions.

Broadly speaking, then, these tests are fine if they give a positive result; which is to say, if an allergy to wheat or egg is found, it exists. Avoiding that food will help with the overall **body load (11)**. But negatives are meaningless (these occur over 95 per cent of the time). Also, a positive reaction on an immunological test only means antibodies are present, *it does not mean the allergy is the one causing symptoms*. Experts often overlook this elementary point.

RADIO IMMUNOASSAY (RIA)

This is the basic immunological test using radioactive labelled molecules for quantifying results.

1. Antigen (a substance capable of stimulating an immune response) is incubated with a plastic plate or tube until it becomes bound by adsorption (adhesion).
2. The plate is washed and the blood serum, with suspected antibody, is added. This naturally locks on to the antigen. Unused antibody is washed away.
3. How much antibody has been 'captured' is measured by labelling it with a radioactively tagged molecule (the ligand), specially designed to latch on to the antibody being sought.
4. After unused ligand has been washed away, the amount that remains behind can be measured using a gamma counter (Geiger counter). This gives an exuisitely sensitive measurement of how much antibody was present in the serum being tested, using only tiny amounts of test solutions.

Enzyme-linked Immunoabsorbent Assay (ELISA)

This is a specialized version of the RIA. At stage 3, the ligand isn't radioactive but is a special enzyme which (stage 4) attacks a substance called chromogen. This releases colour-dye – the degree of the colour change gives a measure of how much antibody is present. The assessment is made accurate by using optical scanning apparatus to measure the colour density.

The Radio Allergosorbent Test (RAST)

This test is another version of RIA with special reference to use in detecting allergic (inappropriate) antibodies of the IgE type. The antigen is covalently (chemically) bound to a small cellulose disc, which means it effectively holds more antigen and this increases the sensitivity of the test.

The ligand used in stage 3 is radioactively labelled anti-IgE antibody. It locks on to the antigen-specific IgE which has been retained by the disc after washing. The gamma counter once again measures precisely how much IgE antibody must have been present in the original serum.

PROVOCATION TESTS

Conventional allergists share with clinical ecologists a respect for using the patient as his or her own test bed.

Ophthalmic Testing

Small quantities of test reagent can be placed into the conjunctival sac of the eye.

Reactions include visible reddening, lachrymation (tears) and (sometimes) sneezing. There is a limit to the number of substances that can be tested at any one time (i.e., very few) and so this has limited application. It is particularly suitable for seasonal reactions (pollens) being tested out of season.

Nasal Provocation Challenge

Potential allergens can be introduced into the nasal passages, either as liquid or powder particles, and the results monitored. The patient is then observed for an arbitrary 5 to 30 minutes (depending on the standard procedure). Reactions can include sneezing, catarrh, a blocked nose and, naturally a clinical ecologist would ask, cerebral and other manifestations as well. One or two initial sneezes are discounted as being probably just a normal response to the irritating effect of the liquid/powder in the nasal passages.

Alternate nostrils are used and up to 20 items can be tested in one session. If severe symptoms develop, a nasal 'washout' using saline (salt water) will normally clear them. If not, testing may have to be discontinued for the day.

Also see **cytotoxic tests** **(24)**

23. Cyclical and Fixed Allergies

Not all allergies are constant and predictable. Many appear to come and go. The key to this shifting pattern is the concept of 'cyclical' and 'fixed' allergies.

Fixed allergies, as the name implies, never really change. Once acquired they are with one for life. In general fixed allergies are severe. Allergies to insect stings, strawberries and shellfish tend to be of this type. These are probably immunologically-induced allergies (see **allergy: a definition (5)**) and, in accordance with our present understanding at any rate, there is no reason to expect them to alter.

Cyclical allergies, on the other hand, vary considerably in the severity of reactions they

produce. The more often the allergen is encountered, the worse the reaction becomes. Conversely, if the allergen is avoided for a period, the reaction tends to dampen down.

The actual period of avoidance varies a great deal. In some cases as little as a few days may result in loss of response to a single mild dose. Other people may have to avoid the allergen for many months. The majority of allergens lie somewhere in between.

The cyclical effect is of great importance when it comes to allergy **challenge testing (18)**. The optimum interval between avoidance and testing for a food is five to ten days. Five days are needed for unmasking (see **hidden allergy (49)**) but, beyond that time, the sooner the tests are carried out the better. After ten days certain allergens may begin to lose their effect and so be missed on a single challenge feed. As a result the patient may consider a food safe, eat it frequently and suffer baffling exacerbation symptoms.

This cyclical nature of allergens means that it is not usually necessary to avoid an allergen for life or, indeed, for more than a few months at a time, before trying it again. However, the patient must understand that returning to a frequent intake of the allergen will *not* work – it will just make the symptoms start up all over again. A hostile food will always have to be treated with some caution.

Rotation dieting (95) is an attempt to prevent the build-up of cyclical allergies. By eating foods in line with a careful timetable, say every four days, it is usually possible to maintain the safe character of a food. Remember also, a food eaten below its 'threshold dose' will appear not to cause a reaction (see **body load (11)**).

Also see **hypersensitivity (53)**

24. Cytotoxic Tests

Use of a 'leucocyotoxic' reaction for in vitro screening for food allergy antibodies was first recorded by P. Black in 1956. The test at that time was crude and produced results that are best described as suggestive, rather than conclusive. Today's method follows 30 years of refining this test.

Since 1960 the test has been researched steadily by W. T. K. Bryan and M. P. Bryan at Washington University School of Medicine in St Louis, Missouri. The technique is simple but depends for accuracy upon a high standard of laboratory technique.

White blood cells (leucocytes), separated by centrifuging, are placed on a microscope slide chamber and mixed with about 10 mg of food extract. The sample is then observed at intervals over the next two hours, using a x 60 lens, and the effect of the food extract on the white cells is noted.

Healthy white cells are mobile and exhibit amoeba-like behaviour. On contact with an allergen, in this case a food sample, the cells lose their mobility and become rounded in shape. Cytoplasmic granules become sluggish and cease to stream. Eventually, damaged cells rupture and die.

A typical test might include several dozen foods, food additives and inhalants such as dust, cigarette smoke and even house gas. Theoretically, hundreds of items at a time can be tested. In practice, the number of items is limited by how many technicians are employed and how many slides they can scrutinize before the samples begin to deteriorate.

REPORTING

It is customary to grade reactions from 0 to 4, depending on severity of damage, observing the following changes:

(a) reduction or loss of amoeboid movement;
(b) intracellular stasis (slow-down or stop-page);
(c) rounding and distortion of cell contour:
(d) vacuolation (the appearance of tiny *vacuoles*, or cavities);
(e) cell lysis (bursting open)

Dr Damien Downing, who first introduced this method into the UK, claims that it has an 80 per cent accuracy. There are many critics however, even among clinical ecologists, who do not take these claims seriously and who point to many well-conducted trials which show that the method is virtually useless.

The difficulty with the test, in common with many other methods, is that it rests in the final analysis on human interpretation rather than objective measurement. This isn't so bad as long as each laboratory is at least consistent with its own standards. But it may, on occasion, lead to patchy quality in results, which can be very misleading for the patient.

Dr Downing comments on the reproducibility of the test:

'If the same blood is examined in two separate preparations simultaneously, or in the same preparation by two technicians, or the same blood is examined at 24-hour intervals under controlled conditions, with any single increase in the degrees of freedom, one generally finds that between one in five and one in six of the test results cross the border from one to another of the four possible results. This is presumably a reflection of the technicians' human limitations. Greater degrees of variability are rare, at around one per cent. That is to say that a technician can manage to get the result accurate to within one degree of reaction 99 per cent of the time!'

This sounds almost too good to be true, until you remember that in this case each 'one degree' of reaction represents 25 per cent of the whole!

BACK-UP

Probably the main drawback of the cytotoxic test method is that it needs intelligent and knowledgeable back-up by a competent doctor. Otherwise the patient is left avoiding certain foods indefinitely, with no clear plan in mind, struggling to keep up an adequate diet on a selection of things to eat that may be pitifully limited.

Unfortunately, this after-care is not always readily obtainable and the laboratories themselves often duck the issue.

Also see **applied kinesiology (9), conventional allergy tests (22)** and **Miller's method (74)**

25. Dermatitis

Dermatitis is a condition of reddening of the skin with itching and scaling that may lead to cracking and weeping sores, when severe. It is not unlike eczema to look at but has important differences. Eczema is an internal disease, that is the skin is damaged from causes within, notably allergy. In dermatitis the result may look the same but is caused by *external* substances coming into contact with the skin. Some of these substances would damage *any* skin, given sufficient concentration or duration of contact. Most cases of dermatitis, however, are caused by a special sensitivity in the patient.

It is easy to tell the difference between eczema and dermatitis if the condition appears on the hands. Eczema usually affects the palms, where the skin is tough and can only be harmed by internal tissue changes. Contact dermatitis, on the other hand, affects the back of the hands first, where the skin is thinnest and most vulnerable. Of course, not all rashes appear on the hands.

Dermatitis should be suspected whenever there are clear areas of demarcation, particularly when these coincide with the pressure marks caused by an article of clothing or are limited to exposed parts of the body. Some sites are classic for dermatitis. The hands are obvious, since these usually handle the offending subtance. But marks under bra clips, where zips touch and around suspenders are also well-known signs of nickel allergy.

Common causes of irritant dermatitis include the following:

- Tap water
- Cleansers: soaps and detergents.
- Alkalis: epoxy resin hardeners, lime, cement, caustic soda, ammonia, trisodium phosphate
- Acids (any)
- Oils: emulsifiers, anticorrosion agents, perfumes, lubricating oil, turpentine
- Solvents: degreasers, paint strippers, hand cleaners, thinners, etc.
- Plants: primulas, orange peel, juices, asparagus

- Animals: cat hair, dog hair, horsehair and danders, or from preparing fish or meats
- Metals: nickel, chromates
- Drugs and medicinal products: lanolin, commonly used in creams and ointments, is a good example. Wood alcohol, from lanolin, may be the culprit in some individuals.

There are several strange versions of this condition. Some people get an increase in the pigmentation (colouring) of their skin when it comes in contact with various substances. Figs produce a substance called *furocoumarin*, which is a photosensitizer. It gets onto the skin of fig-pickers and, in the presence of sunlight, can cause increased pigmentation or even blistering. Celery pickers who are sensitive may experience the same thing, due to an organism growing on the plants producing a photosensitizing chemical. Limes and lemons can do it, too.

Depigmentation is also possible with some chemicals.

TESTS

Contact dermatitis is a good example of a cell-mediated immune response. This condition is very suitable for patch testing.

Sometimes the likely antigen can be guessed at. If not, the patient is tested against a wide range of readily available materials such as rubber, nickel, drugs and household items. However, a positive patch test reaction does not necessarily prove that the reagent is the cause of the dermatitis (see **conventional allergy tests (22)**). Testing must be linked with taking a careful history of the illness.

Chemicals should be diluted before application in testing, since many are primary irritants. That is, they can produce a reaction due to their physically damaging properties which will mask an allergic **hypersensitivity** reaction.

TREATMENT

Avoidance is by far the best policy. If the exposure is an occupational one, the patient may have to consider a change of job, especially if the reaction is severe.

A compromise is to use barrier creams, but these are only of limited value. Rubber gloves may give more protection, but rubber itself is likely to become a sensitizing irritant.

Steroid creams will keep the condition in check temporarily, but long-term use is not to be recommended. A better management plan should be sought.

Also see **target organs (104)**

26. Detoxification

Toxicology is one area of medicine about which clinical ecologists are not in conflict with their more conventional colleagues. We share the same issues, pursue the same phenomena and agree on therapeutic approaches. Toxicologists tend to veer in the direction of epidemiological effects, studying whole-groups, whereas the clinical ecologist takes it more patient by patient, but that's the only real difference.

Toxicology has been around a surprisingly long time. Primitive peoples used natural poisons for hunting. Indeed the word toxicology comes from *toxicos*, the bow from which poison arrows were flung. The ancient Greeks and Romans made a special study of poisons, although more in connection with political assassinations than the pursuit of science. The Persian King Mithridates was so afraid of being poisoned that he took a regular cocktail of known poisons to accustom his body to their effect so that they would no longer work on him. From his name we get the word *mithridate*.

The prolific use of poisons for getting rid of 'inconvenient' people led to a treatise by Maimmonides (1135–1204) entitled *Poisons and their Antidotes*. It summarized all knowledge of poisons at that time.

The Italian fifteenth-century Borgia family were infamous poisoners. Lucrezia's name, in particular, achieved evil notoriety for her nefarious use of chemicals to 'alter' history.

Toxicology finally adopted a more formal scientific footing, and today we are concerned almost entirely with environmental hazards and *unintentional* harm done to human beings. Around 4,000,000

man-made chemicals have been described in scientific literature since 1965. Something like 6,000 new chemicals are added to the list every week and at least 70,000 are currently in production. Only a fraction of this toxic load has been adequately tested for the long-term effects on human health.

We meet chemicals in the air, our food, water supplies and by direct contact. Medical drugs add their share, and even the clothes we wear and the fabric of our homes are mostly artificially made, needing many complex chemical precursors. Some of these emit toxins long after being installed in the home. It is a fact of life in the modern world that indoor pollution can be just as bad, or worse, than the outdoor kind.

The cumulative effect of all these substances may create a total body burden that triggers chemical sensitivity in certain individuals. In the late 1970s Dr E. C. Hamlyn coined the term 'human canary' to describe such people – they are a warning to us all that we are going to be ill if we continue as we are, in much the same way that canaries used to warn miners of impending gas danger. Unfortunately, no one seems to be heeding these canaries.

Most studies done on humans to date have been concerned predominantly with acute massive exposures suffered by workers in industrial settings, but clinical ecologists have been gathering case studies steadily to show that chronic exposure to levels commonly thought to be 'safe' are compromising people's health and may turn out to be a more important hazard in the long term.

MULTIFACTORIAL

The effects of chemical exposure are dependent upon a number of factors, principally:

- the amount and biological activity of the compound
- length of the exposure time
- genetic factors
- biochemical individuality
- the total stress load
- age and sex

- previous exposures
- nutritional factors

The resulting problems can be complex, depending on the **target organs** involved. Misdiagnosis and missed diagnosis are the norm. Safety levels are misleading, since they are based on averages. Some individuals will react to far lower levels than would affect the majority.

The way the body disposes of unwanted and toxic compounds (xenobiotics) we call *detoxification*. In fact, the metabolic pathways discussed here, by which chemicals are inactivated and removed from the body, don't *always* result in a less poisonous end-product. A better term, therefore, is *biotransformation*.

There are several pathways involved. The subject is a vast and burgeoning one; the information given here is necessarily selective.

METABOLISM OF TOXIC COMPOUNDS

To get rid of a toxin effectively it is most important that the body turns it into something soluble in water. At that point the substance or its metabolites (breakdown products) can be removed via the kidneys, sweat, bile and other fluids. There are two principal routes by which the body does this. In Phase I metabolism the molecule is altered by enzymes in a variety of ways, each process assisted by a specific enzyme. These enzymes are found in the microsomes of most cells.

The most important of these enzyme pathways is the cytochrome P450 system, also called the multi-function oxidase system (MFO). Under its influence oxygen is added to the toxic molecule, converting a hydrogen atom in the molecule into a hydroxyl group (hydrogen *and* oxygen). The opposite effect, known as reduction, means that hydrogen is added. Both effects can knock out the toxicity of a molecule.

Two other methods to note are: adding a water molecule (2 hydrogen and 1 oxygen atoms), called *hydration* and knocking out halogen atoms, such as chlorine, called *dehalogenation*.

It is important to note that **magnesium** is essential for Phase I actions, as is a complex co-enzyme called nicotinamide adenine dinucleotide (NADH), a derivative of vitamin B_3. Vitamin C and zinc are also said to help, and possibly other nutrients as well. This is why vitamin and mineral supplements can be so vital for allergics and poor metabolizers.

Phase II detoxification is carried out differently. Here *extra* groups are stuck on to the basic molecule. These change its character and render it harmless and more soluble. We call this process *conjugation*. An example is *sulphation*, the addition of a sulphate group ($-SO_3$). Phenol (carbolic acid), which looks like this:

is converted into phenyl sulphate, which looks like this:

The enzyme in this case is sulphonyl transferase. Phenol sulphonyl transferase may have great importance for food intolerance since it has become clear that a number of foods contain several **phenolic** compounds.

Side Routes

These optimal biotransformation pathways can be blocked for a number of reasons. Certain vitamin and mineral deficiencies could do it; magnesium, for example, has been mentioned. Overload can have the same effect. As the total quantity of xenobiotics increases, we can produce more of the relevant enzyme, up to a point (this is called enzyme induction). But eventually we pass the equalization point and the body can no longer cope.

When the basic system is no longer capable of keeping pace, 'alternative' toxic metabolites may be chosen which may be more stable and can't easily be brought back into the enzyme pathways and broken down.

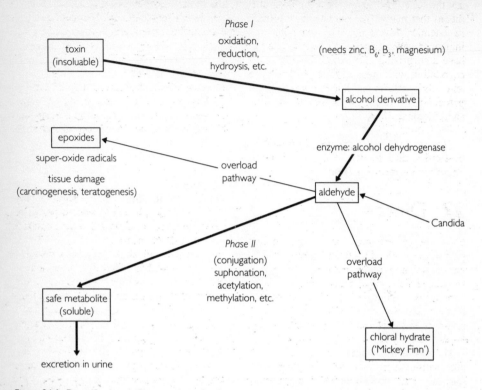

Figure 26.1: Detoxification pathways and overload

Some of these 'alternatives' are capable of causing serious tissue and gene damage.

A Cause of Fatigue

Less serious, perhaps, but troublesome nevertheless is the alternative pathway that yields chloral hydrate. At times of overload, this chemical can build up. It is one of the ingredients of the classic 'Mickey Finn'. If this build-up occurs the patient will begin to feel very fatigued and 'spacey'. These are symptoms that overload patients will recognize.

Candida, incidentally, is capable of producing alcohols and aldehydes, which will add to the overload of these detoxification pathways.

The diversity of routes for xenobiotics and the consequences that they may have for the organism can be represented diagrammatically, as shown in Figure 26.1.

FAST AND SLOW METABOLIZERS

There is a sulphoxidation reaction test that can detect the amount of sulphoxide in the urine following a loading dose of a suitable test substrate.

Those who don't handle xenobiotic chemicals very well produce less metabolite output to the urine. We can call them 'slow metabolizers'. Preliminary results show that the white European population has less than 20 per cent slow metabolizers.

A genetically-determined ability to metabolize in this way could be an important factor in a person's response to toxic environmental chemicals and could determine whether he or she will ultimately contract cancer. It is now held likely that poor metabolizers are the people who suffer from chemical intolerance and are those most likely to become **universal reactors** or to develop 'twentieth-century allergies'.

The implication of all this is startling, to

say the least. If it turns out to be correct it means that many diseases may have a basis in chemical overload. For example, the incidence of Parkinson's disease is found to have a surprising and extraordinarily exact correlation with areas of high pesticide use and also affects a larger-than-expected percentage of slow metabolizers. Could it be an ecological illness?

Work continues.

Also see **enzyme supplementation (37), pesticides and health (85)** and **thermal chamber depuration (106)**

27. Diets

Food allergy and intolerance play a major part in the work of a clinical ecologist. We are not trying to argue that every illness can be traced to food allergy, but so many conditions respond well to a change of diet it makes sense to start with this approach. If a cure is as simple as giving up one or two foods, why do more?

There are two kinds of exclusion or elimination diet: one with a diagnostic purpose and one done for therapeutic reasons. It is important to keep this distinction clearly in mind. Trial diets tend to be rather drastic and should only be kept up for limited periods. Treatment diets are more long-term and would thus avoid severe restrictions. It is essential not to exclude more than a few items and to make provision for nutritional alternatives where this is appropriate. If you find yourself having to exclude many items it is vital you get desensitized in some way so that you may retain as many foods as possible. Consider **Miller's method (74)** and **enzyme potentiated desensitization (36)** (EPD).

ELIMINATION DIETING

The secret of identifying food allergies successfully is to give up sufficient foods to feel well, then to reintroduce these foods one at a time so that detecting a reaction is relatively easy. Guessing culprit foods and eliminating them one at a time rarely ever succeeds.

Here are three levels of structured dieting:

the Stone Age diet, the Eight-foods diet and the Fast. Choose the one best suited to your circumstances and temperament.

The Stone Age Diet

An easy elimination diet (14 to 21 days)

This has been aptly described as a hunter-gatherer's diet, much as our ancestors must have eaten long ago in the forests and on the plains.

Allowed

- Fresh meat: lamb, beef, pork, turkey, goose, duck, pheasant, pigeon, partridge, venison, rabbit, hare, free-range chicken, liver, kidney, heart
- Fresh fish: all kinds (but not smoked)
- Fresh vegetables, including potatoes
- All fresh fruit, except citrus fruits: preferably home-grown or from a farm where sprays are not used. Commercial fruit must be washed and, if heavily contaminated, peeled before eating.
- Drinks: Preferably glass-bottled spring water (some people have trouble tolerating water from plastic bottles). Tap water should be boiled or filtered. Herb teas (camomile, linden flower, peppermint, etc.) can be used. Dandelion coffee (without lactose and not instant). Fruit juices (not citrus): apple, grape, pineapple, cranberry, etc.
- Seasonings: Fresh ground pepper, sea salt
- Olive oil for cooking
- Fructose for sweetening
- Fresh nuts
- Dried fruit, in moderation

Forbidden

- Anything manufactured, processed, sprayed, added to or adulterated chemically
- Cereals: wheat, barley, oats, rice, millet, corn, corn oil, biscuits, bread, cakes
- Sugar, sweets, chocolate, fizzy drinks, fruit squashes
- Dairy products: milk, cream, butter, margarine, eggs, cheese
- Canned meat or fish
- Bacon, kippers, smoked fish

- Crisps, packaged nuts
- Coffee, tea, alcohol

When clear of symptoms on this diet, single items from the forbidden list may be added to the menu, on a test basis, usually one item a day (see **challenge testing (18)**).

It is vital to understand that you must not cheat on this or any other exclusion diet: doing so could prevent your recovery. Remember that it takes several days for food to clear your bowel. If you do slip up you will need to extend the avoidance period for several more days. Later on, when your detective work is complete, the occasional indiscretion won't matter. In the meantime, follow the instructions *exactly*.

Don't forget about addictions. It is quite likely that you will get withdrawal symptoms during the first few days. Usually the effects are mild and amount to nothing more than feeling irritable, tired, or perhaps having a headache, but be warned – it can be tough going and put you in bed for a couple of days.

Note that it is possible to be allergic even to the allowed foods – they are chosen simply because reaction to them is less common. If you are in this minority you might feel worse on this diet, but at least it proves you have a food allergy. In that case try eliminating also the foods you are eating more of (potato is a common offender) and see if you then begin to improve. If not, you should switch to the Eight Foods Diet or to the Fast.

Do not, simply because you don't improve, make the assumption that you could not then be allergic to milk, wheat or other banned foods. This would be a serious mistake which could bar your road to recovery.

Don't worry about special recipes or substitutes at this stage. By the time you have fried, baked, steamed and grilled everything once or twice, the two weeks will have passed. If challenge tests show that you need to keep off a food long term you can begin searching for an alternative. While on the elimination diet try to avoid hanging on to a few favourite foods and eating only those. You must eat as wide a variety of items as possible otherwise you will risk creating reactions to the foods you are eating repeatedly.

My nurse Marion Whiting has gone to the trouble of working out a 7-day menu; it is given in Appendix E.

A Word About Drugs

Drug allergies are not rare and it may be wise to discontinue medications that are unnecessary. However, certain drugs are essential and should not be stopped, such as anti-epileptics, some cardiac drugs (such as digoxin), insulin, thyroxin and others. Other medications, such as cortisone derivatives, need to be phased out gradually.

To be certain, it is better to discuss the implications with your doctor and ask his or her advice on stopping your treatment. You are entitled to know the effect of any drug you are taking and precisely why you are taking it.

The key question that you want answered is, 'Will I come to harm if I stop taking this drug?' Nine times out of ten the answer is 'No'.

Don't forget, tobacco is a drug. You must stop smoking if you are serious about getting well.

The Eight-foods Diet (7 to 14 days)

Not as severe as a fast but tougher than the previous regime, this is a 'few foods' diet. Obviously it is more likely to succeed since you are giving up more foods. Any determined adult should be able to cope with it, but don't subject a child to this diet without his or her full and voluntary co-operation. Fortunately this is rarely a problem: most children don't want to be ill and will assist you, providing they understand what you are trying to do.

The basic idea is to produce one or two relatively safe foods for each different category – meat, fruit, vegetables and starch. Everyday foods are avoided since these include the common allergens. Thus we would choose fruits such as mango and kiwi, not apple and banana; flesh such as duck and rabbit, not beef and pork. The list below contains my suggestions. You can vary it somewhat according to what is available to you locally.

Suggested Foods

- Meat: Turkey, rabbit
- Vegetables: Spinach, turnip
- Fruit: Mango, kiwi
- Carbohydrates: Buckwheat, quinoa
- Sea salt for seasoning
- Drink only bottled spring water

Be prepared to go on for 14 days before you assume this diet isn't working. However, if it does produce an improvement you can begin reintroductions within just a few days. I usually recommend that you spend two or even three days over each additional food when using this method. Be really sure, do it right and you will probably never have to do this again.

The Fast (4 to 7 days)

Fasting is not recommended. It can be very stressful and should not be undertaken lightly. The biggest liability is that patients sometimes unmask numerous allergies at once and find themselves reacting to virtually everything they eat. This is an artificial situation but it can still be confusing and alarming.

Undertake a fast only if you are very determined or if you suspect food allergy even though the other two approaches have failed.

Fasting is emphatically *not* suitable for certain people:

- Pregnant women
- Children
- Diabetics
- Anyone seriously weakened or debilitated by chronic illness
- Anyone who has been subject to severe emotional disturbance (especially those prone to violent outbursts, or anyone who has tried to commit suicide)
- Epileptics

The fast itself is simple enough – just don't eat for four or five days. Drink only bottled spring water. You *must* also stop smoking.

The whole point is to empty your bowels entirely of foodstuffs. Thus, if you have any tendency to constipation take Epsom salts to begin with. If in doubt try an enema! Otherwise your efforts may be wasted.

A variation which I call the 'half fast' is to eat only two foods, such as lamb and pears. This means taking a gamble that you are not allergic to either lamb or pears. It is permissible to carry this out for seven days, but on no account go on for longer than this.

REINTRODUCING FOODS

For best results follow the instructions on food challenge tests exactly.

Do not be tempted to stay on a very restricted regime even if it made you feel well for the first time in years. That is only half the story: we want to know why. What are the culprits? Just because you feel well excluding several foods doesn't mean they are all to blame. The actual trouble-makers need to be pin-pointed; they are the foods you must avoid long term.

Even if you haven't recovered, consider testing foods as you re-introduce them, anyway – you may be in for a surprise.

SPECIAL INSTRUCTIONS FOR THOSE COMING OFF A FAST

Begin only with exotic foods you don't normally eat. The last thing you want to happen is to get a reaction when you begin to reintroduce foods. Instead, for the first few days, you want to build up a range of 'safe' foods that you can fall back on.

Papaya, rabbit, artichoke and dogfish are the kind of thing to aim for – do the best you can with what is available according to your resources.

The other important point is that you cannot afford the luxury of bringing in only one new food a day: you need to go faster than this.

It is possible to test two or even three foods a day when coming off a fast. Pay particular attention to your pulse rate before and after each test meal. It is important to grasp that a symptom, even if not very striking, usually occurs within the first 60 minutes, when coming off a fast. You need to be alert to this or you will miss items and fail to improve without understanding why.

If the worst happens and you are ill by the end of the day and can't say why, condemn all that day's new foods.

The build-up of foods is cumulative: that is, you start with Food A. If it is OK then the next meal is Food A + Food B, then A + B + C and so on.

All safe foods are kept up after an allergic reaction. Therefore, if Food F causes a symptom, while you are waiting for it to clear up, you can go on eating foods A–E.

Within a few days you should have plenty to eat, albeit monotonous. From then on, you can proceed as for those on elimination diets if you wish.

KEEPING A FOOD DIARY

A useful tool in the process of tracking down hidden food allergies is to keep a detailed diary of everything you eat. Mark out the days clearly and note every ingredient (don't just say 'soup', say what was in it). Write down any change in your symptoms. If you feel ill after your evening meal, make an entry. Also, write down the good days, if there are any! A food diary of this sort often becomes a gold-mine of information.

If you seem to have reacted to something look back over entries just before the symptoms started. Was there anything new? If not, did you eat something afresh after an interval of four or more days in which it could have unmasked? Look also for items that are being used too often. Eventually, patterns may become clear. You may discover, for example, that you tend to react about 36 hours after ingesting an offending food. This will help you in later detection work, though don't expect the interval to remain constant. Some foods might have a long lapse period, others could have an almost instantaneous effect.

A word of warning: it is very easy to become obsessive about food while trying to detect food allergies. While keeping a diary you do need to pay attention to what you are eating, but try not to get too introverted and dream up all sorts of vague symptoms. You will lead yourself into total confusion and loss of morale.

A food diary is merely a tool, not a way of life; it should be discontinued as soon as practicable.

ALTERNATIVE EXCLUSION DIETS

If the simple exclusion diet has not worked, you might like to consider alternative eliminations.

For example, you could try following a meat-free diet. Some people do feel better as vegetarians, certainly: but probably more feel ill because of the high incidence of grain and dairy allergies, as grains and dairy products are staple foods for vegetarians.

Organic Food

Some people (only a few) are better avoiding food treated with chemicals. A diet avoiding this sort of commercial produce is called 'organic'. It is easier nowadays to follow such an eating regime than formerly. Try it if you have reason to suspect you may be reacting to chemicals but don't go overboard: many people are convinced that pesticides on food make them ill but fail to detect them when challenged double-blind.

Organic food suppliers belong to various bodies to help promote themselves and their ideas. Try to make contact with these organizations and find out about your local suppliers. The Henry Doubleday Research Organization is a good place to start (see the Useful Addresses section). They have been pioneers in organic farming methods for decades. They can usually supply a list of vendors. The Soil Association even goes so far as to vet produce showing the label 'organic'. Look for their sign of approval but be warned: this is not a legal requirement and anyone can call their wares 'organic' whether they have used chemicals or not.

Your local health food shop should also be able to help find locally-grown supplies.

Nut- and Pip-free

A very useful exclusion diet is the nut- and pip-free diet. This is a wide group of foods and includes a number of common allergens. Some members of this group can come as a surprise: for example, coffee is a nut.

It is an ambitious diet; it is recommended that you don't go on it until you have established a number of alternative safe foods, such as rice, rye, millet or quinoa.

Day	8	9	10	11	12	13	14	15	16	17	18	19	20	21	22	23	24	25	26
rice		✓		✓	✓					✓			✓		✓				✓
apple	✓	✓		✓	✓	✓	✓		✓	✓		✓		✓	✓	✓	✓	✓	✓
banana	✓		✓	✓			✓		✓		✓	✓			✓		✓	✓	
pork	✓		✓			✓				✓			✓			✓			✓
beef		✓		✓				✓			✓			✓			✓		
chicken	✓			✓						✓				✓			✓		
tomato	✓	✓		✓	✓	✓		✓	✓		✓	✓		✓	✓	✓	✓		
lettuce	✓	✓		✓	✓	✓		✓	✓		✓	✓		✓	✓	✓		✓	
onion	✓			✓			✓	✓			✓			✓				✓	
potato	✓	✓	✓	✓	✓		✓	✓	✓	✓	✓	✓		✓	✓	✓	✓		✓
carrot	✓		✓			✓			✓		✓				✓	✓			
cucumber				✓	✓		✓	✓		✓	✓	✓	✓		✓		✓		
fish	✓						✓		✓		✓							✓	
millet	✓		✓				✓						✓			✓			
oats				✓									✓						
egg		✓															✓	✓	
buckwheat		✓				✓			✓			✓			✓		✓	✓	
soya		✓		✓	✓		✓			✓			✓	✓	✓				✓
etc.																			
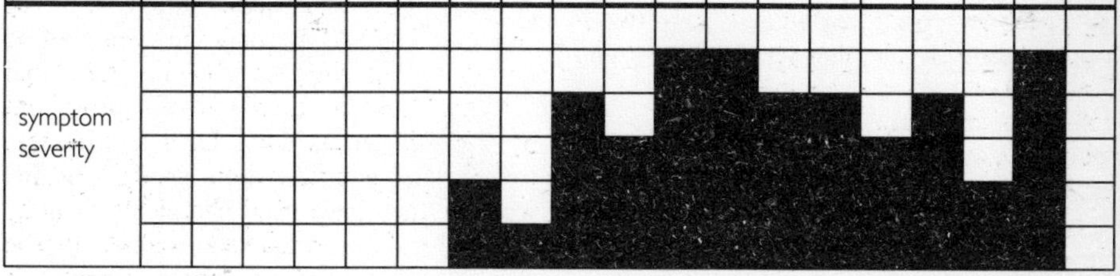 symptom severity																			

Figure 27.1: Example of a tabular food diary

Otherwise you may find yourself with very little to eat.

The following foods must be strictly avoided:

- Tomatoes, sauce, purees
- Apples, pears, plums, damsons, cherries, apricots, peaches
- Strawberries, raspberries, gooseberries, blackcurrants
- Oranges, lemons, other citrus fruits, marmalade and all fruit juices, squash, fruit-flavoured drinks
- All varieties of fizzy drinks, including cola
- Jellies, instant puddings
- Chocolate, cocoa, coffee, and coffee 'creamers'
- Grapes, sultanas, raisins, currants, prunes, figs, dates

- Nuts, coconut, marzipan, macaroons
- Peas, beans, lentils, soya, peanuts
- Melon, cucumber, marrow
- Spices, pepper, mustard, curry
- Cooking oils of all kinds and soft margarines
- All herbs (including mint)
- Bananas, pineapple

Gluten-free

Probably the oldest established allergy to food is hypersensitivity to gluten. It is a sticky protein that is found in wheat, rye, oats and barley and gives rise to the special gluey cooking texture these foods have.

The result of a gluten allergy used to be a very serious wasting condition known as coeliac disease or sprue; the patient simply starved with malnutrition, despite eating adequately. It was eventually discovered that gluten allergy was damaging the lining of the intestine so that it couldn't perform properly. This meant that food was not being digested and absorbed properly.

Another condition known to have a definite connection with gluten sensitivity is *dermatitis herpetiformis*. This is a blistering, intensely itchy rash that usually affects the outer surface of the elbows, buttocks and knees but can occur on any part of the body.

Personally, I think that a lot of the people who get well on a gluten-free diet do so because they are wheat allergic. They can tolerate rye, oats or barley with impunity, so gluten cannot be the offender.

Try a gluten-free diet if you are suspicious, but you must be prepared to stick at it for a minimum of six to eight weeks to be sure of feeling any benefit.

The Feingold Diet

The role of **salicylate (96)** (aspirin-containing) foods in hyperactivity in children was first put forward by Dr Ben Feingold. He claimed dramatic results from a diet free of these foods.

Feingold later improved the diet by eliminating food additives and colourings (the notorious yellow-orange dye tartrazine is related to salicylates). This gives better results. Try the salicylate/colourings-free experiment on your child if you feel like it. However, I think Feingold's approach is over-rated. Some children do improve. But many ordinary foods are capable of causing brain allergy and hence hyperactivity. It is restrictive to confine the evaluation to chemical targets. A much sounder approach is to follow the full elimination/challenge programme given earlier in this section.

Neutralizing **phenolics (86)** can also be very helpful to the hyperactive child.

Special Cases

For most people the problems of exclusion diets are few. Withdrawal symptoms, extra expense or the sloth encountered in changing the habits of a lifetime are the main difficulties. However, certain situations require extra comment:

CHILDREN

Children have more food allergy problems than adults. Yet food is vital to them; their growth will be stunted if nutrition is inadequate. Consider the size of a newborn infant in relation to that of an adult and you will see at once the wisdom in the old adage 'You are what you eat.'

Whatever dietary experiments are undertaken with children it is vital therefore to see they get adequate substitutes. Milk is a problem food. It is by far the most common allergen in children. The important ingredient in milk, I believe, is not really calcium but vitamin D. Fish oils are a good alternative source. Iodine is also vital to prevent stunting and poor mental development. Since most of our supply comes from milk, alternative provision needs to be made for this element also. Kelp or iodized salt should suffice.

If you are faced with complex or long-term eliminations for your child it is important to weigh him or her regularly (at least once a week) and keep a record of growth. Body size can be compared with charts showing average ranges for males and female youngsters and also percentiles for those who are clearly above or below average, showing how fast they too should be gaining weight. If weight gain is affected you *must* get help or discontinue what you are doing. Almost no condition (the possible exception being retarded mental growth occurring because of a food allergy) is worth stunting your child's growth. It is better to defer treatment until the child is older.

Remember that withdrawal symptoms can be experienced by children, too. Be very tolerant for the first few days. He or she may crave favourite foods: just say 'No' firmly and offer an alternative. Eventually, hunger will be on your side.

It's remarkable to watch how a youngster who is a faddy eater (a reliable sign of food allergy) suddenly finds his or her appetite and begins to eat heartily.

DIABETICS

For diabetic patients managed by drugs and diet alone there should be little problem with an elimination diet. Those on insulin, however, must be very careful about embarking on a low-carbohydrate diet and should not do so without medical supervision.

The simplest modification of the basic exclusion diet is to eat rice as a source of carbohydrate. Quinoa is a good food in this context also, if you can obtain it. Better still is to cut down your insulin gradually and reduce your starch intake similarly – under the supervision of your doctor.

The best challenge test to perform (if you have a glucometer and can use it) is to monitor which foods increase your blood glucose. If you haven't a glucometer, just carry out the challenge tests in the normal way.

In the Long Term

'How long must I avoid a food?' is one of the most common questions asked. It's like asking 'How long is a piece of string?' To give some guidance it may be said that major allergens should be avoided for 6 to 12 months and then tried again. If you still react, wait a further 12 to 24 months before trying again.

Beware of sneaking a food back into your diet by taking tiny amounts at first and then gradually increasing the quantity. This kind of self-deception will only land you back where you started – sick.

Some substitute foods are well known. If cow's milk has to be avoided, goat's milk or sheep's milk products may be suitable, but do test them first. Contrary to myth, goat's milk has no medicinal properties. It gets people well by getting them off cow's milk – the real cause of trouble. In fact goat's milk is arguably a health hazard since, in the UK at least, it isn't regulated or tested for tuberculosis and brucellosis.

Evaporated milk can be tolerated by some dairy-allergics. Heating milk changes its chemical nature and this may be enough to render it safe – but do test first, don't just make assumptions.

If wheat is a problem, try flours made from rye, barley, rice or millet. If you find that all the grains give you problems, there are still non-cereal flours such as buckwheat (in the rhubarb family), soya, pea, potato, sago and chestnut flours. Quinoa, a South American plant, is showing considerable promise as a grain substitute for allergics.

For further culinary advice, refer to the available cookery books for allergics (see the Recommended Reading section).

Finally, if you recover on an exclusion diet but can't seem to hold on to your gains you may be developing new allergies quickly. Safe foods are breaking down and becoming reactive. The best answer to this problem is a **rotation diet (95)**.

Also see Appendix A

28. Diseases Caused by Allergies

One of the factors that seems to provoke much of the controversy surrounding allergy and environmental medicine is the sheer diversity of conditions it claims to be able to treat.

The key to the multiplicity of conditions we encounter is **target** or shock **organs (104)**. Simply put, diseases depend not on the allergen or the insult (the toxin, etc.) but on which genetic weak link within the body breaks first. Thus we find allergies affecting the skin, lungs, pancreas, endocrine organs, etc. In fact an increasing number of diseases are turning out to have a basis in immune dysfunction – for example, juvenile-onset diabetes appears to be an auto-immune disease, in which the patient is attacking and destroying his or her own B cells in the part of the pancreas that secretes insulin (the Islets of Langerhans). Myasthenia gravis – a condition characterized by gradual weakness and paralysis but which can be cured dramatically by drugs – also appears to be immunologically-induced. There may ultimately be many similar conditions that come under the same umbrella.

From the purely empirical point of view, clinical ecologists have been accustomed to dealing successfully with a wide variety of conditions. The following list indicates some of the illnesses that respond well to the allergy and environmental medical approach.

CONDITIONS WHOLLY ATTRIBUTABLE TO ALLERGY

Asthma

Eczema

Urticaria

Rhinitis (seasonal and perennial)

Catarrh

CONDITIONS THAT RESPOND WELL TO THE ALLERGY APPROACH

Arthritis (all types but especially rheumatoid)

Behavioural disorders in children

Colitis and Crohn's disease

Eating disorders (anorexia and bulimia)

Haemorrhoids

Hyperkinetic syndrome (hyperactivity)

Hypertension

Mastitis or breast pains

Menière's disease

Migraine

Mouth ulcers

Multiple Sclerosis

Myalgic encephalo-myelitis (post-viral syndrome)

Peptic ulcer

Polymyalgia

Pre-menstrual tension

Psoriasis

Recurring cystitis

CONDITIONS THAT MAY RESPOND TO THE ALLERGY / ECOLOGY APPROACH

Alcoholism

Anxiety

Cardiac arrhythmias (especially tachycardia)

Depression

Diabetes

Frigidity

Hypothyroidism

Impotence

Nephrotic syndrome

Schizophrenia

ATOPY

The atopic individual is defined as one with diverse, acute, Type I **hypersensitivity (53)** reactions. These are usually IgE-mediated, prick test- and RAST-positive, and the individual usually has a rapid and severe onset of symptoms after encountering an allergen. They tend to share a common group of symptoms including asthma and wheezing, rhinitis, eczema and red, itchy eyes.

The word *atopy* (meaning 'strange disease') was coined by Arthur Coca in the 1950s. Atopic patients sensitize easily and are found to react on testing to a whole range of foods and environmental substances including moulds, dusts, danders, etc. Sometimes this sensitization reaches an extreme degree that can be life-threatening. Unburdening (reducing **body load (11)**) is a considerable problem for these patients because it can be very difficult to find safe foods.

Children are more often atopic than adults. However, many individuals tend to have problems right throughout their adult lives, so a wait-and-see-what-happens policy is rarely justified.

Avoidance is the best course and a diet and lifestyle need to be designed that will reduce body load. Nevertheless it is sometimes necessary to resort to drugs for acute episodes of life-threatening bronchospasm or swellings.

Also see **allergy: a definition (5)** and **symptoms table (103)**

29. Dowsing

It seems proper to include a reference to dowsing for allergies in case you should come across it. Usually a lock of hair is asked for and sometimes the term hair analysis is used, but this should not be confused with scientific **hair analysis for minerals (47)** carried out by reputable laboratories using a mass spectrograph. For one thing, these laboratory tests cannot give any information about allergies or even vitamin status from a hair sample. Dowsers claim they can do this.

Typically, the dowser uses a pendulum which is swung over the hair sample. Its swing alters if an allergy is present.

There is no objection to this sort of thing, provided the practitioner makes it clear that he or she uses dowsing as a diagnostic tool (which isn't usually the case). The cost is generally moderate (about £20). Dowsing centres may attract undue criticism if they call themselves clinics or if the dowsers themselves claim to be medical specialists.

Dowsing for **geopathic stress** is covered under that section (**45**).

Also see **applied kinesiology (9)**

30. Drugs for Allergies

Numerous drugs can be used to treat allergics which play no part in altering the underlying cause of the condition. Thus tranquillizers may be prescribed if the patient is distressed; skin rashes may be treated with creams, arthritis with pain-killers and stomach upsets with various remedies aimed at slowing down, speeding up or altering the acidity of the alimentary tract.

These are all what we call 'symptomatic' treatments. That is, they are geared solely to suppressing the symptoms and are not a cure. Basically, this sort of drug therapy assumes less and less importance as the detection of specific allergens and their avoidance is increased.

There are, however, three classes of drugs intended to alter the status of allergic disease and so diminish or eradicate symptoms.

These are a) antihistamines, b) steroids and c) mast cell stabilizers.

ANTIHISTAMINES

Antihistamines are possibly the best known and most widely used of all allergy remedies.

Histamine (50) is released when mast cells break down. It is responsible for the redness, swelling and itching typical of allergic rashes. It also causes tissue swelling as in bronchospasm and pain as in migraine.

Antihistamines are generally very safe; any inherent problems stem mainly from their side-effect of drowsiness. Patients vary in their response. Newer preparations such as terfenadine (*Triludan*) and astemizole (*Hismanal*) have attempted to eradicate the drowsiness and have been fairly successful. Other preparations seek to exploit it and promethazine (*Phenergan*) and trimeprazine (*Vallergan*) are used as sedatives for children.

Other brand-names you may encounter are: *Tevegil, Optimine* and *Fabahistin*.

Antihistamines may provide helpful short-term relief for allergy sufferers. One important point, however: they will mask the effect of skin testing and should be discontinued several days before undergoing any such tests.

STEROIDS

Mention the word steroids and most people now recoil in horror. Yet, apart from antibiotics, probably no class of drug has saved more lives. Why all the fuss? The side-effects can be pretty awful – fat deposits ('moon face'), infertility, loss of skin tissue and osteoporosis (brittle bones) – but they usually only develop when the drugs have been taken long term.

The fact is, steroids may produce dramatic recoveries but, again, no cure. When they are stopped the illness often roars back into view, sometimes worse than before (this is called the 'rebound' phenomenon).

A one-off dose of Depomedrone or Kenalog can prompt wonderful relief from severe and debilitating hay fever or an unbearable rash, for as long as three weeks at a stretch (though usually for about 10 days). Often the use of these drugs amounts to practical logistics – say where the patient is a busy and committed businessperson who cannot for some reason follow a more fundamental plan of avoidance and desensitization as described elsewhere in this book. Naturally, such 'emergencies' should not be repeated often.

The common steroid you will encounter is prednisolone. Other names for it include 'cort', referring to the origin of these hormones (the adrenal cortex – the outer layer of the adrenal gland).

It is often forgotten that the contraceptive pill is steroidal (oestrogen and progesterone). Cholesterol is a distant relative. All are **phenolics (86)**.

MAST CELL STABILIZERS

The breakthrough drug in this class was sodium cromoglycate (SCG). First used in asthma (as *Intal*), it was found to be an excellent prophylactic since it prevented the breakdown of mast cells and the consequent release of histamine. It therefore operates one step ahead of antihistamines. Providing the patient takes it regularly it can diminish the frequency and intensity of bronchospasm, though once the symptom comes on it is useless for relief.

It was logical to try it for rhinitis and a nasal insufflation called *Rhynacrom* was developed. There were high hopes that this drug might be of benefit for food allergics and Fisons (the license holders) brought *Nalcrom* onto the market. Unfortunately, it was a failure. It loses its effect very quickly and has little or no long-term therapeutic benefit. Nevertheless, it does work short-term and can be of great benefit to patients who need to attend special occasion dinners such as weddings and anniversaries, or even to use it before a sinful 'blow-out' when the restrictions of structured dieting become too much. Take 3 to 6 capsules on the day in question and, to be quite safe, on the following day, too.

Ketotifen (*Zantac*) is a newer mast cell stabilizer. Its long-term efficacy is uncertain. It has antihistamine properties and therefore causes drowsiness.

Finally, of course, all drugs can be allergenic. They are all xenobiotics. Just because they are used to treat allergy does not mean they might not be culprits themselves.

Also see **conventional allergy tests (22)**, **enzyme potentiated desensitization (36)** and **Miller's method (74)**

31. The Dynamics of Food

In recent years I have become increasingly interested in what might be called the dynamics of food – that is, the cooking, eating and chemical formulation of it rather than the purely allergic or 'ingredients' phenomenon that is so important to the work at our clinic.

The first clues came from unrelated observations that were simply interesting facts: for example, well-cooked and minced beef is more allergenic than rare steak; pastry is the form of wheat *most* likely to upset a patient; vegetables such as celery, carrots and cabbage when well cooked seem to be far less allergenic; fried potato is more likely to cause a reaction than boiled; stir-frying is a particularly 'safe' way to prepare foods, and so on.

It is easy to hypothesize that processing or cooking food will alter the allergic basis for it and therefore produce a different reaction. Evaporated milk (heat-treated), for example, is tolerated by about half our milk-allergics. Indeed, the discovery of fire had a great deal to do with humanity's ability to feed safely on a wide variety of foods.

Dr Amy McGrath, a doctor of history from Australia, has pointed out that bread is no longer manufactured in the way it used to be and that this could have had hidden effects on its allergenicity. Apparently the change in conditions of work, specifically the hours of shift-working introduced after the Second World War, meant that bread was no longer fermented overnight. Instead it was rushed through the rising process using so-called 'improvers' to fluff up the loaf. The result was a very different bread, chemically, to the traditional loaf.

Dr McGrath hypothesizes that modern bread contains unchanged maltose in large quantities and reckons that is why her family can't tolerate it. The same bread ingredients, baked using the old-fashioned *long dough* are fine for her and her children, since the maltose is removed.

She points out further that it was traditional practice in Ireland to cover oatmeal with water overnight before cooking and that this gave a much finer porridge. The secret seems to be that this allowed a simple fermentation process to take place (there is sufficient yeast present) and once again this would remove maltose and other reactive complex carbohydrates. I'm sure most of the people did not appreciate this point but they had *learned* that it was the best way to prepare that food.

As Dr McGrath puts it, it seems that there is a lot of traditional wisdom that has been passed on from generation to generation simply by trial and error: people have found that certain procedures render food less toxic and harmful and therefore more nutritious. We seem to be in danger now of throwing out this traditional wisdom and replacing it with modern technology, pre-packaged food and the mania for 'instant'.

A BRIEF FOOD ANTHROPOLOGY

Dr McGrath points out that Australian aborigines, Melanesians and Polynesians rarely eat food raw. Traditionally they cook vegetables at high temperatures, steaming them or baking them in earth ovens. Asians, too, seldom eat raw vegetables or brown rice. Vegetables are usually cooked well, as in stir-fry. Rice is soaked, the water thrown away, then boiled, baked or fried. The husks or bran are fed to the pigs. Brown rice, they say, is indigestible.

Indians often cook foods for a lengthy time. Greeks soak and boil beans for some hours. West Africans process corn for days. Taiwanese farmers boil sweet potatoes before giving them to the pigs as food. The Native American Hopi pick corn green and dry it to make bound niacin available.

Finally, my young secretary from Dublin points out that certain Latin American tribes soak maize in lime juice before cooking it; apparently this frees up the niacin (B_3), without which pellegra – the symptoms of which include dermatitis, diarrhoea and dementia – is common (as in the southern USA). They may not know any biochemistry but they *have got* ancestral wisdom, which is what this section is all about.

Also see **bread (13)** and **plant toxins (87)**

32. Electrical Fields and Allergies

Ever since Luigi Galvani sent a kite up into a thunderstorm and found that the lightning discharge caused frogs' legs to twitch when put near the string of the kite, the biological significance of electricity has been steadily increasing. Fascinating work was carried out by Harold Saxton Burr in the USA in the 1930s and 1940s. He demonstrated that all life-forms have an electrical field which he called the 'L-field'. Indeed, this seems to be the principal difference between living and dead tissue.

It should not be surprising, therefore, if electrical fields were found to be capable of causing profound biological disturbances. New scientific evidence points strikingly to this indeed being the case. Furthermore, most background (natural) electricity is chaotic or random, whereas we are subjected to an alarming increase in 'coherent' or directional – and potentially more damaging – electrical fields.

Today we live in a world which, by conservative estimates, has more than a million times the natural levels of electrical radiation. This 'electrical pollution' comes from televisions, radios, telephones, cookers, computers, lighting, heating and a myriad of other appliances with which we have surrounded ourselves in our 'civilized', technological society.

It is becoming increasingly obvious that a number of people are made ill in the presence of electro-magnetic fields. Symptoms include flushing, palpitations, diarrhoea, muscle aches and pains, disorientation, headache, fits and blackouts. Depression may also be a feature. It is known that human brain waves (EEG patterns) alter when an electric appliance is switched on anywhere in the vicinity.

Alarm was spread when Dr Stephen Perry pointed out a high incidence of suicides in locations that could be plotted along a narrow corridor across countryside that followed the line of a high-tension electricity cable. More recently he has carried out studies on residential blocks of flats and shown a correlation between field strengths and a whole host of diseases including myocardial infarction (thrombosis), hypertension and depression. A further provocative finding was that if only those blocks with under-floor heating were considered, the incidence of 'depression' rose by 80 per cent!

Electro-magnetic activity around high-tension cables is easy to demonstrate. If you carry an ordinary domestic fluorescent tube near one on a dark night you will be able to observe it glow while you are still over 100 metres away. People, it seems, are far more sensitive and notice effects even from three times that distance.

Some people are extremely sensitive to external electrical fields. This adds to their **body load (11)** and may be a hitherto-unrecognized contributor to allergic sensitivities. The probability is that allergy itself is an electro-magnetic effect. Most clinical ecologists are familiar with the fact that it is sometimes possible to get a reaction from a patient simply by holding the allergen substance near to his or her body (i.e., within his or her L-field). This cannot be a humoral (chemically-borne) effect.

Dr Cyril Smith of Salford University has pointed out that current environmental exposures might be on the order of tens of micro-amps. Such currents are significant and comparable to those known to be able to produce electro-anaesthesia in dentistry and also to stimulate the production of endogenous opiates (see **endorphins (33)**). One of the leading clinical researchers in this field is Dr Jean Munro; co-operation between her and Smith has resulted in the steady breaking of new ground.

Smith and Munro suggest points to look out for that should arouse suspicion of hypersensitivity:

1. The individual is hard to stabilize with normal allergy desensitizing methods.
2. There may be sensitivity to weather effects, since there are important electrical changes in the atmosphere which precede the arrival of weather fronts, thunderstorms, etc.
3. The patient may demonstrate a poor tolerance of drinking and washing water, though paradoxically sea bathing may alleviate symptoms in electrical sensitives.
4. The patient may be aware of feeling bad in the presence of electronic equipment such as computers, TVs, etc. One of my patients gets an asthma attack every time the TV is switched on. It can be as obvious as this yet people remain unaware of the culprit until it is pointed out to them.
5. Fluorescent lighting often troubles the patient.
6. A curious and fascinating effect is that electrical gadgets often go wrong or fail in the presence of these patients; they are notorious for stopping watches, causing glitches in computers, failure of machinery, etc.
7. Some patients are even aware of giving off static charges and other people get a spark or a shock when touching them or coming close. This is very troublesome, particularly in allergics of this kind. My nurses report an unusually high incidence of highly-charged patients of this type.

TESTING

Testing is particularly difficult since it is virtually impossible to get outside existing fields and be able to have a baseline of zero. Unless that is achievable it is only possible to check for electrical sensitivity in the most general way. Compromises must be sought. It may be possible to dampen ambient electrical fields by placing a bucket of salt water in a central position in the room so as to absorb some of the electrical field energy.

Individuals can only be tested on a good day, well-neutralized with **Miller's** neutralizing solutions if they are needed **(74)**, in a specially prepared room known to be free of **geopathic stress (45)** and any potential chemical triggers that may cause confusing reactions. The room must be free of all electrical appliances and as remote as possible from any such equipment in the same building (extra-sensitive patients can tell with a great degree of reliability when something is switched on even several rooms away).

Various kinds of wave-function generators are available. It is not necessary to connect the patient to these but a trailing wire will emit a field into the room across a space of several metres. It may be possible to test the patient for how he or she feels, noting subjective reactions. Objective changes can also be included such as changes in respiration, heart rate or size of pupils, any reddening, loss of tone, alteration in speech and consciousness; even convulsions have been observed in exceptional individuals. There may be several detrimental frequencies, usually in the 30 – 100 Hz range.

According to Dr Munro it is now possible to measure critical values of magnetic and electrical fields corresponding to the onset of the patient's symptoms. In some individuals these thresholds approach the physical limits set by the laws of physics. More typical trigger levels would be of the order of 30 nanoTessla, roughly equivalent to being a quarter of a mile from a high-voltage power line, and 50 volts/m, about the same as being 3 feet from a hair dryer or food mixer.

Table 32.1 gives some idea of the ambient ranges we are exposed to.

Ambient Alternating Electrical Fields

Location	Range (volts/metre)
Home/office background	0.9–10 V/m
VDU at 50 cm	2–90 V/m
Close to domestic appliance	6–200 V/m
Industrial background	10–400 V/m
Under large power line	500–3,000 V/m
Power station near a generator	1,000–50,000 V/m
Electrical field during a thunderstorm	1,000 – 50,000 V/m

Local 'hot spots' many times the recognized safety levels can exist within a house or other building due to unbalanced ground return circuits. Whole localities can be affected for the same reason, especially where the supply is within a loop (such as at the end of cul-de-sacs).

FIELD METERS

Simple hand-held meters for detecting electrical and magnetic fields are now available, so you can test your own environment. The *Kombi-test* made by Bio-Physik Mersmann GmbH and available from Environmental Diagnostics Ltd is probably the most sophisticated of these and retails at around £200. However, Coghill Research Laboratories have produced a much cheaper version for the mass market, costing around £40. It is called the *E-meter* and simply warns when levels are too high (over 30 V/m.). A push-button resets the sensitivity to react when levels are over 10 V/m. This is an extra safety factor for use around babies and old people. However it should be pointed out that these limits are chosen based on the levels, in the light of recent research, considered to constitute a risk of cancer/leukaemia – *not* levels at which an allergic may suffer symptoms.

WHAT CAN YOU DO?

If you are concerned about electrical levels and think you may have a sensitivity:

1. Remove all unnecessary electrical devices from your bedroom, such as electric alarm clocks, radios and tea-makers.
2. Get rid of your electric blanket.
3. Change your bed for one without any metal in the framework.
4. Get a mattress without springing (a 'futon'-style bed would serve very well for both this and point 3).
5. Avoid electrical equipment as much as possible. If you have to cook with electrical systems, try to have them all down one side of the room. Tests show that being surrounded on all sides by such equipment has a more detrimental effect.
6. Switch electricity off at the mains each night. The 'ring main' (loops of cables around a room) bathes inhabitants in a

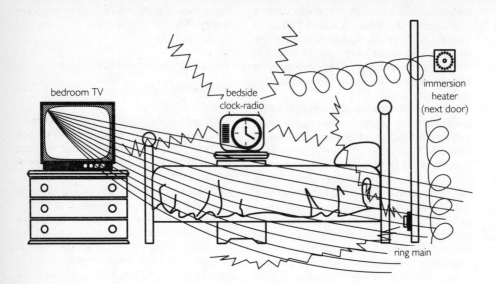

bedroom TV

bedside
clock-radio

immersion
heater
(next door)

ring main

Figure 32.1: Electro-magnetic fields surrounding a bed

pool of electro-magnetic energy, day and night while the mains are switched on. It seems logical that this isn't really good for us.

Coghill Research Laboratories, which specialize in 'electrical pollution', produce a simple EMF demand switch that turns off mains when the bedroom light is switched off last thing at night (but leaves the central heating, fridge and freezer working). Power returns as soon as the light switch is turned on again.

7. We normally recommend that patients who feel the effects of electrical static build-up try to 'discharge' themselves once or twice a day. This is easily done by walking barefoot on the earth or grass in the garden outside. If outdoors is not easily accessible or the weather is inclement, earthing to the water pipes can be tried. Just touching them should be sufficient, in theory. In practice there is more relief to be gained from standing on an earthed plate: *On no account do this while handling any live electrical equipment.* Some patients prefer to wrap a wire connected to the water pipes round their wrist in bed at night.

Synthetic carpets are particularly

hostile to electrical sensitives. Bare floor boards or tiles are far better. At least try to have these in the bedroom, even if not the lounge. A kitchen with tiled floors, and cooking in bare feet, are ideal, so that earthing needs no special time or procedure.

Safety with all electrical apparatus is important. An iron with a faulty wire becomes far more lethal if you are not insulated by a thick carpet and underlay.

Finally, remember that some effects from electricity may be due to low frequency sound vibrations caused by resonance at mains frequencies (50 cycles per second). Buzzing of fluorescent tubes is a case in point. Sound waves have a distinct pressure that is capable of great harm to biological systems. Electric fields from some apparatus are not strong enough to cause symptoms to most allergics but vibrations are capable of harming anyone (see **noise (80)**).

Also see **microwaves (71)**

33. Endorphins

A fascinating pharmacological discovery in recent years has been the recognition of endorphins. These are naturally occurring substances with effects similar to those of morphine. They are capable of affecting thoughts and mood just as morphine does, though in a milder, more biologically benevolent way. Endorphins also seem to have natural pain-killing properties.

Symptoms that could be due to opioids are similar to many that are caused by allergies: lethargy, headache, abdominal swelling or discomfort, depression, tingling, nausea, irritability, anxiety or panic attacks, poor concentration, joint pains, palpitations, dizziness and sleep disturbance, among others.

It has been shown that endorphins have a number of other reactions of interest to allergists and allergic patients. They can suppress immune function and generate direct allergic reactions.

EXORPHINS

Dr F. C. Dohan in his classic studies on gluten allergy and schizophrenia in the early 1970s first suggested the possibility that the pathogenesis of severe mental illness might lie with gluten or possibly peptides derived from it. A number of substances of this type, similar to endorphins but coming from exterior sources, have been identified. These are known logically, if clumsily, as *exorphins*; they can arise during the digestion of several dietary ingredients, particularly wheat, milk and corn. The gluten exorphin is particularly active on brain tissue and may account in part for that characteristic drowsiness felt after a typical heavy meal.

Possibly these exorphins also have some direct effect on the gut, releasing **histamine (50)** ('asthma of the gut'). Once again morphine and codeine have serious effects on the bowel, causing spasm and loss of motility (constipation). Any substances derived from food mimicking these drugs would therefore be likely to disturb bowel transit and mechanical function.

Finally, perhaps exorphins are the reason that patients become so remarkably addicted to their allergy foods and experience such profound withdrawal symptoms when eliminating them, just like junkies.

Also see **phenolic testing (86)** and **plant toxins (87)**

34. Environmental Allergies

This section is devoted to inhalant allergies, sometimes known as environmental allergies, but excluding chemical triggers, which have a section of their own (**chemical cleanup (19)**). Here environmental allergies are taken to mean the sensitizing allergens such as dusts, pollens, moulds, danders etc. **Moulds (75)** are dealt with in far greater detail elsewhere (see also **mycotoxins (76)**) but are of necessity also part of this section.

The one thing all these substances have in common is that they are particles light enough to float in air and so be breathed in. Larger particles of over 100 microns in size easily 'settle out' and are principally present in the air only when they are agitated, as for example by draughts or vacuuming in the home. Particles under 10 microns (most mould spores, house dust mite faeces and cat dander) will stay in suspension, that is, floating in the air. A proportion of aerosol particles are of this smaller size and similarly accumulate. Even foods such as flour during baking can become 'dust' particles.

Environmental allergies are quite common. Indeed, for half a century they were the only kind to be recognized. Probably as much as 30 per cent of the population is said to suffer significant effects (e.g. sneezing) from inhaled substances although many do not consider this an allergy. Since doctors do not see a great deal of these minor reactions, the incidence could be far higher (and probably is).

Environmental allergies can be divided into:

(a) seasonal
(b) non-seasonal, sometimes clumsily called 'perennial'.

Seasonal allergies, of course, are made manifest at particular times of the year, usually summer, and include allergies to pollens and mould. All-year-round allergies are essentially a disease of 'place'. A clue that would lead you to suspect an environmental allergy is that certain locations are bad for you, such as other peoples' homes, particular buildings, specific rooms in your house or particular geographical regions (the countryside or holiday locations).

Sometimes a time factor is helpful in pinpointing an allergy. Allergies that are worse in winter are usually connected with household or office allergens and pollution. We go indoors in autumn, closing the doors and windows, turning up the heating and then living with high densities of dust, danders (if we have pets) and mould (present in all buildings to some degree). Levels of carbon monoxide, formaldehyde and house gas fumes rise 200-fold in concentration; these and other chemical pollutants must be considered in a differential diagnosis.

DUST AND DUST MITE

We put these two together for practical purposes; they are probably the most widely known (and suffered) inhalant allergies. Individuals sensitive to one usually also react badly to the other.

House dust is a mixture of particles of food, human skin scales, hair and grits – but the main ingredient is fabric fibres from carpets, clothing, upholstery and drapes.

House dust mite is a living organism. It has been known about for a long time although it wasn't until the 1960s that the real importance of it as an allergen was recognized. The main species is *Dermatophagoides pterynissinus*. Another representative, *D. fariniae*, is less common. The main allergen is the animal's excrement.

Dermatophagoides ('skin eater') is found mainly in beds but also in bedroom carpets, bathroom carpets, lounge carpets, soft, foam chairs and settees, home and automobile upholstery – in fact, anywhere that human skin scales may be expected to fall.

Rhinitis and asthma are well-known allergic conditions due to dust and dust mite, but they may also be a potent trigger in eczema. Many patients with these conditions improve when hospitalized because the relentless routine of changing bed-linen, sometimes daily, is a major factor in keeping down dust and dust mite.

It is impossible to get rid of dust and dust mite, but reducing it significantly will help reduce your total **body load (11)**. The full routine given here is impossibly burdensome and most patients would not wish to undertake it; indeed, it is doubtful if more than the most exceptional case would need to. The important point is to carry out *some* of the steps, to reduce levels of exposure.

I would suggest that for a serious allergy the very least needed is to cover your mattress and remove your bedroom carpet, though you could try using a mite spray on the carpet first. The carpet can be replaced by lino or tiling, but I would recommend cork, which remains warm and friendly. Rugs can always be thrown over it, providing they are small enough to be washed at least *weekly*. Do not leave floorboards exposed, no matter how much you like the look – dust will travel up between the gaps.

The mattress cover must be dust-proof; these covers are available commercially or you can make your own from polythene. In the latter instance, for comfort, use an underblanket before you make the bed up with sheets. Choose something light and easy to wash for the underblanket, and replace or clean it weekly.

If you are not living somewhere that belongs to you and lifting the carpet is impracticable, consider investing in a good vacuum cleaner. The one I would recommend is the Medi-Vac from Taylor-maid Products Ltd (see Useful Addresses). It has a micro-pore filter that is 99.9 per cent effective down to a particle size of 0.3 microns. The trouble with most other vacuum cleaners is that even when they vacuum dust up efficiently they blow 60 – 70 per cent of it back into the atmosphere due to a leaky bag (*Good Housekeeping* survey, May 1989).

An alternative treatment for carpets is a modern miticide chemical such as benzyl alcohol. These tend to be well tolerated by the 'classic' allergic. Several brands are now available, such as *Acarasan* and *Allerex*. Repeated application every few weeks is needed for any beneficial result. Remember, the treatment itself only kills mites; it does not reduce the allergen pool. Only vacuuming away the mite products can do that.

Claims are being made for an anti-mite paint, but I have no evaluation of its effectiveness available. Logic says it would keep mites from the bedroom woodwork but not from the fabric, where 99 per cent of mites reside.

There are pesticide sprays available with which to treat your mattress. Those containing methoprene are effective and relatively harmless; the World Health Organization has deemed this substance safe enough to add to drinking water in those malarial zones where there is a risk of infection by mosquito larvae. Be sure you don't react to aerosol sprays – or have someone else do the spraying while you are absent from the home (at least overnight). Follow the instructions exactly. *Note:* even after using a miticide spray you must still vacuum the mattress for several more weeks. It is the mite droppings that usually cause a reaction and even when no more are being produced it still takes some time to get rid of all traces. Spray treatment lasts a variable time and needs to be repeated at least every three months.

To go further remove all objects that gather dust – such as pelmets, curtains, lampshades, bookshelves and open wardrobes – from the bedroom. Vacuum frequently – in all corners no matter how hard to reach – at least once a week.

Avoid electric open-bar heaters, convection and especially fan heaters, which all circulate dust. If ducted-air heating is present it should be blocked off to the room and substituted with a radiator. If there is no central heating, the free-standing oil-filled electric radiators are best (such as the Dimplex model).

Finally, air-purifiers (avoid those with scented filters) may help. The HEPA type is best (see **air purification (1)**). Try one and see. Ionizers are inefficient for eliminating dust and should be avoided.

POLLENS AND HAY FEVER

Pollens, the cause of hay fever, were first discovered by Charles Blackeley in 1873, right here in my own city of Manchester. He sent kites with sticky plates attached high into the air, saved up pollens and tried sniffing them in winter (he himself was a sufferer) and rubbing samples into his skin to produce what was a very elegant scientific demonstration of cause and effect.

Pollen to plants can be likened to sperm in humans. They are the male seeds that get carried in profusion to the female gamete. Only one of these myriad male elements can twin with each female spore to make a zygote: the rest are wasted. Many plants are pollinated by insects, birds or animals transferring the pollen to the female spores in their search for food. The problem comes with those plants (chiefly trees and grasses) that rely on atmospheric currents for pollination: they release *huge* amounts into the air at appropriate times.

Hay fever is characterized by red, itchy eyes, sneezing and catarrh – but any seasonal symptom, made worse by pollens (for example, wheezing or a rash) is covered by the remarks that follow.

Certain pollens can be identified because of the time of year when symptoms become manifest. For example, trees begin to pollinate in March and April, grasses in May and June and flowers from June onwards, though there are exceptions to these very broad generalizations. Sometimes the trigger is not a pollen but a seasonal mould. For example, *Cladosporium* (see below) peaks in London during August. This can be suspected if the patient has bad symptoms unrelated to days when the pollen count is high.

Ragweed is the chief pollen allergen in the USA and blankets the country east of the Mississippi, peaking in late summer. Each year it makes millions of people suffer. In Britain we have created for ourselves a new similar allergy hazard: rape. The pretty yellow fields that have brightened up our countryside in the last couple of decades produce an extremely potent allergen. Many people now cannot drive through a country area in summer without feeling extremely unwell because of rape plants. It is affecting individuals who would never have previously admitted to allergies.

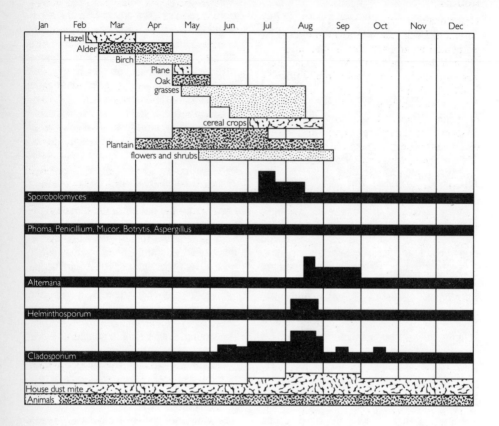

Approximate incidence of seasonal allergens

Adapted with permission from Keith Eaton, Anne Adams and Janet Dukesley, *Allergy Therapeutics* (London: Baillière Tindall, 1982).

The main problem with pollens is that there is nothing you can do to escape them, as you can with dust. Short of taking continuous antihistamines, with their tiresome side-effects, or isolating yourself indoors for the best days of the year, the problem has to be tackled in some other way.

The secret is the total body load. How many people ever think of going on a diet to combat hay fever? The logic is simple. If you eliminate any food allergies, your body will be better able to cope with inhaled allergies. This is particularly true when it comes to avoiding foods in the grass family, such as wheat, corn, rye, etc.; people with classic hay fever (allergies to grass pollens or hay) may find this step especially beneficial. But avoiding milk, food additives, tea, coffee and alcohol can also bring a remarkable improvement.

Follow the simple **elimination diet (27)** at a time when the pollen count is high. Even if you don't clear the symptoms completely, you may reduce your need for medication quite considerably or even eliminate it.

Hyposensitization had a degree of effectiveness but is no longer done (see **conventional allergy tests (22)**). Safest and best desensitization is **Miller's method (74)** of low-dose neutralizing, which can investigate individual pollens and switch off each reaction; or **enzyme potentiated desensitization (36)**, which scores very well against classic inhalant allergies.

Pollens virtually disappear with the first frost.

MOULDS

Unfortunately, mould allergies are very common. Drug reactions to antibiotics such as penicillin are actually mould allergies (*Penicillium notatum*). Most exposures, however, come from mould spores floating in the air. Moulds are rather like an all-year-round pollen, only absent during hard frost or when the ground is covered with snow. Suspect a mould allergy if you are bad on damp, humid days but better in cold weather. Also, if damp, musty buildings make you ill, mould is probably the cause.

Different moulds peak at different times of the year and it may be possible from this to deduce which one is the culprit (see Figure 34.1). Consider mould problems if your house is low-lying in a damp valley (East Lancashire, where the damp valleys favoured the cotton industry, is notoriously bad; so are the Fens). Older houses are especially suspect, particularly those with a condensation problem. Sometimes it is possible to see the mould growing on the walls and carpets.

If there is a damp problem in your home you may need professional advice from a builder and possibly a timber maintenance specialist. Major structural repairs may be required to overcome the defect properly. If the problem is too extensive you should consider moving, if you value your health. In the meantime a dehumidifier should help to reduce the damp. But do keep it cleaned out regularly, otherwise mould will accumulate in the machine itself.

Remember that house plants encourage moulds, which grow in the damp soil. You may need to get rid of them.

Some Common Moulds

Alternaria: Grows on wheat, crop plants and potatoes. Peaks mid-August. Associated with seasonal rhinitis and asthma.

Aspergillus: From hay and straw, compost and rotting matter. Common in winter, probably due to leaf rot. Also common in damp old houses, showing up as black patches.

Botrytis: Grey mould that attacks a number of vegetables and garden crops, especially strawberries. Some people who think they are allergic to strawberries may in fact have a Botrytis allergy. Likes cold and damp.

Cladosporium: Widespread mould, sporing in summer months which may cause it to be confused with a pollen allergy.

Fusarium: A white or colourless fungus that grows on cabbages, tomatoes, potatoes and grains. Its powerful mycotoxin is discussed in the section on **mycotoxins**.

Helminthosporium: Grows on cereals and decomposing matter. Peaks at harvest time, mainly in August and September.

Merulius lacrimans: Dry rot fungus, a potent allergen. Despite the name, it needs a degree of moisture to grow in wood.

Mucor: Grows on stored food, thrives on damp. An important constituent of house dust.

Penicillium: The classic bluey-green mould on stale bread and over-ripe food. All-year-round spores.

Phoma: Characteristic 'black spot' on fruit. Grows on many summer flowers and may be a factor in seasonal rhinitis.

Pullularia: Grows on vegetables, fruit and damp surfaces. Spores in summer.

Scopulariopsis brevicaulis: A household mould that was once responsible for deaths due to Gosio's disease (see **sudden infant death syndrome (101)**). Releases deadly arsine gas from arsenical paint pigment compounds and flame-retardant treatments.

Sporobolomyces: Present in wines and beverages. Spores after light rain and dew. Affects people who live near river banks, lakes and woodlands.

Trychophyton: Grows in human skin and is responsible for athlete's foot and a similar rash in the crotch area. A component of *TOE* (a test mixture for allergists made up of Trychophyton, Oidium and Epidermophyton: Oidium albicans being the former name for Candida).

ANIMAL HAIR AND DANDERS

Not all cultures share the British love of pets. Dogs are looked on as vermin in the Middle East, and trailing one about on a strip of leather as many Britons do is considered crazy.

Unfortunately, dogs, cats, horses, birds and other pets can sensitize their owner, or even other members of the household, and can cause severe allergies. The obvious solution – getting rid of the allergen – is often refused on emotional grounds.

Desensitization will often help. Using Miller's method it is sometimes possible to desensitize for the exact animal that is causing the trouble by collecting its hair and danders and making up serial dilutions which are then the basis for testing and neutralization.

Keep animals out of bedrooms at all costs. Once the fur and dander are present they can be very difficult to get rid of. The principal cat allergen is said to be small (under 10 microns in size), which means it lingers in the air. Opening doors and windows and letting fresh air circulate is a very simple way of getting rid of this particular allergen.

Using the vacuum cleaner often helps to keep hairs to a minimum.

Beware of your diagnosis. One woman we tested was convinced she was allergic to her horse. It turned out to be a reaction to the dust from the corn feed she was mixing for it.

Feathers in pillows and mattresses are not as fashionable as they once were, although Eider down is still favoured for quilts. Direct contact with birds, apart from hardy country folk, is limited to those with a penchant for caged birds. Nowadays there are many more exotic species than just budgerigars and canaries. Allergen to mould from the cage and faecal dust may be just as important as a reaction to the feathers.

So-called 'bird-fancier's lung' is a hypersensitivity condition of the respiratory air-sacs which leads to inflammation, fibrosis and difficulty in gas exchange. It manifests as a shortness of breath (akin to pneumoconiosis in miners, but with a different trigger agent).

SMALL RODENT URINE

The urine of small rodents can be a powerful allergen. Rats and mice are not the problem as much as the pets children sometimes keep such as guinea pigs, hamsters and gerbils. The last two are particularly troublesome since they are often kept in the child's bedroom.

These animals tend not to live very long and pronounced attachments are rare. Don't replace the animal when it dies if anyone in the house suffers from asthma. If you can persuade your child that it's for the best, give it away. If not, ban it from the bedroom and see that bedding is changed frequently.

FABRICS

Allergies to wool are relatively common, also to lanolin, one of its principal ingredients. Avoid sheepskin rugs and untreated wool. Dyed and processed wool may be acceptable in small quantities.

Leather can cause problems but these are more likely to be due to chromates, formaldehyde, dyes or other chemicals used in tanning and finishing rather than to the leather itself.

Cotton, silk and other natural fabrics are generally pretty safe. Sensitive individuals should try and wear these types of fabric next to the skin. Trouble sometimes arises from fabric treatments such as dyes, 'softeners', etc. Wash new clothes once or twice before wearing them if you are super-sensitive.

Synthetic fabrics are often very bad for allergics. This is due in part to the polymerized chemicals involved. A great deal of the trouble, however, comes from static electricity build-ups caused by these materials. Tights are a particular problem, since the whole of the lower body is encased in an electrically-charging mesh that gets more and more charged by being rubbed against other fabrics, such as a skirt. Tights, incidentally, seem to encourage thrush in women. Try to get those with a cotton gusset and cotton soles.

Carpets and upholstery can be major problems. Once again the real offender may be a chemical treatment such as an anti-staining chemical. Formaldehyde used in dyeing, colour fastening or even anti-moth treatment can cause trouble. Suspect this if you get symptoms when you're in a carpet (or any textile) shop.

35. Environmental Control Units

A logical diagnostic approach growing out of ecological theories is a test environment in which the patient's recovery is monitored while he or she is screened from all extraneous chemicals, foods and other triggers. We call these centres environmental control units (ECUs). There is no more comprehensive method for defining which parts of a patient's illness are due to environmental triggers and which are not.

The original ECUs were finished in stainless steel, tiling and hardwood. However plaster walls and wooden varnished floors are usually safe after a few months. Even vinyl tiling is suitable once gassing out is completed. Individual rooms, as well as lounges and common areas, are furnished with wood or metal; natural upholstery fabrics such as cotton, felt or leather are used. Natural fibre stuffings are used for pillows, mattresses, etc. Rubber, foam, feathers, horsehair, nylon and other synthetic substances are excluded.

Most strong cleaning fluids and detergents are banned and only unscented soap and water are used. Aerosols and air fresheners are banned, of course.

Special precautions must be taken so that unwarranted chemicals are not introduced by visitors and staff. Overalls, shoe-covers and hats must be worn; no perfumes are allowed and heavy smokers are banned (their breath can be a source of pollution). Even writing instruments such as felt-tip pens come under suspicion and must be excluded.

Personal effects made of, or containing, plastic are banned. Rigorous procedures must be followed when entering the unit, rather like the decontamination process enacted in isolation wards except that here the procedure is reversed: the idea is to prevent pathogens getting *in* rather than preventing them getting out.

In this specially isolated environment patients will gradually eliminate chemicals in their body over the space of a few days. They will detoxify and unmask chemical allergens and it becomes a relatively easy matter to test them with challenges.

FASTING

Drugs are usually discontinued on admission to the ECU, unless they are life-saving ones. Some may need to be tapered off gradually beforehand. Smoking is strictly banned – the patient must therefore get over this hurdle in advance, or be ready to go 'cold turkey' on entry.

The patient then begins a five-day fast. Special water is supplied (usually bottled spring water or distilled water); a wide range is made available to cater for different needs and tastes.

The patient is monitored by medical staff during this unmasking phase. Baseline readings and attitudes can be established. Unpleasant withdrawal symptoms are common, though usually little more than reassurance is required for the patient to put up with them. Medication is somewhat counter-productive, though **alkali salts (4)** may help.

PSYCHOLOGICAL ASSESSMENT

Almost all patients have psychological symptoms, either primary (cause) or as overlay (due to their health difficulties); thus psychological evaluation is a useful 'before and after' assessment. Usually a battery of such tests is administered, such as the Wechsler Adult Intelligence Scale, Bendagestalt Test, the Minnesota Multiphasic Personality Inventory (MMPI) or similar.

At the same time, aptitude and reaction time tests may be carried out to establish a useful baseline from which to measure improvement in neurological parameters in response to the ECU programme.

CHALLENGE TESTING

During the chemical clearing process the patient endeavours to find some safe waters to drink. Most highly sensitive patients react to one or more spring waters. Boiled or filtered tapwater may be acceptable to some. Occasionally, patients unable to tolerate any of these may need to take distilled water or water purified by reverse osmosis.

After five days or so of unmasking, the patient generally has recovered and is ready to go on to the stage of identification by means of **challenge tests (18)**, beginning with foods. Produce used in challenge testing must be specially prepared in a kitchen belonging exclusively to the unit, avoiding gas and anything else that may contaminate the food. Cooking utensils are either glass or stainless steel, not aluminium. Only electric cookers are used.

Foods are organic and flavourings (apart from sea salt) are not used. Foods are washed with pure water, not tap water, before cooking. Plastic-packaged food is not permitted.

Safe foods are taken cumulatively. Thus if a reaction takes place on the sixth food, the five previous safe foods are continued.

Once the initial building stages of the diet have taken place nutritional supplementation can also be introduced with a careful programme of vitamin supplements and complementary minerals.

Food testing may be done in conjunction with **Miller's method (74)** of provocation/neutralization.

Chemical Challenges

Testing for chemical sensitivities can be carried out using Miller's method. Reactions discovered can be neutralized, ready for the patient's prophylactic use on departure. Recommendations may also be made regarding suitable changes to the patient's home environment.

Alternatively, inhalation testing of common chemicals can be carried out in a special booth. The patient is challenged double-blind – that is, neither patient nor practitioner will know in advance the chemical being tested – using standardized concentrations of formaldehyde, chlorine, phenol, pesticides, ethanol, natural gas and petrol fumes.

STRESS MANAGEMENT

There is a close relation between stress and immune reactions, which goes both ways, so it is important to try to reduce stress or to improve the patient's management of stress. This is part of reducing the **body load (11)**. Counselling may help and group therapy sessions can be established, though full-blown one-on-one psychotherapy is rarely called for. If such a requirement arises it would be best carried out either before admission to the ECU or after the patient leaves the unit.

Behavioural studies often show that patients admitted to the unit have preoccupations with their ill-health and disease, low self-esteem and low energy. Depression, often accompanied by anxiety, may be an important feature. Improved knowledge of the patient's personality will avoid being led to the wrong conclusions by these imagined symptoms.

Exercise, even if of the gentlest kind, has a beneficial effect for most individuals, increasing energy levels and heightening feelings of self-control and accomplishment.

EFFECTIVENESS

Patients who find their way to these units are, by definition, tough cases. Total recovery is thus not always a realistic goal. Bearing this in mind the results achieved are more than satisfactory. Even where symptoms persist, assessment often shows they have dropped from 'frequent' or 'severe', to 'mild' and 'occasional'.

The biggest real stumbling block to this approach is cost: approximately £1,000 per week at the time of writing. This usually puts it well beyond the means of most people. Hopefully, someday ECUs will be available within the NHS.

Also see **chemical clean-up (19), environmental allergies (34)** and **thermal chamber depuration (106)**

36. Enzyme Potentiated Desensitization (EPD)

A bridge between conventional desensitization (see **conventional allergy tests (22)**) and low-dose neutralization is Dr Len McEwen's method of enzyme potentiated desensitization.

It is definitely a vaccine approach, whereas **Miller's method (74)** of neutralization seems to be more akin to the antidote principle. Briefly, in EPD a cup is taped over the forearm (after the skin on the area has been scarified – scraped repeatedly – to remove the waterproof layers). Under this cup is placed a vaccine containing dozens of commonly-encountered food and environmental substances, along with an enzyme to make it work (hence the name). The cup is kept in place for 24 hours and then removed.

Antigens leak into the blood over several hours and this creates a favourable antibody response. Obviously the patient will not be desensitized to every ingredient, but since there are dozens of foodstuffs and most common environmental allergens in the mixture, even if only 20 per cent of the items 'take' this would mean a significant improvement to many patients.

The doses used are extremely small. In fact, more food appears in the blood after eating a meal than from this technique. It is vital therefore that the patient avoid most foods the day before, the day of and the day after treatment.

The treatment takes up to 12 months to produce a worthwhile improvement in complex food allergies. **Environmental allergies (34)**, such as to grass, pollen and house dust, respond much quicker.

McEwen estimates EPD is about 85 per cent successful. It doesn't work for chemical sensitivity or insect bites.

Nowadays we dispense with the cup and administer the dose by intradermal injection, except in special cases.

EPD is a compound vaccine: the user-practitioner mixes the appropriate proportions immediately prior to administering the dose.

The modern vaccine contains:

(a) 1-3 diol, a kind of alcohol which activates the enzyme.

(b) beta glucuronidase, which appears to act as a lymphokine. It occurs naturally in human blood and is present in the vaccine in an amount equivalent to that normally present in 4 cc of blood. This enzyme, which gives the technique its name, is thought to be responsible for stimulating the Langerhan cells (immunologically active cells in the skin) to migrate to the local lymph glands and 'reprogramme' a new population of T-suppressor lymphocytes (those that switch off

immune reactions). In the presence of antigen in the appropriate concentrations, this will result in a satisfactory desensitization. (Conversely, in the presence of antigen at a 'wrong' concentration you may get a hypersensitization, probably by stirring up helper T-lymphocytes and B-lymphocytes.)

The following mixes are used most frequently:

'X' – mixed foods and additives, mixed moulds, mixed pollens, cat/dog, flock, fly mix and bacterial mix.

'I' – inhalants alone. This is used to treat hay fever, cat, dog, horse allergies, pure mould and housedust allergies.

Separate mixes of odds and ends, laboratory animal hair/dander and sawdusts are also available. So far EPD has not provided any useful means of desensitizing for chemical reactions.

Hay fever and rhinitis usually respond to the first dose of inhalant mix. Two treatments are usually given in all. But doses of EPD are cumulative and a few of the more complex allergic patients will not start to improve until eight doses have been administered over two years.

INDICATIONS FOR EPD

A wide variety of conditions respond to EPD, including the following: asthma, eczema, rhinitis, chronic urticaria, angioneurotic oedema, hyperkinetic syndrome, migraine and chronic headaches, irritable bowel syndrome, inflammatory bowel disease, food-induced psychological states – depression, anxiety – post-viral fatigue syndrome and multiple food allergy.

McEwen draws attention to a combination syndrome of psychological disturbance, irritable bowel and migraine, which he calls PIMS.

SET UP
Foods

Desensitization for foods demands that there are no circulating food antigens at the injection site. This means patients have to go on a diet of foods that have been found from experience rarely to upset EPD, such as lamb, sweet potato, buckwheat, carrot (cooked), celery (cooked), cabbage (cooked), sago, fructose and rhubarb; chicory drink or spring water.

Alternatively, the patient may use one of a number of elemental or synthetic food supplements or replacements, such as Elemental-08, Vivonex (still available in some countries), Pregestimil or Pregomin (Milupa). Dairy and grain-based meal replacers are *not* allowed.

Inhalants

Treatment for seasonal allergies should be given at least four weeks before the season begins. Desensitization to animal furs may not succeed if the patient returns straightaway to his or her pets. He or she will absorb pet antigen, which finds its way to the injection site in far greater concentration than that in the vaccine, and this may block desensitization. Fortunately allergy to house dust and mites works well without patients having to leave home, but reasonable precautions against house dust mite must be observed, especially prior to EPD.

Micro-organisms

McEwen points out it is not uncommon to see patients who have become sensitized to their own **gut flora (46)**. In these cases it is necessary to reduce the bowel antigen load starting at least 10 days prior to a dose of EPD. The commonest problem is **Candida (16)** allergy and this must be pre-treated with a suitable antifungal such as Nystatin. Allergy to gut bacteria often goes unnoticed and untreated. Preparatory treatment may be satisfactorily carried out with antibiotics such as tetracycline or nifuroxazide.

FAILURES

EPD can be blocked by a number of factors. If one or more of these factors is present the physician must decide whether to defer treatment until conditions are more suitable:

1. excess exposure to inhalants, foods, Candida, fumes, etc. close to the time of treatment
2. incidental infection such as a cold or flu
3. stress
4. nutritional agents: excess vitamin C, cod liver oil, evening primrose oil at treatment time (or large excess at other times)
5. drugs: paracetamol, aspirin, NSAIDs, high-dose oestrogen (the Pill or HRT implants), progesterone-like drugs, H2 histamine antagonists (notably cimetidine or Tagamet), alpha and beta sympathomimetics (ventolin, bricanyl in large doses), cyclophosphamide, opiates, trimethoprim, Septrin and antimalarials.

SAFETY

Whenever antigenic material is injected into any person there is always the theoretical risk of **anaphylaxis (6)**. Reactions to the 'conventional' desensitizing injections are common because large amounts of antigen are injected. In fact deaths have occurred and this method of injecting large amounts of antigen is no longer considered justifiable.

With EPD far smaller quantities of antigen are used, which greatly increases the safety margin. Over 30,000 treatments have been given by cup since 1966. No patient has been admitted to hospital to treat an emergency provoked by EPD. This includes patients who have severe asthma or who have previously suffered acute anaphylactic reactions to multiple foods.

EPD is now usually administered by intradermal injection, except for the high-dose inhalant vaccine, which must only be given by the cup method. However, the current practice is to retain the cup technique for patients who may be especially at risk of anaphylaxis, even for administering the low-dose vaccine. This bolsters the safety element greatly.

Insect bites have not been included in EPD for safety reasons.

NUTRITIONAL SUPPLEMENTS AFTER EPD

Increasing the short-term availability of zinc appears to improve the effectiveness of EPD.

So does the administration of folic acid and vitamin D_3. The average response to treatment is accelerated by giving additional supplements of these substances for approximately three weeks after each dose. Generally these nutritional supplements are not used after hay fever treatments, although they may be added if the response to a first treatment has been poor. Inadequate patient nutrition must be tackled as a separate problem. As with any other approach, most patients benefit from multivitamin and mineral supplements.

TIMING AND SPACING OF EPD DOSES

EPD is a long-term project and this needs to be clearly understood by the patient. Treatment is begun at intervals of two months. Once the response is established, this can be increased to three months, then four and so on. Usually it is possible to get it down to once or twice a year. Some patients have been able to discontinue regular treatments altogether.

Patient response to EPD varies widely. Typically, nothing happens for about three weeks, then there is a sudden surge of improvement. This usually lasts a couple of weeks and then wears off. After the second dose, this improvement may last three to four weeks; then for longer and longer intervals until improvement is maintained right through to the next dose. This is the signal to start increasing the interval between treatments. Improvement, in this context, may mean either feeling better, or tolerating more foods, or (usually) both.

37. Enzyme Supplementation

Dr William H. Philpott has carried out pioneering investigations into the efficacy of pancreatic enzyme supplementation for people with food allergies. The pancreas is one of the prime but least often identified **target organs (104)** for the allergic/intolerance process. It is also an important endocrine gland for the secretion of the hormone insulin.

Gastric digestion occurs in an acidic pH (1.8 to 2.0), whereas the small intestine functions in an alkaline medium (pH 8.0 to 9.0). The stomach secretes hydrochloric acid to achieve this acidic pH; the small intestine and pancreas produce bicarbonate to neutralize this and achieve the alkaline effect.

In addition, the pancreas secretes important digestive enzymes: proteolytic enzymes (such as trypsin, chymotrypsin and carboxypeptidase) to digest protein, lipase to digest fats and pancreatic amylases to digest starches. These enzyme processes are known to be regulated by tissue hormones called *kinins*.

Lack of proper digestion may cause food to retain its antigenic characteristics – thus it will still have a wheat, milk, banana, etc. character and be capable of generating an antibody response when it reaches the bloodstream. This will aggravate or precipitate food allergy and intolerance in susceptible individuals.

Philpott's approach was to minimize or defeat pancreatic deficiency where it existed. This was achieved by supplementing acids and alkalis to achieve the correct pHs, and by pancreatic enzyme replacement. His recommended regimen in full is as follows:

1. With main meals: 30 minutes before each meal take two tablets of pancreatic enzyme extract.
2. At the commencement of the meal: if the gastric acid (by saliva test) is shown to be low, take betaine hydrochloride or similar acidic replacement. This is best taken in conjunction with gastric enzyme pepsin and pancreatic concentrate.
3. After the meal: take two more tablets of pancreatic enzyme extract.
4. Thirty minutes after the end of the meal: take a further tablet of pancreatic extract, a tablet of bromolain with papain, and a half teaspoon of **alkali salts (4)** mix (sodium and potassium bicarbonate).
5. At bed time: take five tablets of pancreatic enzyme extract and two bromolain with papain tablets.
6. At 2 a.m.: take five tablets of pancreatic enzyme extract, 2 tablets of bromolain with papain.

This programme needs to be maintained for two to four months and then reduced according to the patient's needs.

The approximate amount of acid or alkali needed for each individual can be judged by taking readings of saliva pH before the meal, 30 minutes after the meal and one hour after the meal. Normal saliva pH is 6.4 to 6.8. If it is below 6.4 before a meal this means the patient is producing too much gastric acid; accordingly this acid should not be supplemented. If the saliva is higher than 6.8, the betaine hydrochloride will be necessary.

Patients with pancreatic insufficiency will need an aggressive nutritional programme to restore the balance of lost nutrients, which may have taken place over many years.

Also see **malabsorption (67)** and **nutrition and allergies (81)**

38. Essential Fatty Acids

The proper recognition of the importance of essential fatty acids (EFAs) only occurred this century. We now know them as vitamin-status substances that the body needs but cannot manufacture. They are required particularly in the structure of cell membranes, in **prostaglandin (92)** synthesis and in cholesterol transport. Lack of EFAs is implicated in diabetes, hypertension, arteriosclerosis, cancer and connective tissue disorders (the so-called 'auto-immune diseases').

Most people have heard of the distinction between saturated and polyunsaturated fats. Essential fatty acids (EFAs) are polyunsaturated, but not all polyunsaturated fatty acids are EFAs. In fact, the polyunsaturated fats in many vegetable oils may interfere with EFAs and as such they are **anti-nutrients (7)**.

For example, hydrogenated fats in margarine can markedly inhibit the body's uptake of EFAs. Since EFAs are vital to the smooth working of most body tissues, including the cardio-vascular system, it is now believed that margarine is *not* protective against heart disease. In fact, it may underlie the *increase* in myocardial infarction seen this century.

PROSTAGLANDINS

The importance of EFAs lies in their relation to prostaglandin synthesis. Linoleic acid, which is present in a number of foods, is the precursor of gamma-linolenic acid (GLA). This in turn is metabolized to dihomogammalinolenic acid (don't panic; the names aren't important) and then on to become prostaglandin E1. An alternative pathway takes it to arachidonic acid and prostaglandin E2.

Prostaglandin E1 is noted for reducing swelling, redness and pain at sites of inflammation. Thus it would have a protective effect in arthritis and eczema (among other conditions). Prostaglandin E2, on the other hand, is involved in pathways which directly oppose some of the E1 functions. It may increase redness and pain at sites of inflammation. However it isn't sensible to try to delineate clearly the prostaglandin roles in this way, for a number of reasons. To begin with they are little understood, and that should advise caution. Secondly, prostaglandins are present in almost all body tissues – clearly for a reason. It seems highly probable that optimum health is based on a proper *balance* between E1 and E2 and thus there are no 'bad' prostaglandins.

It will readily be seen that lack of linoleic acid will disadvantage patients with inflammatory conditions. In fact patients rarely lack this fatty acid; it is plentiful in food. But progress to the next stage (gamma-linolenic acid) may be interrupted by a number of factors, such as excess fats, ageing, too much alcohol, viral infections or the lack of zinc.

This is where oil of Evening Primrose comes in. It contains large amounts of gamma-linolenic acid and *by-passes* any block, facilitating the production of E1 prostaglandins. However, vitamin B_6, vitamin C, niacin and zinc are needed for the two intermediate stages, so lack of these could still stall the process.

OMEGA-6 AND OMEGA-3 EFAs

These two groups of EFAs are named on the basis of the number of carbon atoms in their molecular chain. The omega-6 series originate from linoleic acid, as described above. The omega-3 series is derived from alpha-linolenic acid, which is present to some degree in foods such as wheat, beans and spinach. However, its prime source is marine plants and the omega-3 fatty acids are thus plentiful in fish.

EFA metabolism is complicated. The two different series seem to 'compete' to a certain extent. Thus a patient who has poor hair, skin and nails due to lack of omega-3 EFAs will find that oil of Evening Primrose will make his or her condition *worse*. And vice versa.

The optimum ratio of omega-6 EFAs to omega-3 is said to be 4 to 1. The omega-6 series are probably more important in mammals.

Not surprisingly, given the widespread involvement of EFAs in the production of very potent biological materials, deficiencies and imbalance can lead to a diversity of problems. Chief among these are inflammatory and degenerative diseases such as cancer, arthritis, arteriosclerosis and heart disease, obesity, psychiatric disorders (notably schizophrenia), behavioural disturbance in children, PMT, diabetes and allergy.

Aspirin is the oldest medication known to prevent prostaglandin production and it is probably via this action that it has so many valuable effects in the body. Today, many new anti-prostaglandin drugs have been developed.

THE VEGETARIAN CONNECTION

Arachidonic acid in the diet (as opposed to being synthesized from dihomogamma-linolenic acid) comes mainly from meat. Thus diets too high in animal sources *may* favour the production of prostaglandin E2, which is implicated in clotting abnormalities and inflammation. This might explain the connection – if one exists – between eating too much red meat and heart disease, and also arthritis, which sometimes benefits

from avoiding red meat (beef, pork and lamb). This tendency would obviously be exacerbated by a relative lack of linoleic acid and prostaglandin E1.

DOSES

It must be stated clearly that no one knows what the dietary requirements are. Various authorities have suggested from 1 to 15 per cent of dietary energy sources should be linoleic acid. Recommended doses for supplements are therefore largely 'guestimates'.

Evening Primrose Oil is marketed under a variety of names, of which *Efamol* (250 or 500 mg capsules) is best known. Safflower oil also contains significant quantities of linoleic acid. So does sunflower oil, but rather less. The most widely available fish oil preparation is *Maxepa*.

Suggested dosages are 1 to 4 g of *Efamol* per day and 4 to 8 capsules of *Maxepa* per day. Children should receive smaller doses.

These supplements must be part of a programme including proper multivitamin and mineral supplements, especially vitamin B complex, vitamin C, vitamin E, zinc and magnesium.

People with any form of epilepsy should not take Evening Primrose Oil without medical supervision, since it may make the condition worse. Those with blood disorders or bleeding problems should only take *Maxepa* or purified fish oil under medical supervision: prostaglandin E2 reduces clotting.

Also see **nutrition and allergies (81)**

39. Flatulence

On a par with bloating, this is one of the major recurring symptoms of which food and other allergics complain. Bloating is caused by gas in the intestine, mainly the colon. If the gas becomes excessive, flatulence results. It can come and go very dramatically. I have seen patients during challenge tests enlarge in a matter of one or two minutes, putting on as much as 8 in/ 20 cm.

There is no comprehensive physiological

explanation as to where the gas comes from or, if not expelled, where it goes. Perhaps it is reabsorbed – but this seems a bit unlikely in view of the obvious volume involved. One of medicine's great mysteries, but not one likely to attract a would-be Nobel prize-winner!

The fact is, any allergy can cause it but certain groups of foods are particularly associated with flatus: the pulses are notorious for it (beans and wind often being the subject of crude jokes); brassicas are not as widely recognized but are just as much trouble. Remember, it is not necessarily *every* member of a food family that causes a reaction.

Gluten enteropathy has long been associated with bloating, flatulence and bulky, stinking stools – indeed, these are important diagnostic signs. Lastly, the yeast syndrome, or **intestinal fermentation (59)**, causes much flatulence.

40. Fluoride

Fluoride has long been known as a toxin – and, moreover, one that *damages teeth*. It causes mottling and destruction of tooth enamel. Natural springs containing high levels of fluoride are condemned and cannot be used. Between the First and Second · World Wars litigation damages against steel- and aluminium-smelting companies in the US reached enormous proportions due to their contamination of ground water supplies and the resulting health problems.

Then suddenly, as if by a miracle, the health problems were 'solved': not only was fluoride no longer described as harmful for us – we were told it was *beneficial*. Just how the scientific community fell for this piece of absurd, convoluted and immoral logic defies the imagination.

The evidence that fluoridation prevents dental caries (decay) is weak at best and actually downright dishonest in some studies. Yet it is constantly paraded by government advisers and scientific com-mittees as proof that we need to have fluoride added to our water supply. Even if it were true, the amounts we get are more than sufficient.

The history of this is very revealing. Metal industries hired a man to find a safe way of disposing of fluoride. By chance this man had also worked for several years for a big sugar corporation. He was in fact being paid to find a solution to caries so that more sugar could be pushed on the populace. He came up with a solution that pleased both his employers at once: fluoride was suddenly a cure for caries. Now the metal industries could get rid of all their unwanted, dangerous fluoride by adding it to water supplies as a 'medicament'.

Requirements suggest 1 mg per day, but we get this from our general food supply. Remember, plants take it up from the soil. Tea is particularly rich in fluoride and it is said that six cups of tea a day meets the 1 mg of dietary intake. Then there is the amount added to toothpaste. It is not supposed to be swallowed, but in fact most people swallow significant quantities – especially children who swallow large amounts in relation to their size. This may produce a further 1 or 2 mg. Some individuals are, therefore, getting *four times* the amount of fluoride said to be good for them.

Also see **food additives (41)** and **water (110)**

41. Food Additives

In 1984 the average Briton ate over 2.4 kilos of food additives. That's equivalent to a *daily* intake of 6,500 mg (one aspirin tablet = 500 mg). There are now something like 3,500 additives available to food manufacturers in the UK. We are told constantly that these additives are quite safe – but are they? One of the truly shocking aspects of 'democracy' in the UK is that food manufacturing concerns are allowed to invoke the Official Secrets Act – designed to protect the security of the state – in order to shield themselves from public scrutiny of their safety testing data.

Many people claim that they are sensitive to food additives, but on double-blind **challenge tests (18)** they often find they are not. The truth is, allergy to food additives isn't nearly as common as allergy to good whole foods such as yeast, egg, wheat, milk, etc. Nevertheless, there is every good reason for avoiding unnecessary additives, as they are part of a toxic **body load (11)** – and since we don't need them, why have them?

The term 'food additive' is very vague. People usually take it to mean deliberate ingredients but in fact there is much more to this problem than just that. A review of the food chain will show that the chemical contamination of food takes place at many stages:

First, there is unintentional contamination by chemicals such as herbicides, fungicides and insecticides added to crops. These will appear in the flour after milling and be incorporated in all the foods the flour is used to make. Other foods, such as milk, may contain antibiotics, while meats may contain hormones and other artificial chemicals intended for veterinary use, not for humans.

Then there are contaminants that enter at the transportation stage. For example, the breakdown of plastic packaging may affect the product sufficiently to cause reactions in acutely sensitive patients. The chemical treatment may be deliberate though not intended as a food 'additive'. This applies to the artificial ripening of bananas with ethylene while in transit at sea.

Food is sometimes treated during storage. Potato crops are sprayed with tecnazine to prevent them sprouting and grains are often resprayed with fungicides, etc. many times to enable them to survive long-term storage. Fungi, mites (and their faeces) may become incorporated in foods at this stage.

Even hermetically-sealed storage has its problems. Lead solder in food cans may dissolve and contaminate foods. The **phenolic (86)** linings (the bright, golden-coloured resin) inside tins can also leach and present problems for some individuals.

Then there is further contamination for retail purposes, even with 'fresh' and 'natural' produce. For example, cucumbers, apples and other fruit may be dipped in wax to help them maintain their bright, shiny colour. Meat may be treated with niacin (vitamin B_3) to retain its bright red colour. This vitamin is notorious for its side-effect of reddening and burning the skin, rather like excessive exposure to the sun. Not knowing this, patients may feel unpleasant

symptoms after eating meat and wrongly assume that they are allergic to it. I also discovered only recently that it is the practice of some butchers to inject meat with dextrose to give it a sweeter flavour, which would be disastrous for anyone allergic to corn.

Finally, there is the 'manufacture' and odious adulteration of food into products that bear little or no similarity to their counterparts in nature. This often reduces its nutritional worth to next to nothing and some 'food' could be described as little more than flavoured plastic or junk.

In order to make this alimentary rubbish into something appetizing, the food industry has to resort to what is a cosmetic operation, using texturizers, colourings, flavour enhancers and so on. It's a fraud and all about Big Business profits.

A few words of advice. First of all, try not to get into a lather about 'E's: remember, not all are bad. For instance, E102 is the notorious yellow dye tartrazine, cause of hyperactivity and asthma attacks in susceptible individuals. Yet E101 is also a yellow dye, riboflavin – vitamin B_2! Similarly, E127 is erythrocine, a red dye many doctors would rather not see used, but E167 comes from beetroot red.

Don't go too far the other way, either. What are often called 'natural' additives can come from insects, crab shells, bird feathers, seaweed, cotton, wood and other substances found in nature. Chalk is 'natural'; its chemical name is calcium carbonate and it is used in white flour and baby foods in order to 'fortify' them!

In general the early 100 E numbers are azo-dyes and should be viewed with the utmost suspicion. Avoid them altogether if you can, including caramel (E150). The early 200s are bad news also, being the benzoates and sulphites (preservatives). Children, asthmatics and urticaria sufferers should avoid these particularly. E320 and E321 – butylated hydroxyanisole (BHA) and butylated hydroxytoluene (BHT) respectively – are not recommended for children, whatever manufacturers claim.

LABELLING

The problem is labelling. The EEC has laid down guidelines to cover the packaging and labelling of food, but it keeps changing as the conflict of interest between Big Business and the consumer see-saws backwards and forwards. In 1970 regulations required manufacturers to state what kind of additive was being used but did not require them to provide any details. Thus 'preservative' could mean benzoates, which might cause unpleasant reactions in allergics, or sorbate (E200) from the rowan tree (*Sorbus*), which is a lot less toxic. At present the rules require that all additives, with a few exceptions, are listed by E number or by name, and that the uses to which they are put are stated.

The trouble is that so many additives are still not shown because they are contaminants, as outlined above. There are also problems with 'secondary' sales. Thus BHA (an **anti-oxidant (8)**) may be used to treat vegetable oils which are then sold to manufacturers who fry in it and then, in all good faith, describe their product as having no artificial additives.

Metabisulphite is a preservative and antioxidant commonly used in seafood and wine. It is the cause of life-threatening bronchospasm in sensitive individuals yet there is no onus on people such as restaurant proprietors or seafood vendors to make it clear that such a product has been used. This may put allergic patients at risk.

Also see **antinutrients (7)**, **chemical cleanup (19)**, **diets (27)**, **fluoride (40)**, **hyperactivity and minimal brain dysfunction (52)** and **water (110)**

42. Formaldehyde

There is probably no chemical so ubiquitous in our modern world, nor one so insidious and complex in its effects, as formaldehyde (commercial name: *Formalin*). Its very toxicity we exploit as an antiseptic. Its vigorous chemical aggressiveness we harness to participate in many chemical reactions, such as polymerization (stringing together long chains of molecules). The trouble is that we ourselves are also subject to its effects.

It is an ingredient of fertilizers, fungicides, insecticides, glues, laminates, certain varnishes and lacquers, medicated shampoos, germicidal soaps, mouthwashes, antiperspirants and deodorants. Burning organic matter causes formaldehyde to be given off in variable quantities. This includes bonfires, internal combustion engines, cigarette and pipe smoke, coal fires, gas fumes, incinerators, open fires, stoves and barbecues and the roasting of coffee beans and the toasting and browning of food.

Textiles are often treated with formaldehyde to improve the fastness of dyes, to make garments crease-proof, shrink-proof and waterproof and as part of the bleaching pre-treatment of wool. Workers in the textile industry or clothing shops are particularly at risk, but you may be able to recognize the characteristic odour from your own wardrobe if you are familiar with it.

Formaldehyde is given off as a vapour by many plastics and polymers, especially polyvinyl chloride (PVC), foam rubber (carpet backing, furniture padding) and expanded styrene. At present, cavity wall insulation in the UK is carried out by using expanded urea-formaldehyde foam in situ (UFFI); this insulation continues to give off formaldehyde fumes for many years, especially when heated.

Food may be directly contaminated if formaldehyde has been used as an insecticide or fumigant, in storage or shipping or for sterilizing food containers. The tanning of leather and vulcanization of rubber also involve the use of formaldehyde.

Formaldehyde occurs in newsprint, especially coloured inks, and may be to blame if reading 'fresh' newspapers and magazines makes you sneeze.

Finally (no pun intended!), formaldehyde is used in embalming.

It is among the most common environmental sensitizers. Its effects can be dramatic. I have patients who can't go into a textile or carpet shop without completely losing track of what they are doing or why, often within seconds, so bad is the brain disorientation this chemical causes.

Formaldehyde may even be carcinogenic (the evidence is inconclusive).

Also see **detoxification (26), environmental allergies (34)** and **sick building syndrome (99)**

43. Garlic

Garlic (*Allium sativum*) is a member of the Lily family, which contains over 6,000 species including well-known edible plants such as onion, chives, leek and shallot.

The ancient Egyptians, Greeks, Chinese, Indians and Romans all advocated the therapeutic value of garlic in the treatment of ailments ranging from eye disorders, sore throats and headaches to old age. It was even known as an aphrodisiac.

More recently, garlic was used in the First and Second World War both as an oral medicine to treat battleground infections and as a wound dressing. It was a great success in both applications.

Modern medicine is now investigating garlic's traditional properties and, surprisingly, several of them are standing up to scientific scrutiny. Clinical ecologists are particularly interested in it as an antifungal, detoxifier and immune-system regulator.

ANTIBIOTIC ACTIVITY

Louis Pasteur commented on the bactericidal (bacteria-killing) effect of fresh garlic juice when dropped onto growing bacterial colonies. Over the years studies have shown that fresh garlic juice inhibits the growth of *Staphylococcus* (wound infection), *Brucella* (**brucellosis (14)**), *Salmonella* (Typhoid) and several other bacteria. The action was comparable in vitro (in the laboratory) with that of several antibiotics including penicillin, streptomycin, chloramphenicol, tetracycline and erythromycin.

The action of garlic on yeast and fungi is perhaps even more dramatic. One study showed that growth of *all* soil fungi was totally inhibited by an aqueous garlic extract. Medically-important fungi and yeasts (notably **Candida** albicans **(16)**) are also inhibited and then killed by increasing concentrations.

This is particularly useful, since the range of antifungal agents available to the practitioner is far smaller than the range of antibacterial agents, resulting in fewer alternative treatment regimes if complications occur. Garlic, of course, has far less risk of side-effects than most antifungals and can be used indefinitely in quite large amounts (the patient's nearest and dearest permitting!).

IMMUNE-SYSTEM MODULATOR

New scientific data shows that garlic can be a potent immunoregulator. Researchers used mice implanted with transitional carcinoma (cancer) and introduced garlic extract both systemically (into the whole body) and into the actual tumours. They found that the tumours were reduced and/or eliminated and that the degree of beneficial effect corresponded with the dosage level and length of garlic treatment.

In humans, garlic has been shown to enhance the activity of natural killer (NK) cells. These are cells that act as part of the **immune** defence **system (56)** and can destroy some types of tumour cells.

DETOXIFICATION AND ANTI-OXIDATION ACTIVITIES

Garlic contains significant amounts of vitamins A, C, B_1, iron, copper, zinc, calcium and sulphur. It is a rich source of organically-bound selenium and germanium. Nutritionally, selenium is known to aid in detoxifying heavy metals and this may explain why garlic has been shown to be effective in countering lead, mercury, cadmium and arsenic poisoning.

There is a growing awareness of the damaging contribution that free radicals make to many degenerative conditions including cancer and ageing (see **antioxidants (8)**). Garlic has been shown to have a free-radical scavenging activity, probably because of the oxidation potential of many of the free sulphur compounds in garlic and also from the selenium, zinc and glutathione found in garlic and known to enhance the concentration of certain antioxidant

enzymes superoxide dismutase and glutathione peroxidase.

Garlic's antibacterial and antifungal
activities come from allicin and ajoene
respectively. Allicin is also responsible for
the characteristic odour of garlic.

GARLIC SUPPLEMENTS

There are a variety of garlic supplements
currently available from health food shops
and chemists. Most of these take the form of
'garlic pearls' containing various amounts of
garlic oil. There are also garlic tablets that
contain dried powdered garlic.

Garlic oil contains little allicin and ajoene,
due to the heat extraction process: thus a
great deal of the antimicrobial function is
lost. This type of preparation does not seem
to be logical in the light of scientific studies.

Garlic powders and tablets offer greater
reliability in ensuring that at least some of
the antimicrobial substances are still
present. These products can be very variable
and some are useless. The best powders are
those where the freshly chopped or pureed
garlic has not been heated or dried for long
periods, thus preserving the antimicrobial
components. Best of all are freeze-dried
preparations.

Also see **alkali salts therapy (4)** and
drugs for allergies (30)

44. General Adaptation Syndrome

No book on allergy and environmental
medicine could be complete without some
reference to Hans Selye's hypothesis of
stress adaptation. It is something that
environmental medicine doctors have taken
very much to heart, because it seems to fit
our daily observations and explains a great
many of the phenomena we encounter. The
fact that so much experience matches the
theory suggests that it is 'true'.

Hans Selye, a Viennese by birth who
moved to Canada and practised medicine in
his adopted country, began with the
observation that many people ill from
different causes had similar symptoms.

These were general symptoms, which
seemed common to all afflictions, such as
pallor, fatigue, loss of appetite, vague pains
and a coated tongue. Selye, still a medical
student, likened this to the 'syndrome of
being ill' and he couldn't understand why his
teachers didn't pay more attention to these
symptoms: they were obviously important,
since everybody got them, no matter the
illness.

Selye eventually pursued his interest to the
point of describing a mechanism of stress
and adaptation that seems to be universal. It
is not just applicable to humans but *to all
life*: any organism, any stress – from an
amoeba crawling into tainted water to a busy
executive having a tough time at board
meetings. The stages of 'adaptation' to
outside stress he called the General
Adaptation Syndrome, or *GAS* for short.

Briefly, stage one is the first encounter,
when the body reacts and alarm signals
herald the onset of some adversity (a
stressor). These signals we know as
symptoms: pain, discomfort, etc.; some
unpleasant response that entails a desire to
limit the exposure by escaping from
whatever is causing the symptoms.

Avoidance brings the reaction to an end
and the symptoms go away. But if the
individual does not desist and instead keeps
on, eventually he or she might learn to
tolerate the stressor and find it doesn't worry
him or her too much. For example, someone
moving to a much hotter climate might feel
very unwell at first, but with persistence
learns to tolerate heat at a level that would
have been dangerous to him or her on first
arrival. We call this *adaptation* process stage
two.

It might be possible to go on coping with
a stressor to which we are adapted for a long
time, perhaps indefinitely. But circumstances may come about where there is too
much load at one time, or something might
cause resistance to run down (a virus
infection, too many late nights, intemperate
drinking or even the gradual process of
ageing). The adaptation is then lost and the
stressor begins to produce symptoms once
again. This is stage three.

But this time, the consequences are more
serious. The individual concerned no longer

has any powers of resistance. His or her body has run out of fight and the stress can become overwhelming. This is the stuff of coronary heart disease, perforated ulcers, cancer and strokes. When the effect is less threatening to life, increased allergies can certainly be a possible outcome. If stage two is 'adaptation', this stage could be termed *maladaptation* to a substance (the word I prefer for someone who has an allergy or an intolerance – see **allergy: a definition (5)**).

We can illustrate this with an example from an allergy doctor's experience: milk. If an individual, as a child, is allergic to milk, he or she will experience unpleasant symptoms when ingesting it, such as mood changes, rashes, hyperactivity or whatever (stage one).

If the parents insist that the child must continue to drink milk 'because it is good for you', not knowing that it is the cause of the condition affecting the youngster, the child may get used it and learn to tolerate it. The rash or other symptoms may even clear up. Doctors often say that a patient can 'outgrow' an allergy this way. He or she is now adapted to the milk allergen (stage two).

As the years go by, little of note may be observed; perhaps just the occasional bout of illness or digestive disorder, probably made worse at examination times and other periods of stress. But gradually the clock is running down. That individual's intolerance of milk is slowly wearing out the body's resistance. Trouble will inevitably follow.

Either because of ageing or at a specific trigger, the milk allergy will return and symptoms start up all over again. This time it could be asthma, migraine, arthritis or any one of dozens of conditions (see **diseases caused by allergies (28)**). The patient may be quite unwell and yet never suspect milk – because he or she has always drunk it and has never had any previous trouble.

In fact, patients often become addicted to their allergy food and may find that avoiding it for any period results in unpleasant withdrawal symptoms. This encourages further ingestion of the food; the patient may even feel it 'does me good' since it tends to relieve the symptoms. At this stage eating the food 'masks' unwanted symptoms; it keeps them at bay. Providing he or she eats the food

regularly, ill effects are kept at a minimum. This is what we mean by a **hidden** or masked **allergy (49)**.

You probably know that milk is often said to soothe stomach ulcers; patients who suffer this complaint are encouraged to drink it in great quantities. It does sometimes appear to work – you now know why!

One other example might serve, and that is smoking. Those who smoke will doubtless remember that their first attempt was accompanied by unpleasant consequences: headache, dizziness and nausea are not uncommon (stage one). But by persisting, the would-be smoker gets used to tobacco and the symptoms are no longer experienced (stage two). Finally, as the addiction takes hold, the individual will find that unpleasant symptoms come on with a vengeance when going too long without a 'fix' for the nicotine craving. This is stage three and one of the hardest of all addictions to break.

SIGNS OF DANGER

Selye published a list of warning signs that patients should look for when they are under stress and about to become *maladapted* to foods and other stressors. It is remarkably similar to the lists that allergy doctors have arrived at, travelling via a different route. I reproduce them here without any comment:

1. General irritability, hyperexcitation or depression
2. Pounding of the heart
3. Dryness of the throat and mouth
4. Impulsive behaviour, emotional instability
5. The overpowering urge to cry or run and hide
6. Inability to concentrate
7. Feelings of unreality, weakness or dizziness
8. Predilection to become fatigued and loss of *joie de vivre*
9. 'Floating anxiety' – afraid but not knowing what causes the fear
10. Emotional tension and alertness, feelings of being 'keyed up'
11. Trembling, nervous tics
12. Tendency to be easily startled by small sounds, etc.

13. High-pitched, nervous laughter
14. Stuttering and other speech difficulties which are frequently stress-induced
15. Bruxism, or grinding of the teeth
16. Insomnia, usually a consequence of being 'keyed up'
17. Hypermotility (technically known as hyperkinesia), the inability to relax
18. Sweating
19. The frequent need to urinate
20. Disturbed gastrointestinal function – diarrhoea, indigestion, queasiness in the stomach and sometimes even vomiting, irritable bowel
21. Migraine headaches
22. Premenstrual tension or missed menstrual cycles
23. Pain in the neck or lower back
24. Loss of or excessive appetite
25. Increased smoking
26. Increased use of legally prescribed drugs, such as tranquillizers or amphetamines
27. Alcohol and drug addiction
28. Nightmares
29. Neurotic behaviour
30. Psychoses
31. Accident proneness

Altogether this is a most satisfying theory. It is simple and easy to understand. It explains a great many observations that would otherwise remain puzzling. It is very much in accord with the idea of **body load (11)**, allergies and **target organs (104)**. Patients should understand it and use it to avoid making obvious and avoidable mistakes in interpreting their condition.

Also see **challenge tests (18)** and **symptoms table (103)**

45. Geopathic Stress

It is a new idea that location can be a factor in disease. There seem to be certain spots on the Earth's surface that are unhealthy. People who live in the countryside have known for centuries that there are places in which cattle and other livestock sicken and die inexplicably. If there were dangerous 'Earth currents' running, these places would be as harmful to humans as they'd been to animals.

In 1990 a significant study was carried out by Christopher MacNaney of the People's Research Centre in Cumbria. Assisted by his wife Sheila and five interviewers, he surveyed approximately 750 families of gypsies at the Appleby Horse Fair. It was found that the incidence of cancer among 'travelling' families was a startling 0.6 per cent – lowest in the Western world. Yet the survey also showed their lifestyle – smoking, drinking, etc. – was no healthier than that of the rest of the population. Moreover, of the families with one or more members who had contracted cancer, all had succumbed in the two years *after settling down in a static location*.

We call this proposed phenomenon geopathic stress. No one as yet knows what the danger factor is but it seems very likely to be a disturbance in the Earth's magnetic field.

The problem is definitely *not* **radon** gas **(94)**, which affects granite areas. In any case, unusual geographical distributions of disease do not necessarily indicate radiation. Areas where bracken contaminates water supplies have a well-documented high incidence of cancer. In some areas of Wales farmers are advised to wear masks. Professor Jim Taylor of Aberystwyth University is reported as saying 'I regard bracken as a present-day Triffid.'

In my view, geological aspects of terrain could also be an important factor. I refer to the writings of George Lakhowsky and others. Lakhowsky surveyed Paris in the 1930s and discovered interesting geographical variations in the prevalence of cancer. Areas where the incidence was high (Auteuil, Javel, Grenelle and St Lambert) were sited on clay; areas where the incidence was low (Port Dauphine, Champs-Elysées and La Muette) were on sand and sandy limestone.

The disturbance phenomenon may account for 'cold' spots in houses, which as many people are aware do not always relate to draughts. The positive or 'friendly' side of this gives rise to the idea of 'good' places, and **dowsing (29)** shows that many ancient buildings, such as churches and temples, were built on positively-charged zones, as if the builders were aware of safe, enhancing radiation present in the locality.

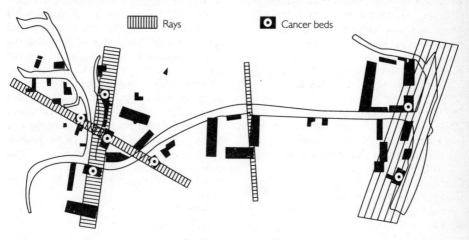

Dr Viktor Rambeau, 1934

Figure 45.1

Modern evaluation of the hazards of Earth radiation began with experiments in 1929 by the German baron, Gustav Freiherr von Pohl. He was an expert dowser and dowsed a town called Vilsbiburg. He used an arbitrary scale of 0 to 16 and reckoned anything at 9 or over was potentially a cancer hazard. He marked all the zones of this dangerous radiation he could find, then went to the town hall to check the records for everyone who had died of cancer in the town, and found, remarkably, that every single person who had died of cancer, without exception, had been living over one of the radiation lines.

Some doctors were astounded by this discovery; others remained sceptical and asked von Pohl to repeat the experiment in another town. He did and the results were exactly the same.

Dr Hager, in Stettin, president of the local Medical Scientific Association, tried it the other way around. He took the records of over 5,300 cancer victims and dowsed their homes. He found that in every single case there were dangerous radiation spots. Even more startlingly, some buildings turned out to be extremely dangerous: five houses had resulted in over 120 cancer deaths.

Another German physician, Manfred Curry, also a dowser, took along impartial witnesses to his experiments and showed that he was able, by dowsing a person's sleeping place, to say with accuracy which part of his or her body was affected. His predictions were right every time, to the astonishment of the onlookers. One bed which he said was 'dangerous in the pelvic area' had seen two successive women with cancer of the uterus.

Dr Viktor Rambeau also dowsed; the results of one of his surveys in 1934 is shown in Figure 45.1. Note that he dowsed the danger zones *before* investigating where the cancer beds lay. Convincing? I think so.

The modern-day leading exponent of dowsing is Kathe Bachler, an Austrian teacher. She became interested in how Earth radiation might be affecting the health of her pupils and causing behavioural and study problems. She wrote a book called *Earth Radiation: The Startling Discoveries of a Dowser*, which became a bestseller in Austria and Germany and started a health revolution.

Her work was so respected that she was given a grant by the authorities to carry her studies further. Ultimately Bachler dowsed

11,000 cases in 3,000 homes in 14 different countries, and has made a phenomenal contribution to this field of study. Her files show case after case of Earth radiation, particularly affecting the sleeping place, making people ill with such diverse conditions as arthritis, cancer, allergies and mental illness.

The use of sophisticated electronic detector equipment is just emerging as an alternative to traditional dowsing skills. It is possible to show that body resistance and other biological parameters change when individuals are sited over hot spots. Professor Hugo Hubacek has invented a machine for measuring electrical changes in the body and correlation with the findings of dowsers is remarkably high – almost 100 per cent.

WHAT IS EARTH RADIATION?

There seems little doubt that an earth radiation phenomenon exists, but what is it? It's possible it may be a distortion of the Earth's own magnetic field; underground

caverns may diminish it and underground ridges and streams intensify it.

Corroborative evidence for the harmful result of interfering with the Earth's own magnetic field comes from the problems experienced by early astronauts. They became inexplicably sick out in space. Eventually it was realized they were lacking the Earth's magnetism. When an artificial field was placed in the rockets their sickness disappeared. We were naïve to assume the Earth's magnetism was so weak as to be insignificant or that its effects only applied to migrating birds and animals.

THE GRIDS

In addition to geophysical influences such as streams and rock strata, there have been defined a number of grids detectable only to dowsers. The *Hartmann Net* (described by Dr Ernst Hartmann) consists of a grid of north-to-south lines, crossed by east-to-west, alternatively charged positive and negative. The grid lines are 2–3 m (6–9 ft) apart and some 15–20 cm (6–8 in). The

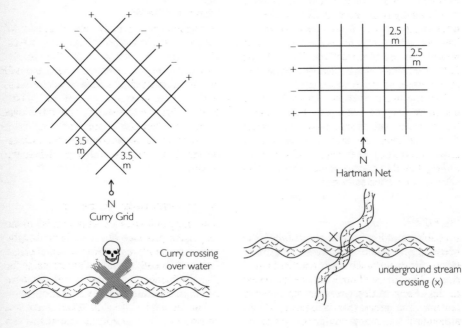

Figure 45.2: Geopathic stress crossings

Curry Grid (described by Manfred Curry) runs diagonal to the Hartmann Net at approximately 3½ m (7 ft) apart and 80 cm (2½ ft) wide, but unlike the Hartmann Net it doesn't vary. There are the same positive and negative bands and, where positive intersects with positive or negative with negative, these are particularly dangerous spots known as *nodes*. If these fall over underground water, they are said to be even more dangerous.

PLANTS AND ANIMALS

Plants and animals are sensitive to geopathic stress: stunted trees with peculiar growths are often shown to be growing over areas of geopathic stress. It is as if their branches are trying to get out of the way of the harmful 'rays'. Horses, dogs, cows, sheep, pigs and mice would not willingly settle over areas of geopathic stress, so if the dog has a favourite spot in your house, it can be identified as a safe zone.

On the other hand, certain plants seem to like geopathic 'stress', particularly oak trees, firs, elderberry, peach, cherry and mistletoe. Studies in woodland areas show that lightning is far more likely to strike oak trees than, say, beech, which is known to hate geopathic stress zones. Is this telling us these areas are electrically polarized? Von Pohl is emphatic that lightning only strikes at underground water crossings.

Cats too like disturbance zones; so if the cat likes sleeping with you, better move! Some insects such as ants, wasps and beetles thrive over geopathic stress areas; look for ants' nests along the outer walls of your home. Finally, bacteria and viruses also seem to like affected zones.

DISEASES

Probably any disease can result when the body is put under any kind of stress. Geopathic disturbance is just another kind of stress. Allergics will obviously be interested in the effects of this stress on the immune system. The great fear is cancer which, although it has many predisposing factors, may only come to fruition in the presence of geopathic disturbance.

Probably the most common single finding on a geopathically stressed individual is that he or she is resistant to other forms of treatment. Either there will be partial success followed by a relapse, or treatment will fail completely until the individual is removed from the source of stress.

The sleeping place is particularly important; most of the trouble seems to come when the bed lies on a dangerous spot, and although there are theories about protective devices such as amulets, iron bars outside the house, etc., there is little doubt that Kathe Bachler's advice is best: simply move from the danger zone.

A number of artefacts have appeared on the market supposedly designed to protect from Earth currents. Some I consider frankly fraudulent. If you *cannot* relocate your bed to a safer place however, try a *Biophoton Mat*, developed by R. Wiggenhauser GmbH, Multipolaris (see Useful Addresses) or the *Geolphil Mat* developed by Professor Hugo Hubacek and marketed by Sanoway International (see Useful Addresses).

SCHUMANN WAVES

A phenomenon closely related to that of geopathic stress is that of Schumann waves. These run vertically from the Earth's surface. They are diminished by tall buildings and virtually absent in city areas with tall buildings, such as New York's Wall Street. Yet authenticated scientific data shows that they are important to us.

Experiments are continuing with systems designed to supply missing Schumann waves.

THE ARCHITECTURAL MOVEMENT

Safe siting of houses and buildings is now no longer the province of the Chinese 'dragon men', as traditional dowsers were called ('dragon's breath' being a Chinese name for good influences). Western architects have begun to take the matter very seriously.

The Ecological Design Association is a consortium of architects interested in furthering knowledge about geopathic stress. Gaia Environments Ltd is a commercial organization with the same end in view. Safe House is a UK mail-order firm dealing in products for an ecologically better way of life. (See Useful Addresses.)

Also see **electrical fields and allergies (32)** and **microwaves and the electromagnetic spectrum (71)**

46. Gut Flora

HYPERSENSITIVITY TO BACTERIA AND PARASITES

A great many allergy patients are sensitized to organisms growing within their own intestines; so-called 'gut flora'. **Candida (16)**, which has risen to prominence recently, is just one aspect of this important and at times baffling phenomenon. It is as if the patient had a permanent 'on-board' food allergen and is unable to get rid of it. Unless the diagnosis is suspected, it can block all progress and interfere with treatments such as **enzyme potentiated desensitization (36)** (EPD) and **Miller's method (74)**.

In 1962 Dr Len McEwen started to investigate the medical histories of 'intrinsic' asthma patients. He identified a group who were improved by taking tetracycline. These patients could have their symptoms made worse by challenge with old-style bacterial vaccines and made better particularly reliably when treated with Enterovioform, making it clear that the offending antigen had something to do with gut flora.

Interestingly, careful stool sample studies from patients taking tetracycline, ampicillin or Enterovioform showed no detectable change when compared to controls. In particular, McEwen found no increase in the Candida counts, which is what might be expected to happen. He deduced that although the antibiotics did not kill the bacteria they somehow prevented the release of antigenic substances and he hit upon the idea that the trouble might be coming from the upper gut, in particular the stomach. He reasoned that since this area is normally sterile, the mucosa would not be adapted to antigens from bacterial flora. Thus if organisms *were* to be found there, it might be that the normal defence mechanisms were being by-passed and that allergic reactions were being set up.

Thus there are patients who will be improved allergically by taking antibiotics, in contrast to the majority, who get worse.

In the late 1970s Orion Truss was working with allergic symptoms associated particularly with psychological illness. Gradually it became evident that people with Candida seemed to develop multiple food allergies. A possible mechanism for this effect, apart from the Candida itself acting as an antigen, was that hyphae from the yeast cells penetrated the gut wall and caused it to become permeable to food products. These food products could then reach the bloodstream in much larger quantities than normal. This in itself would increase the likelihood of an allergic reaction without the Candida acting as a 'bystander antigen'.

All these are no more than hypothetical explanations. Regardless of the theories, the fact remains that many patients improve with either antifungals or, in some cases, antibiotics. It may even be that the effect is not achieved by means of reducing the flora at all. Perhaps these remedies act by stabilizing cell membranes in the gut. This might explain why some practitioners have noticed that although routine therapeutic quantities of the antifungal Nystatin have no effect, very substantial doses may keep the patient's allergic symptoms in check. Alternatively, in these large doses the Nystatin may be having a stabilizing prophylactic effect on the mast cells of the gut mucosa in much the same way that sodium cromoglycate protects the lungs (see **drugs for allergies (30)**). McEwen says: 'The real effect of Nystatin may have fed a myth.' We shall have to wait and see. In the meantime, as McEwen allows, it makes sense to go on using it, since manifestly it works in many cases.

ANTIBIOTICS

Note: Enterovioform has been withdrawn for safety reasons. It led to 10,000 cases of disastrous sub-acute neuropathy in Japan. A possible replacement is nifuroxazide. It is licensed in France, Germany and Belgium, where it is sold under two trade-names: *Ercefuryl* and *Pentofuryl* (currently the drug is not licensed for use in Britain or approved by the US Food and Drug Administration).

In the meantime, according to McEwen, the most effective treatment is a 10-day course of *De-Nol* (two tablets, twice daily, about 30 minutes before food), which eliminates the gastric flora, combined with one of the systemic antifungals to reduce colon Candida. Remember De-Nol and Nystatin (or amphotericin) interact and so should be taken separately.

Tetracycline can be considered as an alternative (500 mg twice daily).

PARASITES

This allergy-sensitizing effect may also been seen with gut parasites such as *Giardia lamblia* (see **parasites (83)**). Once again, the argument goes that if these are found higher in the gut than they should be, normal immunological mechanisms may be by-passed.

Obviously, if the infestation is over-whelming, parasites anywhere within the bowel can cause this type of 'cryptic allergy' and negate other treatment. The presence of Giardia in the jejunum may also predispose to food allergy.

Treatment of Giardiasis will often reveal that the patient's other allergies have disappeared.

Also see **intestinal fermentation (59)**

47. Hair Analysis for Minerals

Using argon torch photospectrometric analysis to measure minerals in human hair continues to be a highly controversial technique. Its advocates have perhaps been a little over-zealous in extolling its accuracy and too willing to ignore the paradoxes and inconsistencies in results. Matters came to a head (no pun intended) when, some years ago, a cynical journalist sent off samples of the same hair under two separate names and was sent two entirely different results.

The method will probably establish itself when used in conjunction with whole-patient evaluation and other techniques such as sweat testing (see below) and serum or red blood cell complementary estimations. A certain amount of intuition and judgement still appears to be called for. Some, like Dr Stephen Davies, seem to be very good at it and can deduce things about the patient from his or her hair analysis, rather Sherlock Holmes-style.

Examining hair biopsy specimens is not new. Forensic scientists have long known that substances such as arsenic can be concentrated in the hair, even after death. Earlier this century, archaeologists began to study mineral compositions present in the hair of mummies thousands of years old.

TRACE ELEMENTS

In recent years it has been realized just how important are a number of elements if we are to attain, or maintain, optimum health. Often these are required in only the most minute quantities and yet are vital to the integrity of the organism as a whole. Hence the name *trace elements*. These should be distinguished from minerals, which the body needs in substantial quantities – for example calcium, **magnesium (66)** and potassium. Examples of important trace elements are **zinc (112)**, copper, cobalt and iodine. Lately this list has grown, with chromium, selenium, molybdenum and other contenders being added. Some of the claims for these elements are dubious and seem to have a great deal to do with commercial interests and pressures rather than credible scientific studies.

CONTROVERSY

The difficulty with interpreting hair analysis results lies in being sure exactly what we are measuring. One source of conflict is that hair biopsy results don't always correlate very well with blood serum levels of a given element. Proponents of hair analysis are not deterred and argue, rightly, that we have no justification for assuming that blood levels are an accurate guide to the total amounts of any substance in the body, let alone of trace elements. Since the body tends to regulate carefully the levels of substances in the blood, these levels could be high while in fact the body is depleted of the substances. This is certainly true of a substance such as calcium, for which the body would rob the bones and cause them to become soft and weakened rather than allow blood levels to fall. So why should the same not be true of copper or selenium?

In any case, workers in this field are quick to point out that the picture given by the blood, which changes almost from hour to hour, could hardly be expected to reflect results in the hair, which represent changes over many months.

ADVANTAGES AND DISADVANTAGES

One of the great advantages of hair as a biopsy material is that it is easy to collect, the method being non-invasive and therefore painless. Hair also keeps indefinitely under normal conditions without deterioration and its mineral content can be measured relatively easily. Only about one gram is needed, which most people can spare without any visible sign of loss.

Another important point is that the substances being measured may be anything up to two hundred times more concentrated in hair than in the bloodstream. This makes relative measurements (see 'The Ratios', below) much more accurate and minor variations less significant statistically.

Some obvious problems present themselves when using hair in this way. One is contamination. The hair of someone who lives in the city, for example, may contain lead – has this lead come from the body *or* been deposited by traffic fumes? Of course, the samples are washed carefully to minimize extraneous elements, but vigorous washing may leach out quantities of the minerals that are truly present, rendering any measurements inaccurate.

Cosmetic hair treatments are also a problem. Selenium is believed to be a very important trace mineral and measuring it accurately is of vital concern. Yet it is the chief 'gimmick' ingredient of a number of shampoos, such as *Selsun*. Similarly, hair-darkening compounds such as *Grecian 2000* may add spurious lead levels due to their utilization of lead acetate. Bleaching and cold waving will also alter considerably the true picture of chemicals present in the hair.

MOST USEFUL AREAS

Those who use the method frequently generally agree that hair analysis is accurate and informative enough to be useful in three main areas: identifying exposure levels, indicating malabsorption and providing valuable ratios to be examined.

Identifying Exposure

Hair analysis can identify exposure to potentially toxic metals such as **lead (63)**, nickel, cadmium, **mercury (69)**, arsenic and aluminium. It has been shown that we have several hundred times the amount of lead and over a thousand times the amount of mercury in our bodies that primitive people had. Some workers, such as the highly respected Professor Bryce-Smith, are convinced that we are already, most of us, exposed to fully toxic amounts of lead. This is especially true of children, many of whom have smaller body weights and yet the same *ambient exposure* (higher body concentrations). Routine screening consistently brings back results of lead levels higher than required to affect mentation, and in many cases much higher than could be regarded as safe.

Aluminium is also a toxic metal. Aluminium cooking pans are the principal source of exposure to this metal. The association of Alzheimer's disease with aluminium levels is now widely accepted. Abdominal pains are common with high aluminium levels.

Raised cadmium levels may also be noted; in smokers levels are often double that of the rest of the population.

Mercury is discussed at length later in this book. A raised level of mercury in the hair is held to be quite meaningful.

Malabsorption

Conventional medical thinking only recognizes severe degrees of **malabsorption (67)** – that is, defective utilization of food passing through the bowel so that proteins, vitamins, minerals, etc. are lost despite being present in the diet. Coeliac disease, caused by an allergy to gluten, usually presents as frank malnutrition. The bowel is so damaged by the allergic reaction that it ceases to perform adequately.

In fact malabsorption is very common and probably affects about a third of the population, especially those over 35, on whom the stresses of life have begun to leave their mark. It is easily detectable on hair mineral screening by a flattening of all or most results. The minerals are simply not being absorbed correctly and, by inference, vitamins and their co-factors.

The Ratios

Although the actual values found by hair analysis may be of debatable accuracy, ratios – that is, the relative proportion of one element to another – are much more reliable. Even though there may be differences in technique from one laboratory to another, this would not affect a ratio.

Again, knowledge is still in its infancy, but it does appear that certain ratios may offer guidance to the performance of certain aspects of physiology. For example, the measured ratio of calcium to phosphorus can provide an important pointer to the possibility of bone deterioration. Sodium and potassium ratios can indicate malfunctioning of the adrenal gland, so-called 'adrenal stress syndrome' found in allergic conditions and **hypoglycaemia (55)**.

Most important of all seems to be the zinc/copper ratio. High copper/low zinc is common in a number of diverse conditions such as schizophrenia, criminal and violent behaviour, allergic diathesis and eczema. Conversely, if zinc supplementation is too vigorous or prolonged there may be an apparent lack of copper, leading to deficient blood production, possible impaired liver performance and arteriosclerosis.

SWEAT TESTING

It is probably true to say that it is far easier to interpret hair analysis results in conjunction with other corroborative tests such as sweat analysis for mineral content. If the results of these tests are then combined with a recording of ordinary blood serum levels an even better grasp of an individual's mineral status is possible.

The main drawback with sweat testing is that patients must present themselves in person at the laboratory, unlike the case for hair analysis. Since there are very few centres equipped to carry out this procedure, for the majority of patients this means considerable travel. It is possible that sweat testing will become more widely available in the future, but until it does its use is confined to those living near a laboratory or for whom distance is not a deterrent.

Also see **nutrition and allergies (81)**

48. Hay System

William Howard Hay, a US physician, was born in 1866. Of staunch Presbyterian Scottish ancestry, he must be reckoned an unlikely rebel. Yet he was one of the great pioneers in medical thinking – among the first to make a study of the nutritional approach to disease. Despite his apparent success, he was ostracized and reviled for showing that patients could be cured of a wide variety of ills, simply and cheaply, by changing their eating habits.

His approach was twofold: eat more wholesome foods and pay careful attention to *when* the foods are eaten. I suspect a lot of his recoveries probably had more to do with the first than the second point, but there is no doubt in my mind that what I call the **dynamics of food (31)** and nutrients holds the key to a lot of nutrition problems.

The main rules for the Hay System, as it is now known, are as follows:

1. Starches and sugar (carbohydrate) foods should not be eaten with proteins and acid fruits at the same meal.
2. The diet should consist largely of vegetables, salads and fruits.
3. All food categories are to be eaten, in small quantities.
4. Unrefined carbohydrate is substituted for the refined kind – especially *no* white

flour or white sugar. Fats should be unmodified and so margarine is banned, butter being preferred, for all its higher fat content.

5. A minimum of four hours is to be allowed between meals of different character.

It should be noted that points 2 and 3 go a long way to meeting the allergy exclusion principle, which may be the reason his success has sometimes been misinterpreted. His main innovation is embodied in item 1: not mixing acid- and alkali-forming foods.

Again, there is often misunderstanding. By 'acid' and 'alkali'. Hay meant foods that *metabolize* to become acidic or alkaline as residues. Thus citrus fruit, highly acid in nature, actually forms alkaline products when broken down in the body.

The principal alkaline foods are milk, fruits and vegetables (with a few exceptions such as plums and cranberries); acid foods are the reverse of these – meats, fowl, sea food, grains, sugar and nuts (except almonds, which are really fruit stones). For more comprehensive lists, consult a book on the Hay System but beware, there are a lot of lists of acid and alkali foods that are *wrong*.

The Hay theory states that combining foods incorrectly leads to adverse effects. Thus fruit should not accompany starches or they might appear to disagree. This will give an apparently adverse reaction to the foods when, eaten apart, both could be tolerated. This has important implications for allergics, and those who can apply it often report success.

The ideal proportion of alkali to acid foods is said to be 4 to 1. To achieve this balance the recommendation is one protein meal only, one starch meal only and one or more wholly alkaline meals in a day.

The typical 'Hay day' would thus be:

● a fruit breakfast with maybe yoghurt (no toast, no cereal)
● a starch lunch (baked potato or a sandwich, with no protein)
● a protein evening meal. The main meat, fish or poultry dish eaten here. Wine is allowed on this regime (to the relief of many gourmands).

Also see **diets (27)** and **rotation diets (95)**

49. Hidden Allergy

One of the dividing principles between conventional allergy and clinical ecology is the concept of the hidden or 'masked' allergy. Conventional allergists and immunologists don't recognize the existence of the phenomenon. Clinical ecologists use their understanding of it all the time to treat many patients and many diseases.

Basically, a hidden allergy means that a substance is capable of making a person ill *but* that constant exposure to it (as with a frequently eaten food) mutes the person's reaction to it. A masked allergy is a variant of this, whereby exposure to the substance diminishes or 'masks' the symptoms. Both phenomena make diagnosis very difficult.

If a hidden allergy suddenly becomes active, overload is usually the cause (see **body load (11)**). As described in the section on **general adaptation syndrome (44)**, allergies may be tolerated for years – then some trigger causes a crisis and the allergen can no longer be tolerated. Such triggers include stress, illness and pollution.

Symptoms

As the clinical ecologist and practitioner Dr E. C. Hamlyn points out, the symptoms of a hidden allergy can be protean, perverse, bizarre, changeable or paradoxical.

PROTEAN

By protean he means that the foremost characteristic of an illness caused by a masked allergy is the incredible variation in the pattern of patients' symptoms (see **symptoms table (103)**).

PERVERSE

Symptoms are perverse because a twisting of the patient's perception is a prime ingredient of this form of illness and constantly endangers his or her credibility, especially in the eyes of doctors.

Symptoms tend to bear no relationship to anatomical structure; they are unique to the individual and defy description in ordinary terms: individuals speak of 'cobwebs over the face', 'legs full of boiling water', 'a feeling of floating outside the body', etc.

CHANGEABLE

Symptoms come and go without apparent reason and move from one body system to another, causing, for example eczema, then asthma, migraine, spastic colon, etc.

PARADOXICAL

These are illnesses full of contradiction: lethargy that swings in and out of hyperactivity, anorexia with bouts of bingeing, tachycardia (fast heart) alternating with pseudo-heart block, feeling miserably cold or tormented by heat.

Obviously, a hidden allergy is a complex and mysterious phenomenon. No wonder recognition was so long in coming.

In fact the first person to uncover the hidden allergy effect was Dr Herbert Rinkel, one of the founders of clinical ecology. It was by observing his own responses that led him to postulate the mechanism of 'masking'.

Rinkel suffered greatly from catarrh. This was at a time when he was studying medicine as a mature student. Like all students, he was permanently broke. To help out, his father regularly sent crates of eggs from the family farm in Kansas. Inexplicably, Rinkel became more and more ill as time went by. He blamed the eggs but necessity prevailed. He graduated successfully.

Years later, Rinkel noticed that eating several eggs at once made him feel very ill. So he tried eliminating eggs from his diet altogether. This was the first time he had ever gone without eggs for any significant period and he was gratified to find that he felt much better. But then a few days later he ate a cake with eggs in it, quite by mistake. He fell unconscious! Rinkel realized at once that he must have been allergic to eggs for years but that eating them constantly had masked the allergy.

The body seems to get accustomed to an allergen, in a sickly sort of way. Only when too much is encountered at one time do symptoms break through. This also seems to happen when the body's resistance is lowered temporarily, such as due to stress or acute illness. Age can have the same effect, so that an allergen that may have been harboured unwittingly for decades gradually comes to the surface.

Also see **allergy: a definition (5)** and **hypersensitivity (53)**

50. Histamine and Mast Cells

Mast cells are large granulated cells found in the lymph nodes, the skin and in mucous membranes such as those in the gut and lung linings. In fact mast cells found in mucous membranes appear to be slightly different from those found in connective tissue. When a Type I **hypersensitivity (53)** response takes place, the mast cell granules release a number of chemical mediator substances into the blood and the surrounding tissues, which results in the classic allergic reaction – and sometimes true **anaphylaxis (6)**.

Best known of these mediator substances is histamine. Others include heparin, serotonin, kinins, arachidonic acid and **prostaglandins (92)**. Apart from histamine and heparin (which prevents blood clotting), not much is known about the pharmacological effect of these substances.

HISTAMINE

Histamine has two modes of action on the body. This presupposes two kinds of 'receptors', which we call H1 and H2. H1 reactions are related to the classic allergic reaction and include increased capillary permeability, vaso-dilatation and smooth muscle contraction. Capillary permeability and vaso-dilatation can lead to massive fluid loss from the circulation, resulting in anaphylactic shock. Smooth muscle contraction is responsible for bronchospasm, as seen in asthma. H1 receptors are blocked

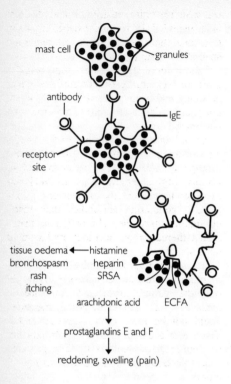

tissue oedema ← histamine
bronchospasm   heparin
rash   SRSA
itching

arachidonic acid   ECFA

↓

prostaglandins E and F

↓

reddening, swelling (pain)

Figure 50.1: Mast cell degranulation

by *antihistamines* (see **drugs for allergies (30)**).

H2 receptors lead mainly to the increased secretion of stomach acid; they are blocked by drugs such as cimetidine (*Tagamet*).

Histamine in Food

Many foods contain histamine, usually in only small amounts. Red wine has many times more histamine than white, which may be why it is more prone to cause headache and somnolence. Histamine levels in food can rise while the food is in storage. This results from the conversion of histidine to histamine in the food by bacteria.

Foods that may contain histamine include 'mould' foods such as cheese and sauerkraut as well as a number of manufactured foods, including sausages. Large amounts of histamine usually occur only in old, fermented products or those that have undergone spoilage.

Scombroid fish poisoning (or scombrotoxin illness) is a condition that arises from eating badly stored scombroid fish (such as mackerel) containing high levels of histamine. The symptoms, which cannot be distinguished clinically from an allergic reaction, may be provoked by canned, uncanned and smoked fish; they include urticaria (raised, itchy patches of skin), nausea, vomiting, facial flushing, intense headache, epigastric pain, a burning sensation in the throat, dysphagia (difficulty swallowing), thirst and a swelling of the lips.

For asthmatics and those who suffer from giant urticaria, it might be best to avoid cheeses and certainly no aged or suspect food should be eaten, especially if it is fermented. Patients may interpret reactions incorrectly as meaning they are allergic to these foods, when in fact they are not. However, the unpleasant and potentially dangerous end-result is the same. With care, it may be possible for some individuals to retain such items in their diet, providing they buy and eat them fresh.

Other food toxin reactions, such as shellfish poisoning, can also be mistaken for an allergy.

51. Hormones and Allergy

Hormones, specifically hormone dysfunction, have become an important part of any comprehensive overview of the environmentally sensitive or allergic patient. We now recognize a number of auto-immune *endocrinopathies* (diseases that affect the endocrine glands, such as the thyroid and pituitary). Best known of these is Hashimoto's disease, affecting the thyroid gland, but similar conditions can also affect the pancreas, ovaries and other endocrine organs.

These conditions should be suspected if there is a family history of thyroid disorder or endocrinopathy. In the female patient, the onset of allergic illness may coincide with various hormonal triggers. Thus, for example, puberty, pregnancy and the menopause; many women also describe a cyclical variation in their condition that matches their menses. These conditions should be sought particularly in individuals who show a limited response to various modes of allergy management including proper desensitization, chemical avoidance and nutritional supplementation. So-called 'universal reactors' (107) may easily become desensitized to their own hormones and begin manufacturing antibodies.

THYROID

Dysfunction of the thyroid gland may induce a temporary hyperthyroid state before it burns out and the condition turns into the more characteristic hypothyroid function, often seen in our clinic. The symptoms include gradual changes in the patient's personality coupled with a slowing of speech, thickening and puffiness of the hands and face, mental apathy, drowsiness, sensitivity to the cold and constipation. The woman patient's menses become extremely copious; rarely there may be psychotic depression or dementia.

The trouble is that tests of the patient's thyroid function (thyroxin levels (T3 and T4), thyroid stimulating hormone levels, etc.) usually prove normal. Excessive reliance on the value of laboratory tests, however, may prompt many physicians to pronounce the patient normal and he or she is then denied further treatment when needed.

A simple test the patient can carry out for him- or herself is to keep a *basal temperature chart*. This means recording one's daily temperature first thing in the morning (in bed before getting up). The readings should ideally be taken rectally. If readings are taken sublingually or under the armpit, the thermometer should be held there for at least three minutes to get a reliable reading. If the basal temperature averages more than half a degree centigrade low (36.5 or less) or more than one degree Fahrenheit low (97.4 or less) this is good presumptive evidence of a low metabolic rate and therefore poor thyroid function.

A better laboratory test is to assess the patient for anti-thyroid and anti-thyroxine antibodies. This is done by an immuno assay test which is quite sensitive. But such a test isn't included in routine thyroid function tests and therefore needs to be requested specially by the physician.

Examination of the patient may reveal a goitre and a characteristic thyroid gland that is lumpy and grainy. If still in doubt about the diagnosis, a thyroid scan may be necessary.

According to Dr Phyllis Saifer, a US physician specializing in allergy endocrinopathy, she has on occasion had to arrange surgical removal of the thyroid gland in order to prevent the patient from continually generating antibodies that attack circulating thyroxine. The patient is maintained thereafter on hormone replacement tablets.

Obviously this is a drastic step and, thankfully, rarely seems necessary. It would only be called for if all intermediate measures fail. However, these measures could not be expected to succeed in the absence of a comprehensive environmental programme; it is no use treating just one aspect of body load (11) and ignoring all others.

OVARIAN HORMONES

Clinical ecologists have long observed that women patients outnumber men by about five to one. This means either women complain more or women are genuinely more commonly ill. I am convinced it is the latter and I believe the reason is that women are subjected to the extra body stress of varying hormone levels which must keep at least some of their tissues in a biological ferment.

Whether this speculation is correct, the fact is that women with allergy problems suffer worse at period times and at the menopause. Their illnesses also change dramatically when they become pregnant. *Progesterone* has a significant immunosuppressive effect and the illness often clears up for the whole nine months – only to recur, sometimes worse than ever, shortly after delivery. Occasionally, however, the illness deteriorates during the pregnancy and then disappears post partum.

We think there are two kinds of effects in

relation to hormones and allergy, and usually resort to **Miller's method (74)** of serial titration to sort out which is which. It may be possible for a woman to be allergic to her own progesterone or oestrogen – therefore, if symptoms, once provoked, can be neutralized in a straightforward way, we suppose that this is what has occurred.

If, however, it is difficult or impossible to neutralize a provoked reaction, some kind of imbalance is held to be the likely cause of the observed difficulties.

Correcting the problem can sometimes be achieved by comprehensive environmental management alone; B_6 and magnesium therapy are particularly effective, and a change of diet is vital, especially during the pre-menstrual period. Neutralizing hormones, a proper diet and a **chemical clean-up (19)** may be the key to successful therapy.

If none of this is successful, or if the hormonal disregulation seems to be of the imbalance type, hormone replacement therapy (HRT) may need to be considered. Natural products, as opposed to synthetic progesterone, are recommended.

It is worth noting that certain foods contain natural oestrogen and progesterone substances; these are best avoided in order to help uncomplicated management. Progesterone is contained in beef, beer, cheese and milk (cow's and goat's); oestrogen is contained in beef, beer, cheese, milk (cow's and goat's), watermelons and yeast.

OTHER ENDOCRINOPATHIES

Other auto-immune allergic-type endocrinopathies are now recognized. For example, there may be antibodies to Islet's cells in juvenile-onset diabetes, resulting in reduced insulin protection. Antibodies to the adrenal cortex may result in Addison's Disease. The pituitary gland itself, the master of all other endocrine glands, may be affected, leading to disorders of various kinds.

Other auto-immune possibilities include pernicious anaemia, myasthenia gravis and general organ involvement in systemic lupus erythematosus (SLE).

Specific therapies may be called for but

diminishing body load is almost always helpful and may at least reduce the need for medication.

Also see **premenstrual tension (90)**

52. Hyperactivity and Minimal Brain Dysfunction

If you refer to the list of the stages of excitation and depression during allergic and hypersensitivity reactions drawn up by Dr Theron Randolph (see **brain allergy (12)**) you will probably be able to predict that some individuals will be markedly 'accelerated' and made restless, irritable and badly behaved because of marked stimulatory effects from food. In fact this seems to happen mainly to children and we call this state hyperactivity or sometimes hyperkinetic syndrome or even 'attention deficit' syndrome. Where there are learning and co-ordination difficulties but no real brain damage, the term *minimal brain dysfunction* suggests itself.

It is said to affect predominantly boys, with a ratio to girls of about 5:1. However, I think that girls are affected just as often but that their response tends to be different: they are more moody, withdrawn and unhappy. A certain amount of reserve is conditioned into females, whereas boys are encouraged to be more boisterous and extrovert.

There has been much controversy about the connection between diet and hyperactivity and many doctors, particularly those with a psychiatric leaning, often refuse to accept the existence of this link. Instead they prefer to blame mother as 'neurotic', insisting that the child's difficulties are imaginary or, if not, that they are being *caused* by maternal concern.

Of course, the contributing factors can be complicated. Children who behave badly, for dietary or other reasons, develop certain personality traits. Offensive behaviour can become a habit. Even when the cause is found and eradicated the results may not be obvious because of this. And there are certainly children who are disturbed solely because of psychological factors.

BACKGROUND

Proof of the connection between diet and brain dysfunction has been very slow in coming. It began with experiments by Dr Ben Feingold, very much a 'conventional' allergist. He tried the effect of excluding aspirin-containing foods from the diets of hyperactive children. He claimed that the results were very good. Others tried to reproduce what he did and said it made no difference. However, Feingold went on to improve his results by also banning food additives, such as colourings, many of which are chemically related to aspirin (**salicylates (96)**). You may have heard of this 'Feingold diet' (see **diets (27)**). The hyperactive children's support group (see Useful Addresses) still recommends it.

Then, in 1983, a trial on migraine in children at the Great Ormond Street Hospital was conducted by a team under Professor John Soothill. It showed that 93 per cent of migraines were caused by food allergy. Even more interestingly, the children on low-allergy diets showed a dramatic decline in their behavioural disorders – 100 per cent, in fact. The important point about this trial is that it was conducted with vigorous scientific protocol and is impossible to dismiss, though some doctors still try.

One of Professor Soothill's team, Dr Joseph Egger of Munich, later went on to study hyperactivity on its own. In his most recent study, again *all* hyperactive cases responded to a low-allergy diet (part of a double-blind challenge study on low-dose desensitization vaccines). There can now be no argument as to the connection between diet and hyperactivity.

To assess your child you can try the Conners' rating scale, used by professionals (Table 52.1).

Table 52.1 Conners' Abbreviated Rating Scales

Observation	Not at all	Just a little	Quite a bit	Very much
Restless or overactive				
Excitable, impulsive				
Disturbs others				
Fails to finish things				
Short attention span				
Constantly fidgeting				
Inattentive, easily distracted				
Demands must be met immediately				
Easily frustrated				
Cries often and easily				
Quick, drastic mood change				
Temper outbursts				
Explosive, unpredictable behaviour				
Scoring:	**0**	**1**	**2**	**3**

Degree of activity

Score: over 15 = Hyperactivity is likely

TREATMENT

Not surprisingly, doctors who don't understand the diet and nutrition connection in hyperactivity and disturbed behaviour often resort to treating with drugs. This was so much the fashion that 10 years ago in the

USA as many as 20 per cent of some groups of children were taking *Ritalin*, a sedative. *Vallergan* has been the routine here in the UK. Yet often drugs are the last thing these children want and chemicals may make the condition worse.

You will gather that the right way to approach this illness is through a vigorous dietary exclusion programme, followed by challenge feeding. Get special testing done such as **Miller's method (74)** or **phenolic testing (86)**, if you can. The vast majority of cases will respond dramatically to a hypoallergenic diet, such as the simple exclusion programme given in the section on diets; the eight-foods diet is even more likely to be effective.

OTHER FACTORS

Vitamins and minerals can also play their parts. Children deficient in **zinc (112)**, for example, tend to experience more behavioural disorders and these can extend into their adult lives. Research has established that a link exists between a zinc deficiency and violent crime.

Also see **mental retardation (68)** and Appendix D

53. Hypersensitivity

Hypersensitivity may be classified into reaction Types I to IV. These divisions are useful for discussion but may not necessarily occur as single entities in an individual.

There is good evidence that Types I and III hypersensitivity can cause food-allergic symptoms, and some evidence that Type III mechanisms can be associated with gut disorders such as colitis. However, it is vital for doctors to appreciate that reactions to food and environmental substances may occur, proven empirically, without any of these mechanisms appearing to be invoked.

TYPE I

Type I reactions are basically antigen-antibody reactions. Mast cells sensitized with IgE antibody degranulate and release chemical mediators such as histamine, bradykinin, anaphylotoxin, slow-reacting substance-S and others. This gives rise to severe local inflammation, which may cause bronchiospasm (asthma), sneezing (rhinitis), urticaria (or other skin rashes) or diarrhoea and vomiting if the gut is the **target organ (104)**.

The occurrence of Type I reactions to foods is undisputed and is what most doctors mean when they refer to 'food allergy'. Typical offenders are milk, eggs, fish and nuts, though any food can do it. Reactions normally occur shortly after food ingestion and are usually associated with positive skin prick tests and generally a positive radio allergosorbent test (RAST) to the relevant food (see **conventional allergy tests (22)**).

Type I reactions are more common in children and have a tendency to disappear as the patient gets older.

Reactions to insect bites and stings are Type I in nature and can be fatal, if severe, though this is rare.

TYPE II (CYTOTOXIC)

This type of reaction occurs when an antibody is directed against a cell-surface or tissue antigen. Complement activation (see **the immune system (56)**) leads to the generation of inflammatory mediators, with resulting tissue damage. **Cytotoxic tests (24)** probably rely on this process.

Diseases caused by Type II hypersensitivity include certain haemolytic (cell-destroying) anaemias, purpura (bruising) and systemic lupus erythematosus; it is also usually to blame in incompatible blood transfusions.

Diagnosis is done by detecting serum antibodies. A number of techniques exist that depend on the ability of serum to agglutinate (unite) red cells, or even latex particles, previously treated with a likely antigen.

Raised levels of circulating serum antibodies are seen in many cases of bowel disorder thought to be due to food sensitivities but, unfortunately, they are also seen in healthy individuals and their role in food allergy seems confusing and unclear.

TYPE III

Type III reactions result from the deposition of antigen/antibody complexes in the tissues. These complexes are commonly produced after eating, and indeed would be expected. Normally they are removed by the reticulo-endothelial system. But if the formation of immune complexes is excessive, the quality of the complex is abnormal or the reticulo-endothelial function is impaired, then this normal process is unworkable and disease results.

Tissue damage occurs as a result of the inflammation surrounding these abnormal deposits. Rheumatoid arthritis is an example of a Type III process. There are many other such hypersensitivity reactions documented.

TYPE IV (THE ARTHUS REACTION)

This is often called the *delayed hypersensitivity reaction*, so-named because of the fact that in skin testing the reaction may not show up for 12 to 48 hours. Antibodies are not involved. Contact dermatitis is one clinical condition caused by this process.

Conventional allergists say this reaction has little to do with food allergy. Clinical ecologists disagree: it quite commonly causes food allergy. Many patients react late after **challenge testing (18)**. The reason the patients' reactions are considered irrelevant is that most doctors do not see them (the patients have gone home) and, since some doctors are not in the habit of listening to information from their patients, they miss it!

IS FOOD ALLERGY A SERUM SICKNESS?

It has been suggested that patients with delayed onset food allergy (as opposed to the IgE type) have a form of chronic serum sickness caused by (possibly undetected) circulating immune complexes of the sort described above. This is an attractive theory and would explain the widespread organ involvement responsible for the characteristic multiple symptoms.

It would also lend an explanation to the well-known effect of 'withdrawal symptoms' when patients go on a exclusion diet. As long

as the patient is eating the food, excess allergen means immune complexes remain soluble and relatively harmless. The result, at worst, would be mild, chronic symptoms. But when the food is excluded from the diet, antigen concentrations will fall, causing the immune complexes to deposit in the tissues, with well-recognized and predictable pathological effects.

This could be behind the paradoxical effect most of us have observed, that if a patient eats *more* of an allergy food, the reaction sometimes switches off. It is possible to construct a sort of dose-response curve (hypothetical) showing this effect (see Figure 53.1).

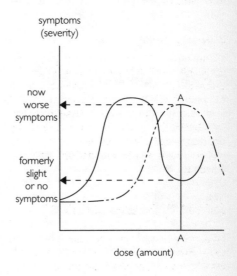

Figure 53.1: Dose response curves

The graph line, showing symptoms (effect) in response to the dose (quantity), shows that small amounts cause little effect, larger amounts produce an exacerbation of symptoms. Then, if the patient is desensitized, the whole response curve shifts to the right (the dotted line). In general, tolerance has improved. But a food customarily ingested at level A–A and well tolerated at that level is now unmasked and starts to cause trouble. All the patient observes is that treatment has 'made things worse'; he or she does not see this hidden mechanism. The answer, of of course, is to eat more – or less – of the culprit food.

What governs the selection of the target organ by these immune complexes is still a mystery.

Also see **allergy: a definition (5)** and **anaphylaxis (6)**

54. Hyperventilation

The subject of hyperventilation is of considerable importance to many allergics. Opinions seem to divide doctors into two distinct groups: those who believe that hyperventilation – and not allergy – is the real cause of the patient's symptoms and those who think that allergies trigger hyperventilation, which then leads to symptoms, but that allergies come first.

WHAT IS HYPERVENTILATION?

The word means overbreathing: that is, breathing in excess of physiological requirements.

In the normal course of events air is drawn into the lungs, oxygen is removed into the blood and, at the same time, carbon dioxide is given off as a waste product in the exhaled breath. We call this process respiration or, more correctly, external respiration.

The uptake of oxygen need not concern us here. The oxygen is tightly bound to haemoglobin (the red blood pigment) and remains at a fairly constant level provided the lungs are working normally. Carbon dioxide, on the other hand, dissolves directly into the plasma. A simple chemical reaction takes place, which may be represented by the equation:

$$CO_2 \quad + \quad H_2O = H_2CO_3$$
carbon dioxide + water = carbonic acid

Carbonic acid dissociates into H+ ions and HCO_3-(bicarbonate) ions and this affects the acidity of the blood (the blood's pH, for those with scientific knowledge).

Both the kidneys and the lungs control bicarbonate levels, the kidneys by selective excretion and the lungs by blowing off extra carbon dioxide. There are chemicals called *buffers* present in the blood that are able, to

a certain extent, to 'mop up' excess acidic and alkaline ions, but there is a limit to how much they can regulate the body's acid-alkali equilibrium.

You will now readily see that over-breathing will lower the carbon dioxide levels excessively, which will deplete blood bicarbonate and will in turn upset the body's acid-base equilibrium enough to cause symptoms in susceptible patients.

Of course, we are talking about unconscious involuntary overbreathing now, not something indulged in temporarily in order to play the bagpipes or some similar act. It is a bad habit that has become elevated to the status of a disease process.

SYMPTOMS

The brain is susceptible even to tiny drops in carbon dioxide levels. It is not surprising, therefore, that a number of subjective symptoms can be produced, as well as objective responses. Table 54.1 lists the common symptoms that may be attributable to hyperventilation.

Hyperventilation Symptoms

For each category score I point for each symptom even if only one symptom within the category applies to you. Do not increase your score if you suffer from more than one of the symptoms in a category.

Mental States

Sensation of floating (feeling 'spaced out', 'unreal' or 'distant')

Difficulty with memory

Difficulty concentrating

Mental confusion ('racing thoughts')

Tension

Anxiety

Panic attacks

Fear of crowds, shops, queues, stuffy places, artificial lights, lifts, trains, underground trains, etc.

Feel physically ill/tight chested/prone to collapse when faced by the above situations

Temporary delusion

Seeing things that are not there (hallucination)

Quick temper

Quick/easy tears

Coma, stupor or convulsions – if hyperventilation is severe

Sleep

Vivid/frightening dreams

Waking in morning feeling 'drugged'/headachy/
fatigued/lethargic/with aching muscles

Waking in the night choking/breathless/panicky

Waking repeatedly soon after going to sleep

Eyes

Blurred or double vision

Distortion of perspective ('the room tilts away')

Sensitivity to bright lights

Ears

Vertigo (dizziness)

Tinnitus (ringing/buzzing in ears) which varies from
hour to hour

Sounds seem distant or unusually loud

Sensitivity to loud noises

Nervous System

Lack of co-ordination/bumping into things/clumsiness

'Tension headache'/thick head/hangover-like state for
large part of many days

Headache during 'attacks'/caused by exercise

Migraine attacks

Numbness/'deadness'/tingling in extremities, limbs,
lips, face, tongue

Touching certain objects causes a tingling or unpleasant
sensation

Feeling 'electric' – but not the electric shock one can
get by making contact with an object

Unpleasant sensations in skin/just below surface of the
skin

Cold/burning/aching/'creeping' feeling, commonly in
the thighs/buttocks/feet but maybe other parts of
body

Autonomic Nervous System

Emotional sweating/sweaty palms/armpits

Easily blushing or going very pale

Cold hands/feet (when rest of body is warm)

Raynaud's disease

Respiratory System

Unreasonable breathlessness/air hunger/feeling of
restricted chest

'I do exercises to improve my breathing'

'I do not breathe enough/breathe deeply enough'

'Sometimes I stop breathing/have to remember to
breathe'

Frequent sighs/yawns

Cigarette smoke provokes other symptoms listed on
this chart

Singing voice becomes off-key/tuneless/husky

Speaking/singing loudly provokes symptoms listed on
this chart

Speaking voice goes husky/feels strained

Throat dry/'rough'/sore

Asthma attacks now/in the past

Heart

Rapid, slow or irregular heartbeat

Blood-pressure changes easily

Dull pain/ache in centre of chest

Angina/coronary pain, but medical investigations prove
negative

Profound/frequent fainting spells

Muscles

Weakness/fatigue

Exercise has to stop due to sudden unreasonable
exhaustion

Sudden loss of strength

Hard exercise improves symptoms

Muscles feel stiff or 'in spasm'

Muscles ache (feeling 'beaten up' or as if 'been in a
fight')

Tense jaw muscles (may cause headache)

Muscle tremors

Muscle twitching

Tightness around eyes/mouth

Throat

Globus (sensation of pressure or lump in throat or at
root of neck)

Sensation of restricted throat

Difficulty swallowing

Gastrointestinal System

Excessive belching, swallowing air

Discomfort/tension/sinking feeling/distress just below
tip of breast-bone

Distended stomach

During attacks of other symptoms: urgent/
uncontrolled bowel movement

Urinary Tract

Frequent need to pass urine

Discomfort at neck of bladder

Severe urge to pass urine/incontinence, when
accompanied by any of the other symptoms in this
table

Reproductive System

Orgasm during cult activities ('unusual' sexual
practices)

Premature ejaculation
Sex provoking prolonged exhaustion
Sex improving all symptoms for a few hours

Interpretation

Less than 15: Unlikely to overbreathe
15–20: Symptoms may be caused by hyperventilation

TESTS

There are no laboratory tests to detect hyperventilation, though patients subject to it may have chronically low serum phosphorus and this is well worth checking. The only real way to diagnose it for certain is for the patient deliberately to overbreathe by way of a test. This should be done with the patient lying down and preferably accompanied by someone who understands his or her condition. The overbreathing needs to be kept up for several minutes; the patient should be quite tired as a result. If the familiar group of symptoms appear, the diagnosis is obvious.

It is often a source of great satisfaction, and of course relief, to a distressed patient to find that the symptoms that have been troubling him or her so persistently and perhaps frighteningly are caused by nothing more than faulty breathing.

TREATMENT

Drug treatment is quite inappropriate.

The real answer lies in retraining the patient to breathe correctly. Help from an expert physiotherapist is invaluable but beware: many physiotherapists make the problem worse by teaching the patient how to breathe deeply and efficiently, which is fine for someone with asthma but the exact opposite of what is wanted here.

During severe panic attacks the old trick of breathing into a paper bag is as valid as ever. Or, if the patient can be reasoned with, get him or her to breathe out, count for six long seconds, then breathe in slowly, out again, hold for six more seconds, and so on. It should be possible to slow the respiration down to about ten breaths per minute or less.

Also see **alkali salts therapy (4)** and **stress (100)**

55. Hypoglycaemia

The word hypoglycaemia simply means 'low blood sugar'. Glucose circulating in the bloodstream is a vital metabolic nutrient: all organs combust it with oxygen to release energy for life processes. The brain is especially susceptible to a lack of it, and the consequences if glucose levels fall too low can be almost as serious as those resulting from a lack of oxygen.

The symptoms of hypoglycaemia mimic many conditions including multiple allergy and psychiatric problems. In fact hypoglycaemia often exists side-by-side with other conditions and more exactly can be inextricably linked to them. For example, one of the effects of an allergic reaction may be to induce a sudden drop in blood glucose supply.

The pancreas gland, a key organ in food allergy syndromes, is probably implicated. Hypoglycaemia is often described in terms of insulin abnormality and indeed it may very well be a pre-diabetic (a precursor of diabetes). But the real culprit organs are probably the adrenal glands. They too secrete glucose-regulating hormones (*glucocorticoids*) and are part of the front line of our response to shock. Thus hypoglycaemia is sometimes known as *adrenal stress syndrome*.

SYMPTOMS ATTRIBUTABLE TO HYPOGLYCAEMIA

Almost any symptom can result from hypoglycaemia, particularly if it causes neurological impairment. Some of the more common symptoms are listed in Table 55.1.

Symptoms that May Be Caused by Hypoglycaemia

As with all such lists, the reader is warned that many symptoms can have other causes and many do. But taken overall these may give you some clues as to the presence of hypoglycaemia:

- Sudden hunger pangs
- Urgent desire for something sweet
- Feeling tired late morning
- Feeling exhausted late afternoon
- Waking in the night to raid the refrigerator

- Panic attacks
- Rapid heartbeat and palpitations
- Shaking and inner trembling
- Double vision
- Incoherent speech, tendency to slur words or gabble
- Outbursts of temper
- Extreme depression
- Drowsiness
- Negativism
- Difficulty concentrating
- Personality changes
- Lack of co-ordination
- Emotional instability
- Mental confusion
- Light-headedness
- Insomnia
- Poor academic performance
- Premenstrual tension
- Headache or migraine
- Frequent nightmares
- Suicidal thoughts
- Addictions
- Alcoholism
- Antisocial behaviour
- Pain in joints
- Anxiety
- Manic or restless behaviour
- Irritability
- Leg cramps
- Symptoms relieved by food, especially something sweet

As well as diverse symptoms, there are several disorders that may be caused or made worse by hypoglycaemia. These include schizophrenia, epilepsy, depression, migraine and asthma.

A characteristic feature of this condition is the way symptoms are relieved by **sugar (102)** and sweet foods. The relief may only be temporary but the need drives the patient mercilessly. Many feel guilty for succumbing to their cravings – but they needn't: it is not simply a matter of will power. The desire for sugar is sometimes so overwhelming it cannot be resisted. I have on occasion heard a patient claim 'I could kill for a bar of chocolate'. These words alone are sufficient to tell me that hypoglycaemia is at work.

THE MECHANISM

Ironically, the consumption of too much carbohydrate food causes hypoglycaemia. The exact progress of events is as follows:

1. Consumption of excess sugary food.

   Typical hypoglycaemia sufferers eat a poor breakfast, such as cereal with sugar, sweetened coffee and toast with jam or marmalade (or even worse, no breakfast at all, which moves the patient straight to step 3).
2. This raises the blood sugar level rapidly.

   The body responds by releasing insulin and other glucose-regulating hormones from the adrenal glands.
3. Blood sugar is lowered, but usually too fast.

   There is an overcompensation and the level falls too low. This is hypoglycaemia.
4. There is a craving for more sweet food, soon after the previous meal.

   By mid-morning sufferers need a snack – usually cake, biscuits or sweetened drinks – and this triggers hypoglycaemia in a matter of 10 to 60 minutes (remember the '11 o'clock gap' promoted by a well-known chocolate manufacturer?).
5. The new intake sets off the cycle all over again. Blood sugar levels roller-coaster up and down many times a day.
6. Eventually the body's ability to cope with these continuous rushes of sugar becomes exhausted. It cannot cope with or regulate the ever-circling demand and so the regulation mechanism breaks down completely.

Even doctors sometimes get it wrong and advise the patient to eat sugar, or will prescribe dextrose tablets. These methods are incorrect and only exacerbate the condition although appearing to bring temporary relief.

DIAGNOSIS

Any doctor should be able to diagnose this condition purely on the basis of the patient's history: it is glaringly obvious if you know what to look for.

Laboratory confirmation, where

warranted, can come from a six-hour glucose tolerance test.

The Six-hour Glucose Tolerance Test

The patient fasts overnight and a preliminary blood sample is taken to measure a baseline blood sugar level in the morning. He or she is then administered a loading dose of glucose, usually 50 to 100 g, according to body weight. Theron Randolph argues that this may turn into a corn sugar **challenge test (18)**, so care must be taken with corn (maize) allergics and the symptoms must be evaluated accordingly.

Repeat blood samples are taken every half-hour for six hours and in each case the blood glucose concentration determined. *Note:* in hospital, the test is normally carried out for a period of two-and-a-half hours; this is sufficient to detect a diabetic response but is not long enough when hypoglycaemia is suspected because the characteristic reaction takes place long after the two-and-a-half hour mark.

The results of a GTT are usually represented graphically; three typical responses are shown in Figure 55.1a, b and c.

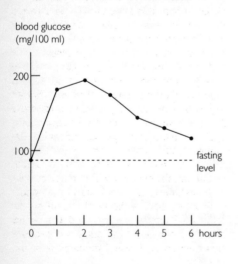

Figure 55.1a: A normal response curve

Note that the blood glucose started with a sharp rise to over 50 per cent of the starting

value within one hour. Then it fell steadily, but at no stage did it fall below the fasting level, which is taken as the baseline.

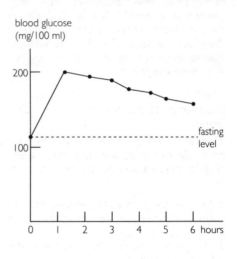

Figure 55.1b: A diabetic curve

The characteristic of a diabetic curve is that it goes high and stays high, falling only very sluggishly, because the body has lost the ability to deal with carbohydrate.

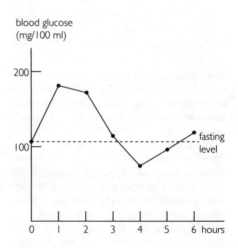

Figure 55.1c: A hypoglycaemia curve

Note that the graph rose as it should during the first hour and appeared to be normal until the third hour when it suddenly fell very steeply. Within an hour it had dropped by over 70 units. Moreover, from then onwards it remained below the fasting level for a considerable time before returning to 'baseline'. The rapid fall in the third or fourth hour is often accompanied by pronounced subjective symptoms.

Diagnosing Hypoglycaemia from GTT Results

There are several possible responses to a six-hour glucose tolerance test that would suggest hypoglycaemia, either actual or latent:

1. The blood sugar fails to rise more than 50 per cent above the fasting level (this is rarely encountered).
2. The glucose curve falls to 20 per cent below the fasting level.
3. The blood sugar falls 50 mg per cent or more during any one hour of the test (usually following a rapid rise of 50 mg per cent in the first half hour).
4. The absolute blood sugar level falls in the range of 50 mg per cent or lower (anything below 65 mg per cent is suspicious).
5. Clinical symptoms such as dizziness, headache, confusion, palpitations, depression and so on appear during the course of a glucose tolerance test – regardless of what the blood sugar readings may be.

Bear these criteria in mind if you ever have a GTT. Your doctor is not likely to be familiar with them, and it may help you to interpret your own results.

TREATMENT

Treatment depends on three key changes you should make in your eating habits. Results may be slow in coming; you need to be patient and work at it for a few weeks, the rewards will come.

I. Eat Less Carbohydrate

You must stop eating and drinking *all* refined carbohydrate forthwith. This means sugar, white flour and corn sweeteners (as used in cordials, squashes, colas, doughnuts and so on). These are stress foods in just the same way that allergens are, and with all the same liabilities. Honey, fruit sugar (fructose) and untreated raw sugar are much gentler on the system, but for the time being avoid these also.

Limit your carbohydrate intake to 60 to 80 g per day, depending on your size; a child should be able to manage with 50 g. The simplest way of working out your intake is to buy one of those excellent little books on the market with the title *Carbohydrate Counter* or similar. You will soon learn to regulate your diet without looking up every item. Many foods have a zero carbohydrate content and can be eaten freely without affecting the daily score: for example, any meats, cheese, most vegetables, fish and so on.

2. Eat a Substantial, Cooked Breakfast

There is no doubt that breakfast is crucial if you want to avoid hypoglycaemia. The average British morning intake – corn-flakes, toast and marmalade, plus tea or coffee (often also sweetened) – is a recipe for disaster. It will rocket your blood sugar and trigger the compensatory plunge by mid-morning, which results in symptoms.

A good breakfast will release glucose slowly from the stomach and so sustain blood levels for a number of hours, without any spikes or dips. By a good breakfast I mean a meal such as chops, liver, kidneys, egg or fish, perhaps accompanied by tomatoes and mushrooms, with fruit to follow. Oatmeal is allowed, also whole cereal muesli, but only within the stipulated carbohydrate-intake level you are allowed.

The fatty part of the meal should not be omitted. There is a very good reason for this: fat slows down digestion and causes a slow release of digested products from the intestine.

Naturally, you will only breakfast on foods that are safe in allergy terms, but that will still leave you plenty of scope for a good, sound meal.

A lot of patients complain they are unable

to face a large meal in the morning. Persist anyway. The usual cause of a poor appetite at breakfast-time is a big meal the evening before. Cut it down; you don't need it then if all you do is sit around watching TV.

3. Eat Little and Often

Don't go more than about three hours without food, preferably not more than two hours. Eat *something*. That doesn't mean chocolates or sweets but, for example, a piece of fruit, some nuts, some ham or other meat, a carrot or whatever you like to nibble.

Learn to take in fewer, smaller meals – hardly meals at all, really. The Americans have coined the term 'grazing' for this type of eating. I like this expression, since it helps to fix in the patient's mind what is wanted.

SUPPLEMENTS

Certain dietary additions will help to combat the effects of hypoglycaemia. Chromium, sometimes known as the glucose tolerance factor, is vital: take 400 mcg. Niacin is also helpful but doses over 100 mg often cause unpleasant flushing.

Zinc competes for receptors with chromium, so make sure you don't cause a relative deficiency by supplementing one without the other.

TOO LITTLE CARBOHYDRATE

It is not wise to continue on a restricted carbohydrate diet for too long. Eventually this will cause problems. The body only has limited resources for making carbohydrate from protein. If you chronically starve yourself of carbohydrate you may find yourself getting hypoglycaemic for the opposite reason. The same symptoms of tiredness, weakness, shaking, etc., will begin to return.

The correct thing to do, after you have defeated the addiction pattern to refined sugar, is gradually to allow the carbohydrate levels to rise. However, it is important, as before, to stay off refined sugar and flours. Eat only whole grain starches. These are digested slowly in the stomach and do not precipitate the rush of glucose to the blood,

which would trigger the hypoglycaemia response.

Suggested levels are 120 to 150 g of carbohydrate daily. You can allow more if you are engaged in heavy physical work.

Also see **dynamics of food (31)** and **hormones and allergy (51)**

56. The Immune System

Any guide to allergies would be inadequate without information on the working of the immune system. For those of you who want to know a little about this fascinating defence mechanism, take a deep breath and here goes!

First of all, *immunity* is the ability to fight off unwanted pathogens. There is *natural* (innate) immunity and *acquired* (adaptive) immunity. The former has been known about for a long time and relies on non-specific processes taking place within the body designed to repel intruders.

For example, in normal circumstances the skin is impenetrable to nearly all micro-organisms and is therefore a very good line of defence. The nasal and respiratory passages have minute hairs (*cilia*) for their defence: these cilia beat constantly to and fro, sweeping out a stream of mucus to the back of the throat, which in turn washes away bacteria. This mucus, along with other secretions such as tears and saliva, contains *lysozyme*, a chemical substance that inhibits the growth of bacteria and breaks down their protective coating.

pH (acidity) regulation can also be a crucial factor. For example, the vagina contains malic acid, which keeps the pH too low to be suitable for most organisms to flourish or grow comfortably. Caprylic acid seems to serve the same function in the bowel.

If all these fail there are *phagocytes* throughout the body to eat up mould spores, dead bacteria, carbon particles and any other rubbish. Note that this *phagocytosis* takes place whether or not a fully-fledged immune response is being mounted.

Finally, the inflammatory process itself

(reddening, swelling, tissue oedema) has important preventive effects in keeping foreign matter from leaving the site and reaching the rest of the body.

All the above processes are common to everyone. They are not dependent upon the exact nature of the invading organism. Hence the term natural or 'innate' immunity. Cellular memory is not involved. Table 56.1 summarizes innate immunity.

Factors Operating in Innate Immunity
- Skin and other physical barriers
- Ciliated epithelium
- Lysozyme in secretion
- pH regulation
- Phagocytosis
- Inflammation containment

The rest of this section concerns itself with responses of the all-important *acquired* or adaptive type of immunity, since it is disharmony in this mechanism that leads to troublesome allergies and other problems considered in this book. In contrast to innate immunity, acquired immunity is all about cell 'memory' – the cells' ability to recognize an invader that they have met before. In fact there are two aspects to acquired immunity: the cellular response and certain chemical activities that supplement this. Table 56.2 summarizes acquired immunity.

Factors Operating in Acquired Immunity

Humoral
- Antibodies
- Complement cascade
- Opsonins

Cellular
- Macrophages
- Granulocytes
- B-lymphocytes
- T-cells
- Natural killer cells
- Memory cells
- Intercellular messenger chemicals (lymphokines)

CELLULAR RESPONSE

Several groups of cells are involved in a cellular response to 'invasion':

1. Phagocytes of various types, that is, cells that eat bacterial and viral particles and other debris. Principal among these are the *macrophages* – wandering scavengers found in all parts of the body and particularly geared to respond to immune system signals.
2. T-lymphocytes, which have a complex role, described below
3. B-lymphocytes, which secrete the antibodies
4. Natural killer (NK) cells

T-cells are so-called because they are recruited and trained by the thymus gland. B-cells are generically the same as a group of lymphocytes in birds which are matured in the bursa of Fabricius, hence B-cells. (Humans haven't got the bursa of Fabricius, a small organ situated at the far end of the intestine, close to the bird's cloaca, but the name persists.)

T-cells

Two main types of T-cells are recognized: so-called *helper T-cells* and *suppressor T-cells*. Helper cells work with macrophages to generate the immune response and elicit antibodies that partly paralyse the invader and so help the macrophages lock on to the enemy cells or particles.

Suppressor T-cells come into play towards the end of an infection to bring a halt to this process. They effectively terminate the battle with the invaders. Balance between the two types of T-cell helps to keep the reactions orderly and stop them getting too fierce or going on too long.

The natural killer cells, as their name implies, destroy cells – but in a regulated, specific way. They are taught to recognize sick body cells, such as cancerous tissues or cells invaded by viruses, and to puncture and destroy these cells, thus releasing their contents which can then be attacked by antibodies and cleaned up by the macrophages.

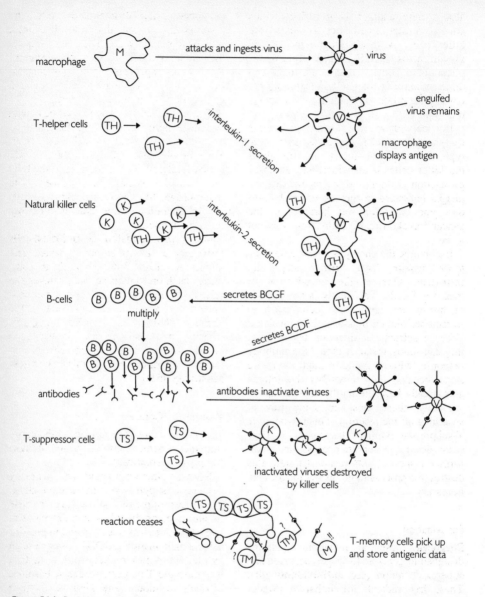

Figure 56.1: Basic immune response

MOUNTING AN IMMUNE RESPONSE

When a infective organism invades the tissues, a precise series of events are set up to limit spread of the foreigner and ultimately to destroy it and its progeny (Figure 56.1). Note that the same process applies to cancer cells.

First a macrophage will encounter the intruder. It engulfs it and then 'displays' its antigenic matter on the surface of the cell. By means of chemical language (a sort of local hormone called a *lymphokine*), the macrophage attracts nearby T-helper lymphocytes. They 'read' the antigenic matter and go off to programme B-cells to produce antibodies to this pattern. T-helpers also secrete another lymphokine, which attracts further T-cells and summons the killer cells. A third lymphokine, B-cell growth factor (BCGF), causes rapid multiplication of B-cells; and a fourth, B-cell differentiation factor (BCDF), steps up the consequent production of antibodies against the invader.

In fact there are many of these lymphokines, or chemical messengers. One type, called gamma-interferon, stimulates the killer cells. It also increases antibody production further and keeps the macrophages interested in the site of trouble. At one time interferon was heralded as the cancer 'breakthrough'. Sadly, this was not to be.

Eventually, the enemy is overwhelmed by *force majeur*. Two further steps are important. One is the introduction of memory T-cells. This really is the essence of lasting immunity. The cells learn to 'remember' the particular antigen involved. When a subsequent infection takes place, they can almost instantly mount the antibody response, without going through the above steps, because they remember the antigen and already have the antibodies 'on tap'.

Finally, there must be some way of switching off the reaction. This is where the T-suppressor lymphocytes come in. They scale down the whole process and limit further response. Nature doesn't want this destructive process to go on any longer than necessary.

Peroxidation

Phagocytes use a metabolic pathway designed to generate hydrogen peroxide and superoxide anion (see **anti-oxidants (8)**). These free radicals are lethal to invader cells.

From a nutritional standpoint, the phagocytic cell must contain high levels of antioxidants to prevent itself from being destroyed by the process.

Other Cells

The *eosinophil* is a cell mobilized especially against parasites and allergens. The *monocyte* is a short-lived circulating phagocyte that differentiates into the macrophage, a cell that may live from months to several years. The macrophage is the 'sanitation plant' of the immune system. It is not only capable of engulfing pathogens, but of removing circulating cell debris and aggregations of immune complexes.

These cells tend to reside in various organ systems, where they selectively differentiate according to the needs of their host organ. For example, macrophages in the liver are called Kupffer's cells, and those in the lung are termed alveolar macrophages. The macrophage, like the granulocyte, depends on the generation of free radicals to destroy its target matter.

Mast cells (see **histamine and mast cells (50)**) play a part in immunity which isn't altogether clear. Antibody-antigen complexes latch on to their surface, causing the release of histamine and other pharmacologically active chemicals. When the immune system is triggered inappropriately, mast cell release of histamine is one of the inconvenient effects that leads to allergic reactions (Type I **hypersensitivity (53)**).

Working in Concert

The T-cells serve as regulators of the entire immune system, modulating and orchestrating all responses.

Normally there are about twice as many helpers as suppressor cells in circulation. The helper/suppressor ratio tends to increase in auto-immune disorders, and decreases in some types of virus infection and in protein-calorie malnutrition. AIDS is characterized by the loss of all lymphocytes, but the first to go are the T-helpers, so that it becomes difficult to mount any kind of immune response since the T-suppressor cells are free to work unopposed.

Complement

The complement system tends to amplify many types of immune reactions. Complement consists of a series of enzymic proteins that trigger each other in sequential fashion. They are generally identified in the laboratory as C1 to C9.

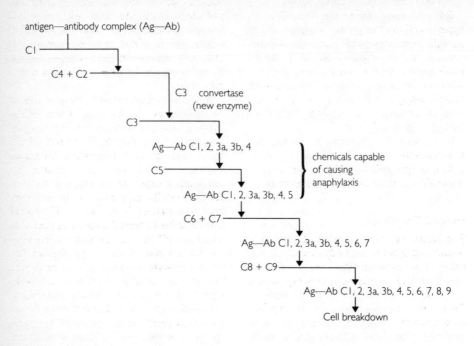

Figure 56.2: So-called 'classic' complement cascade

The antigen-antibody complex combines with C1, which in turn acts on C2 and C4. This acts on C3 and so on, in what is called a *cascade* effect, each step leading to the next (Figure 56.2). The resultant enzymes act on the invader in a variety of ways and also participate in a local tissue reaction, familiar to us as inflammation. Although this is unpleasant and can be painful, it does serve a purpose in containing the attack.

Humoral Immunity and Immunoglobulins

Antibodies are circulating chemicals tailor-made to knock out selectively any foreign substances invading the body, whether live organisms such as viruses and bacteria or inert matter such as pollens. If the body has met the foreign protein it may already have the 'blueprint' for manufacturing the antibody and can get on with it at once. If it is a new intruder, a learning curve must be gone through, as described above under cellular immunity.

The invading chemical substance we call an antigen (since it *gen*erates a response). The time has come to consider what is meant by the term antibody. The functional role antibodies play has already been described. What exactly are they?

Antibodies are large protein molecules circulating in the plasma. These molecules are known as *immunoglobulins* and several different categories are recognized. These have various labels and an incomplete alphabetical scale, leaving us with IgG (Immunoglobulin-G), IgA, IgM, IgD and IgE. The first three occur in quite large amounts. The last two are present only in small quantities.

IgG is the most abundant and is concerned with antibody production against micro-organisms such as bacteria and viruses, giving us long-term immunity.

IgA plays a role in the immunity of mucous membranes. Some is also found in breastmilk.

IgM is concerned with blood-group types and also the 'early' response to an infectious or foreign agent.

No one knows much about IgD.

IgE is responsible for the Type I hypersensitivity response seen in acute allergic reactions and causing asthma, eczema etc. in atopic individuals (which some people would call a 'true allergy'). Abnormally large amounts are seen in acutely allergic individuals but the overall amount, relative to the amounts of IgG or IgM, is still small.

It is possible to measure serum immunoglobulin levels. Individual levels of IgA, IgD, IgE, IgG and IgM are now readily obtainable at most clinical laboratories.

Immune Complexes

The immune complex consists of an antigen bound to a specific antibody, usually in the presence of complement. These complexes may form large aggregates in the circulation and if so are measurable in the laboratory. They serve as one index of an ongoing inflammatory reaction. There is now evidence that food allergens may be a component of some circulating immune complexes.

SELF AND NOT-SELF

One of the mysteries of immunity, still unsolved to date, is how the body can tell its own proteins from those coming from other sources. If the immune system did not recognize 'self', no one would survive beyond infancy. In fact conditions where the body attacks itself are rare and are known as *auto-immune diseases*. These include conditions such as multiple sclerosis, rheumatoid arthritis and systemic lupus erythematosus (SLE). Recent research has come up with two possible explanations as to how the body recognizes 'self' and 'not self'.

One is called *clonal deletion*. This takes place in the thymus gland during maturation of the T-lymphocytes. The basis of this theory is that self-reactive immune cells are weeded out before they can harm the body. Early in life immune system cells are probably non-specific and can, potentially, react to any and all antigens. This includes the ability to react to self, but gradually, for reasons which are not well understood, immature T-cells that bind with presented self antigens die and are removed. Possibly this is because the cells are exposed to massive amounts of the antigen which overstimulate the immature cell in a way that kills them.

A second postulated mechanism is that of *clonal anergy*. In the mid-to-late 1980s, Mark K. Jenkins, now at the University of Minnesota, and Ronald H. Shartz of the National Institute of Allergy and Infectious Diseases noticed that under certain circumstances exposure to antigens did not activate T-cells appropriately. In fact they became permanently unreactive. The signal that should have turned them on appeared to turn them off instead. Further studies have led Jenkins and Shartz to hypothesize that the lymphocyte receptors had to recognize two antigens at the same time, a double signal. If the second signal, possibly a chemical trigger, was absent and the T-cell bound only with antigen, it somehow lost its ability to produce the lymphokine essential to T-cell proliferation. The T-cell would not be deleted as in clonal deletion but it would no longer be able to be activated by any antigens it encountered.

Clonal anergy has interesting possibilities for transplant organ rejection. If scientists can identify and somehow block the necessary second signal, cells will not be triggered to react antigenically to the foreign transplant tissue and consequently will be unable to reject it.

These few pages are just a glimpse of what is a huge and complex subject. If you are interested in reading more, you must study a dedicated text. Also keep your eyes on journals like *New Scientist*; new discoveries are happening all the time.

Really, we have come a long way to fulfilling my prophecy in *Allergies: What Everyone Should Know* (Unwin Hyman, 1986), that the more we learned about AIDS, the more it would teach us about the immune system and the true nature of allergies.

Also see **anaphylaxis (6)** and **urine therapy (108)**

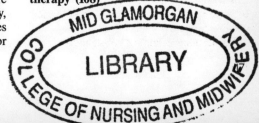

57. Inborn Errors of Metabolism/Enzyme Deficiency

There are a number of genetic conditions in which the individual is unable to metabolize one or more constituents of food properly. One of the best known is *phenylketonuria*: the child is unable to break down the amino acid phenylalanine which, in sufficient quantity, is toxic enough to cause severe brain damage and mental retardation. These disorders are christened 'inborn errors of metabolism'. Symptoms are due to the accumulation of toxic by-products that are not present to any significant degree in normal individuals.

Obviously, the manifestation of such diseases will be not unlike a food allergy or intolerance. There is ground for confusion. Indeed, it might be argued that almost all food intolerance (as opposed to the true Type I **hypersensitivity (53)**) might ultimately turn out to be some kind of 'error of metabolism'; it's simply that, at this stage, we don't know what the metabolic error is.

Most of these conditions are very rare and turn up in early childhood. They tend to be the province of the paediatrician, not the allergist. But sometimes the diagnosis gets missed. This is particularly liable to happen if the condition is marginal. The result will be an older patient who manifests grumbling ill-health until a proper diagnosis is made or, more likely, he or she comes across an allergy or environmentally-orientated doctor who, by trial and error, works out which foods the patient should avoid. The result is the same (a recovery) but both doctor and patient may miss what the real source of the trouble was.

CARBOHYDRATE DIGESTION

Lactose intolerance (62) is usually an inborn error of metabolism, that is, genetic.

Other sugars may be badly metabolized. Primary sucrase-isomaltase deficiency means that ordinary invert sugar and starches in foods cannot be digested. The resulting symptoms can be very diverse but usually include marked digestive disturbance such as abdominal bloating, discomfort or pain and diarrhoea of varying severity. The condition may easily be mistaken for irritable bowel syndrome.

Some patients cannot handle fructose (the sugar in fruit). Trehalose deficiency is much rarer. The sugar trehalose is found in lower plant orders and fungi. Inability to digest this substance would lead to severe symptoms after eating mushrooms, which could easily be mistaken for fungal poisoning. Probably there are other similar conditions and we are not diagnosing them nearly often enough.

ALCOHOL

Inability to metabolize **alcohol (2)** safely is caused by an inherited deficiency of the enzyme aldehyde dehydrogenase. The first stage of **detoxification (26)** of ethyl alcohol is that it gets turned into acetaldehyde. If the second stage is impaired in any way, this toxic chemical accumulates in the body and makes the individual feel very bad. The drug *Antabuse* (disulfiram), aimed to prevent alcohol abuse, does so by blocking aldehyde dehydrogenase; the patient simply cannot drink without unpleasant consequences while taking the drug.

PROTEIN AND AMINO ACID METABOLISM

Protein digestion disorder can come about through an inherited deficiency in the appropriate enzymes, notably trypsin and enterokinase. Even on a good diet, food is wasted since it passes through the body unutilized. The result (in a child) would be a failure to thrive, offensive, bulky stools, low blood protein levels and poor resistance to infection. We call this condition **malabsorption (67)** and it is seen classically in coeliac disease, where there is a failure of fat digestion also (steatorrhoea).

Probably the most important and dangerous inherited disorders of metabolism are those connected with amino acids and their breakdown products. Phenylketonuria has already been referred to above. Homocystinuria (deficiency of cystothionine synthetase) also causes mental retardation. It can also lead to vascular and eye disorders. The condition occurs in two forms, one of which responds to megadoses of pyridoxine (vitamin B_6), the other calling for a restriction of methionine intake and folic acid supplements.

Alkaptonuria, on the other hand, attacks the joints. It is caused by a lack of homogentisic oxidase, which works on tyrosine. Lack of another tyrosine enzyme, tyrosinase, leads to albinism, a bizarre condition in which the patient has no melanin pigment and whose skin appears pure white, with white hair and pink eyes.

Some metabolic errors are so severe as to be rapidly fatal. Hyperammonaemia, caused either by a lack of carbamylphosphate synthetase or ornithine transcarbamylase, results in the accumulation of ammonia in the blood, which is very poisonous.

There are dozens of such conditions, very much a specialist province, with thunderous-sounding names and complex biochemical explanations that are way beyond the boundaries of this book. The important point to grasp is that many disorders respond to diet and, where mild in presentation, they overlap the field of food allergy and intolerance.

TRIMETHYLAMINURIA

This strange condition is worthy of note. Trimethylamine is a tertiary ammonium compound which gives rotting fish its characteristic odour. It is produced by the breakdown of the amino acid choline in the intestine. Most of us oxidize this unpleasant chemical rapidly. Some luckless individuals, however, lack the oxidative enzyme. Thus trimethylamine builds up in their body and they stink of rotting fish. The only answer is to avoid choline-containing foods such as eggs (and, of course, fish).

Also see **allergy: a definition (5)**, **phenolic testing (86)** and **plant toxins (87)**

58. Insect Stings

Insect stings can be serious and even fatal for allergics. Evidence suggests that the ancient Egyptian king Menes of Memphis died this way.

Possibly the first authenticated death from an insect bite allergy came in 1765. A Dr Debret from Montpellier University published *Observations on Epidemic Diseases* in which he mentioned that a 30-year-old man in his local village was stung by a bee and died within minutes. 'He had been stung by bees on two separate occasions, and each time he had collapsed in a dead faint. He feared these insects and assuredly not without cause.'

This account describes perfectly the classic road to fatality. The first sting is not serious but may sensitize the individual. The effect of subsequent stings gets more and more severe, until eventually the reaction becomes dangerous and life-threatening, due to **anaphylaxis (6)**. A fatal outcome is more likely to result with older people, whose cardiovascular performance may not be what it once was. Fortunately it is a rare occurrence, but that is little consolation for the victim and his or her family. Deaths in the USA are estimated at 50 per year, though this could be too low, since such events in older people would be quite likely to be registered as heart attacks.

Thankfully, the vast majority of people, even sensitive allergics, experience nothing more than an unpleasant acute reaction to insect stings. Probably as many as 4 per cent of the population feel unwell after bee stings due to the toxins in the venom.

Only female bees of the order *Hymenoptera* have true stings. Bees are also relatively docile and only sting when provoked. Wasps and hornets are more aggressive. It might be thought that bee-keepers are especially at risk, yet in fact recurring stings may protect them due to the development of IgG-blocking antibody. This is similar to the mithridatic principle (see **detoxification (26)**).

TREATMENT

Treating an acute attack is quite straightforward. If it is a bee sting and is still present, it should be removed forthwith. Hornets and wasps do not leave the sting behind.

After cleansing the wound, applications of ice may be soothing. If the irritation is intense, antihistamines may help.

If the patient at any stage experiences a sharp drop in blood pressure, widespread urticaria (a rash), asthma or laryngeal oedema (throat becoming constricted with fluid), or collapses after a sting, he or she should be considered a candidate for a potentially fatal attack.

At all times during the appropriate season, such patients should have a kit to hand for self-administration of an antihistamine. If a severe reaction has already been experienced, only adrenalin will act fast enough and becomes the preferred drug. The patient must learn how to perform an injection *rapidly*.

If the insect is clearly identified, the RAST is positive (see **conventional allergy tests (22)**) and the reaction is known to be immediate (IgE), some form of hypo-sensitization treatment must be given consideration. In the 1940s, Dr Mary H. Loveless was treating those at risk from insect stings with small doses of the venom of the offending species, a technique similar to **Miller's method (74)**. Typically, she was regarded as a crank by more 'scientific' colleagues. Today she is hailed as a pioneer because we know that what she was doing made sense.

Classic prick test and hyposensitization methods are potentially dangerous; the risk would have to be weighed against the potential gain – i.e. the patient may be so frightened of being stung that his or her quality of life is considerably impaired. In any case, these methods should not be attempted unless full cardio-respiratory resuscitation equipment is to hand, with people who know how to use it. Extreme care must also be taken not to administer the wrong dosage inadvertently.

Also see **hypersensitivity (53)**

59. Intestinal Fermentation

Dr Orion Truss of Birmingham, Alabama first brought the **Candida (16)** hypothesis forward in 1978. Dr Truss is a psychiatrist with a special interest in clinical ecology; his seminal papers in the *Journal of Orthomolecular Psychiatry* ('Tissue Injury Induced by Candida Albicans', vol. 7, no 1, 1978, pp 17–37 and 'Restoration of Immune Competence to Candida Albicans', vol. 9, no 4, 1980, pp 287–301) certainly revealed an extensive and fascinating area of personal investigation. His work was taken up enthusiastically by Dr Bill Crook, who has done more than any single individual to popularize the Candida hypothesis, or what has now become known as 'the yeast connection', taken from the title of his book (*The Yeast Connection*, Professional Books, 1983).

Since that time, the whole theory seems to have gripped the public's imagination and clinical ecologists have been keen to extol the existence of the problem and the enormous benefits to be gained from tackling it vigorously. The fact is there *are* health gains to be made by following an anti-Candida programme, taking antifungal drugs and excluding sugar and yeast foods from one's diet. Yet Truss's idea is no more than a theory.

If there is one valid complaint that members of the medical profession have against clinical ecologists it is their tardiness in backing up ideas with research. It has been 15 years now since Truss's innovative papers – ample time to carry out detailed studies that would validate his claims. Yet they are singularly lacking. A catalogue of startling recoveries does not constitute scientific study. We may be getting the right results for the wrong reason.

Despite a degree of 'brand identification', Truss was in fact far from being the first investigator in this field. His ideas were anticipated almost 70 years earlier by Turner, who presented a paper on what he called 'intestinal germ carbohydrate fermentation' (Proceedings of the Royal Society of Medicine Symposium on Intestinal Toxaemia, 1911). In 1931 Hurst was in his footsteps, writing about 'intestinal carbohydrate dyspepsia'. In the 1930s and 1940s this dyspepsia was being treated with *Lactobacillus acidophilus*, B vitamin supplements and a *low-starch diet* (remarkably like modern anti-Candida treatment except that legumes are no longer banned, as they were at that time).

Medical literature has tried to define the patient-type who suffers with this syndrome. A major text on gastroenterology in 1976 described victims as 'Essentially unhappy people . . . any suggested panacea or therapeutic straw is grasped . . . no regime is too severe and no programme too difficult . . . with the tenacity of the faithful, they grope their way from one practitioner to the next in the search for a permanently successful remedy.' This disparaging description shows a lamentable weakness on the part of doctors for blaming any patient they cannot help.

The 'problem patient' attitude was probably what sank the condition in the 1950s. At that time, the psychosomatic theory of disease was enjoying a great revival. The tendency was to dismiss *all* patients with vague, ill-defined symptoms as psychiatric cases. Unlike today, there were no physical findings to disprove the psychiatric label and so it stuck. It's still with us, to a large degree.

ON-BOARD BREWERY

So the idea of a yeast-like organism that lives on starches and sugars and causes bowel disturbance is far from new. It seems to enjoy a vogue in medical circles every few decades and then lapses out of sight once again. The reason is probably that, as in the 1980s, some doctors become *convinced* they know what causes the syndrome, but then can't seem to find a workable proof that affords a satisfactory explanation. This casts doubt on the basis of the theory. So it is today with 'Candida'.

The success of antifungal drugs may have fed a myth. In some cases, anti-Candida therapeutic agents such as Nystatin seem to work only in very high doses (10 to 100 times the usual dose). This has led to the speculation that it may be helping by some other mechanism than just that of eradicating the yeast micro-organism; possibly by blocking bowel permeability (see **leaky gut syndrome (64)**).

One thing is certain, there is virtually no correlation between Candida in the stool sample and the existence of the 'yeast syndrome'. Indeed, Candida albicans is rarely identified in specimens, despite its known very wide occurrence. This lack of correlation is disappointing but hardly surprising, especially if we are looking for the wrong culprit.

It is true: treatment directed towards this type of organism can be highly effective in selected individuals, so clearly a real phenomenon exists. But that doesn't prove that Candida is to blame. In fact I'd like to set the debate alight with the claim that the culprit may *not* be Candida at all, or that Candida is only one of many potential suspects.

Other available flora that might be at work include the yeasts of the genus *Saccharomyces* (food yeasts), the bacteria *Torulopsis glabrata* and, most fascinating of all, *Sarcina ventriculata*.

Historically, Sarcina is an important organism. In the old days, when surgeons operated in frock coats and quite often smoked cigars at the same time, once in a while they would literally blow up their patients!: as the alcoholic gases generated by Sarcina were released from the patient's stomach when cut open, the cigar would ignite the fumes and a fireball was the disastrous result.

These 'on-board breweries' are probably quite common. Dr Keith Eaton called my attention to the speculation that so-called 'spontaneous combustion' may be due to this microbe. Puzzling cases have been documented of human beings literally vanishing in a sheet of fire, for no apparent reason. Perhaps Sarcina, or some other organism, and its inflammable gaseous excreta could be to blame.

Incidentally, just as Candida isn't the only contender for the role of pathogen, ordinary ethyl alcohol is not the only product of fermentation we seem to be dealing with. Many other products can be derived from the breakdown of sugars and starches, including short-chain fatty acids such as acetate, proprionate, succinate and butyrate, and other alcohols such as iso-propanol, butanol and 2,3-butylene glycol. Testing for these substances is now available commercially in the UK under the expertise of Dr John Howard at Biolab UK (see Useful Addresses).

Further, if detoxification pathways are blocked due to overload, other unwanted metabolites are produced, such as epoxides, aldehydes and even chloral hydrate, ingredient of the classic 'Mickey Finn'. Typically this chemical produces a tired and 'spacey' feeling. Here is at least part of the reason these patients can't take alcoholic drinks. Naturally, these by-products too have a bad effect on the patient; most are quite toxic.

For treatment of this condition, all that is written about Candida is probably valid, at least until we know the truth about what we are dealing with. Antifungals usually help, but probiotics are more logical. Avoidance of fermentable sugars is important.

Paradoxically, antibiotics occasionally solve the problem; presumably when the culprit is a fermenting bacillus.

Also see **gut flora (46)** and **moulds (75)**

60. Ionizers

It has been observed that people often feel better and more zestful when they are near mountain streams or the seaside. At least one possible cause for this is the presence of excess *negatively charged ions* in these places.

The earth is positively charged and so attracts these ions, yet they tend to be diminished in buildings such as homes and offices. In fact, for comparison, the average negative ion concentration near a waterfall is 50,000 per cubic centimetre, in mountain air 5,000 and in the countryside 1500 or so; yet in a modern office, this figure can fall to as low as 50.

What happens to the ions in buildings? They are electrically precipitated by particles in the air, notably dust, cigarette smoke and fabrics such as synthetic carpet fibres. Modern closed ventilation systems and of course the ubiquitous office computer make the problems many times worse, because of static build-ups.

Accordingly, therefore, it seems a good idea to try and supplement your environment with negatively charged ions. This is done by means of so-called *ionizers*. Studies are poor to date but at least one trial carried out by an insurance company in the UK using ionizers 'double-blind' showed a remarkable 78 per cent drop in the incidence of headaches and other minor symptoms.

The atmosphere in ionized spaces is generally cleaner and 'feels fresher' because there is an increased rate of precipitation of particulates, thus reducing cigarette smoke clouds and circulating dust. The potential benefits for allergics seem obvious.

Additionally, ionizers may remove harmful bacteria from the air. Since droplet spread from exhaled breath is a potent method of cross-infection, this may mean less illness. Ionizer trials in a Swiss bank reputedly showed a dramatic fall in absenteeism due to coughs, colds and other infective complaints.

However, a note of caution must be sounded. Mains-operated ionizers generate adverse electro-magnetic fields pulsating at 50 to 60 hertz. Some individuals will be highly sensitive to these fields. At least one of my patients did a blind controlled trial study with his ionizer. His wife would switch it on only on certain nights, without telling him which. It didn't take long for them to realize that on the nights when the machine was switched on he had angina-like symptoms and felt quite ill. Indeed at one point he felt ready for hospital. So the effects are not always necessarily beneficial.

As with so many environmental considerations, individual experimentation is called for.

Also see **electrical fields and allergies (32)**, **microwaves and the electromagnetic spectrum (71)** and **weather and health (111)**

61. Irradiation of Food

The earliest commercial use of food irradiation was in Germany in 1957 to sterilize the spices used in sausage manufacture. The Soviet government was the first to permit irradiation, for the purpose of inhibiting sprouting of potatoes in 1958 and the disinfestation of grain in 1959.

The purpose of irradiating food is to sterilize it. This is considered particularly useful if it kills off bacteria which cause degeneration, rotting and putrefaction of meat, fruit, vegetables, etc. Food that has been so treated remains 'fresh', often for a period of many weeks instead of just a few days. Even meat can be prevented from putrefaction for a remarkable period by this process.

Three stages are defined in respect of food irradiation:

1. Low dose: Sprouting of vegetables such as potatoes and onions can be inhibited so that they keep longer.
2. Medium dose: Ripening of fruits can be delayed so that they keep longer and can be transported over longer distances.
3. High dose: Insect pests in grains such as wheat and rice, or in spices and some fruits can be killed. This might replace current methods involving gas storage or fumigation treatments that are hazardous to workers.

HEALTH HAZARDS

There are a number of potential health hazards associated with the irradiation of food. The most obvious is that bombardment with ionizing radiation may actually create radioactivity within food. A low-energy ionizing radiation is supposed to reduce the chances of this occurring, but it's not possible to be sure it is eliminated altogether. This is simply an unknown risk, but chromosomal changes in animals have been observed, which must give rise to reasoned concern.

There is also a worry that chemicals produced by radiation, so-called *radiolytes*, may in fact be harmful.

Then there is the possibility of radiation producing mutations in virus insects and bacteria, leading to more dangerous or resistant strains. Also of concern is that irradiation may kill living organisms but not remove their toxic waste. Many micro-organisms produce poisonous by-products of their own metabolism. Botulinus toxin, for example, one of the most deadly substances known, is produced by the bacteria *Clostridium botulinum*; *Escherichia coli* may produce a potent exo-toxin, often implicated in outbreaks of food poisoning; and many moulds produce toxins such as the well known *aflatoxin*, a powerful cancer-causing agent. In fact, there is evidence that aflatoxin may be increased by irradiation.

Finally, a less obvious hazard is that food maintains its pristine appearance for far longer than normal and though it may *look* fresh it could be weeks old and have lost most of its nutrients. If food irradiation were to become widespread, a healthy, protective diet of fresh natural produce might in fact turn out to lead to significant mineral and vitamin deficiency, such as scurvy and beri-beri, even in a 'well fed' population. To make matters worse, radiation damages or eradicates most vitamins. The extent of the loss depends on the vitamin, the type of food and the dose given.

A specious claim by proponents is that irradiation will reduce the need for additives (meaning preservatives) to food. However, this glosses over the fact that the irradiation process may require the addition of special chemicals, for example, dipping food in sodium tripolyphosphate, a de-greasing chemical known to cause skin irritation and also used as a purgative.

Also see **food additives (41)**

62. Lactose Intolerance

Lactose (milk sugar) accounts for a startling 25 per cent of all carbohydrate in the average Western diet. It is present as 40 per cent of milk solids (cow's, goat's and ewe's). This percentage rises to over 50 per cent in skimmed milk and whey but is less in whole cream and yoghourt. Butter and cheese have almost no lactose.

Commercial buttermilk is usually made by fermenting skimmed milk, which effectively reduces the lactose level of the skimmed milk by some 10 to 15 per cent. However, buttermilk may have added dried or condensed milk, which would of course alter the proportion of lactose.

ALACTASIA

The enzyme that digests lactose is called lactase; lack of it (alactasia) is likely to cause diarrhoea, abdominal pain and discomfort, bloating and wind. *This is not the same as milk allergy or intolerance:* the two conditions should not be confused, as the treatment and effects are different.

There is a belief that milk in the diet prolongs the secretion of lactase and that a sustained period with little or no milk intake will lead to a loss of lactase; this is called secondary alactasia. However, this cause and effect relationship has not been proven to date.

The difficulty comes when new-born babies suffer lactose intolerance. They may experience profuse diarrhoea which can lead to life-threatening dehydration and loss of vital electrolytes (body chemicals). Early research into this problem was carried out in Manchester by my old professor Aaron Holzel and we now understand the condition a lot better. Special formulas are available for these infants and usually treatment is begun even before they are discharged from the obstetric unit.

Lactose Intolerance Test

Where the onset is less serious and the symptoms less dramatic, alactasia may go undiagnosed for years.

The simplest proof of lactose intolerance is a lactose **challenge test (18)**. However, results are not always reliable and several repeat testings may be wise before the diagnosis is dismissed outright.

More sophisticated testing may include a biopsy of the intestinal mucosa and an analysis of its lactase activity.

TREATMENT

For the majority of people, avoiding lactose is the best course of treatment. Most adults, with a little attention to detail, can get all the nutrients they need without recourse to milk, though since the problem is less serious than an allergy this exclusion need not be comprehensive. The following tips may be helpful:

1. Whole milk is better tolerated than skimmed (this is the opposite of what holds for most allergics).
2. Derivative products such as buttermilk, yoghourt, cream and cheese are usually better tolerated (again, allergics often feel *worst* if they eat cream).
3. Frequent small quantities are better than taking a large amount.
4. Milk is better taken with other foods. The digestion of lactose, even when alactasia is present, is very much influenced by the presence of other carbohydrates.

HIDDEN LACTOSE

It isn't always easy to recognize lactose in manufactured foods. Whey is obvious, but sometimes even this is disguised as 'emulsifiers'. Lactose may also be present in 'milk-free' infant formulas, in sweets and fudges; even in bread.

Conversely, hard cheeses and cream may be well tolerated, as may be plain chocolate. However, cottage and cream cheeses do contain significant amounts of lactose, since they are not fermented.

Prolonged boiling reduces the lactose content of milk. However, pasteurization is too short a process: these days just 15 seconds (minimum) at 162°F/72°C.

Also see **enzyme supplementation (37)** and **sugar (102)**

63. Lead

'The dangles with dry colic' is how we used to remember the effects of lead poisoning as medical students; meaning weakness in the wrists and feet due to peripheral nerve damage and abdominal pain without diarrhoea. Less often remembered are the symptoms of headache, depression, fatigue, confusion, lack of coordination, kidney defects and a blue-black line around the gums.

However, the gross effects of this important pollutant are not as common as the symptoms that arise from a slow build-up of lead in the system. The neurological damage can be very insidious in its onset and effects. Children are especially at risk because their body weight-to-pollutant ratio is higher and their immature brains are more prone to damage. Intelligence tests have shown that elevated levels of lead in the blood can restrict children's mental development; it can also pass the placental barrier, so maternal lead levels are a potential risk to the unborn child. It has been estimated that toxiciological damage can occur at any detectable level of lead. In other words, *there are no safe levels*.

Some researchers describe a condition called *behavioural teratogenesis* – teratogenesis being the medical term for damage to a foetus during development. The idea is that, rather than producing a physically damaged infant, lead, mercury and other toxins can result in a child who at birth already has *functional* (as opposed to actual) brain damage and behavioural disorder.

SOURCES OF CONTAMINATION

Lead is absorbed via food, drink, inhalation and through damaged skin. Adults absorb 5 to 10 per cent of ingested lead; children, up to 50 per cent. Unfortunately, lead is a pollutant that accumulates steadily in the environment. It has been estimated that we are now exposed to over 500 times the natural environmental dosages that were current in prehistoric times, before the onset of lead mining.

Sources are many and include motor vehicle exhausts, lead plumbing, lead-containing paints, food supplies contaminated by passing traffic, imperfect pottery glazes, lead crystal, newsprint, pencils, cosmetics, car batteries and the equipment for certain hobbies (such as stained-glass making). There are also occupational exposures in smelting, pottery, battery manufacture, soldering (electronics), scrap disposal, etc.

Probably the most significant source of lead is that dissolved into drinking water from supply pipes. The problem is worse in areas with soft water. It is important if you want to eradicate the risk of lead in the water supplies to have piping changed to the copper type. In the meantime, allow taps to run for a short time before drawing water for drinking or cooking.

TREATMENT

Once you have lead in your body it is difficult to get rid of. It is better to avoid it in the first place. That having been said, the simplest and safest method for getting rid of lead is to take kelp or apple pectin. Ethyl, diamine, tetra-acetic acid (EDTA) is better but is toxic and should only be handled by doctors, as should DMPS and DMSA, described in the section on **mercury toxicity (69)**.

Homoeopathic lead, 30C, is also said to increase lead excretion, but I have no confirmation of this.

Also see **hair analysis for minerals (47)** and **metal allergy (70)**

64. Leaky Gut Syndrome

Leaky gut syndrome is a hypothesis that has been brought forward to explain certain aspects of food allergy and intolerance. The theory is that for some reason the gut wall allows abnormally large-molecule food residues – particularly those which haven't been digested to their proper constituents – to pass through it. Normally, carbohydrates are reduced to glucose and simple monosaccharides such as galactose and fructose; fats are split to fatty acids and proteins are broken down to a handful of amino acids. In this chemically simplified form, foodstuffs are transported across the cell barrier of the gut wall and so into the circulation.

These small molecules are supposedly too insignificant to cause an allergic reaction. But if the foods are escaping too early, before they are sufficiently broken down, they may be capable of acting as antigens. The molecules will retain the characteristic of the food – in other words, the essence of 'carrot-ness', 'wheat-ness', etc. Note that this is very similar to the mechanism postulated for the pancreatic insufficiency idea in food allergy (see **enzyme supplementation (37)**).

There are a number of conditions that might lead to a so-called leaky gut. Basically, these are inflammations. Thus, we're talking about infections with pathogenic organisms, such as **Candida (16)**; parasites such, as Cryptosporidium; and, last but not least, allergic inflammatory reactions on the gut wall itself. These inflammatory conditions, along with the gut's increased penetrability to abnormal substances, would be expected to lead to a breakdown of the cell barriers and at the same time a decreased transport mechanism for nutrients such as vitamins and microminerals, leading to **malabsorption (67)**.

Leaky gut syndrome is purely a hypothesis, but if it is true it would be nice to devise a suitable standardized test to estimate whether or not it is taking place. Work is now being done on the permeability of the bowel to polyethyleneglycol (PEG).

PEG TEST

The patient is asked to take a standard dose of polyethyleneglycol with graded molecule sizes of known molecular weight and quantity. A urine sample taken six hours later is collected after this loading dose and is evaluated for content of PEG at different molecular weights. According to the sizes of the molecules which have 'got through', we have an idea of just how much leakage is taking place.

This test sounds fine in theory but in practice it soon began to fall out of vogue. However, John Howard of Biolab in London is convinced that some of the test's anomalies can be traced to the fact that baseline statistics are wrong, thus throwing out the estimations of abnormal or pathological states. If he is correct, ultimately this test will re-establish itself and become a valuable tool to the clinical ecologist.

Also see **gut flora (46)**

65. Lectins

Lectins are plant molecules of non-immune origin that act like powerful antibodies, even though this is not their function in Nature.

The important difference between this type of agglutination and that due to true immunity is that no prior challenge is necessary. The study of lectins is now very advanced and includes such surprises as the finding that lectins can be used to test for a person's blood group.

Over a hundred common foods have been shown to carry lectins and the list continues to grow. To be sure, most lectins are destroyed by cooking, but many are not. For example wheat, carrot, maize and banana contain lectins that survive heating and may even be enhanced by it. Kidney beans that have been heated for several hours in slow cookers are likely to retain enough lectin to cause severe gastro-intestinal disturbance, especially if they are not pre-soaked before cooking. Interestingly, sprouted kidney beans have a very low lectin content. This is probably true of all pulses. The average American ingests an average of 200 mg of lectin yearly from tomatoes alone.

Having survived cooking, or evaded it by having been consumed raw, many lectins are then destroyed by digestion. About 2 per cent of the ingested dose of wheat germ agglutinin reaches the faeces intact.

We do not yet understand in full what diseases can be caused by lectins. As Dr David Freed says, lectins are still 'causes in search of diseases'. In addition to their immunological effects, many lectins are powerfully poisonous or inflammatory, or both.

Finally, not all the effects of lectins are bad. They might be beneficial, for example, in the management of diabetes mellitus since, apart from slowing the absorption of carbohydrates, some food lectins extend the effect of insulin.

Also see **phenolic testing (86)** and **plant toxins (87)**

66. Magnesium

Magnesium seems to be involved in several hundred enzyme pathways, all essential for optimum health. Not surprisingly, therefore, a lack of magnesium can lead to a great diversity of symptoms.

Many of magnesium's important functions

are connected with the nervous system. Lack of magnesium causes a state of over-excitability, with twitching, tremors, anxiety, hyperactivity, cramps, convulsions and insomnia. Because it counters such symptoms, magnesium has been christened 'Nature's tranquillizer'. Correction of some of these symptoms due to magnesium deficiency may be vital to the allergic patient, who may mis-assign them to an allergy.

Paradoxically, a lack of magnesium is a major factor in fatigue (a depressed, rather than excited state). This is almost certainly because magnesium is essential for phase I xenobiotic **detoxification (26)** pathways. Lack of it can lead to an increase in unwanted metabolites such as chloral hydrate ('Mickey Finn', giving rise to a 'spacey' and tired feeling.

Another mechanism that could implicate magnesium in fatigue is that it is vital for splitting adenosine triphosphate (the body's principal energy-carrier molecule) into adenosine diphosphate. Without magnesium, this tissue energy is not bio-available.

A lack of magnesium can also lead to raised blood-pressure and heart abnormalities. PMT seems to benefit greatly from magnesium supplementation, probably because it is needed in metabolizing **essential fatty acids (38)**. So does musculo-skeletal pain: magnesium can be a *great* help to backache sufferers.

Despite its importance, there is no known test to substantiate how much magnesium is in a person's system. What is recognized is that the average diet provides only about 40 per cent of even the Recommended Daily Allowance (RDA)! Soils are depleted of magnesium due to acid rain; food processing removes a great deal of magnesium and high phosphates in the diet interfere with its absorption (colas and other fizzy drinks are high in phosphates).

Those especially at risk are alcohol drinkers, individuals with inflammatory gut disease, whether due to infection or allergies, and joggers and health buffs, who sweat a great deal. Overdoing it in the gym, without supplementing magnesium, may not be so healthy.

Orthomolecular levels: 200 to 400 mg daily. Care may be needed in supplementation as it can lead to diarrhoea and a worsening in magnesium status, due to a loss of electrolytes from the colon.

MAGNESIUM STATUS TEST

Dr Sherry Rogers of Syracuse, New York has devised a test to check for magnesium status in individuals. The test presupposes that the body retains magnesium if it needs it.

1. Urine samples are taken over a 24-hour period, to measure a baseline level of magnesium.
2. The individual is dosed with magnesium chloride tablets, 62 mg (two tablets) three times a day (372 mg daily).
3. After 48 hours a second urine sample is taken. The patient can report subjective changes (i.e. feelings of any improvement) at this time.
4. Percentages are found by dividing the baseline magnesium by the second level. Results of over 50 per cent suggest the person is absorbing magnesium poorly or that the magnesium is being retained because the patient is deficient.

Intravenous Magnesium

If the patient's status warrants it, intravenous administration of magnesium may be recommended by a physician. One gram is administered in a 2-ml solution, slowly into a vein in the arm.

A recent article in the *Lancet* by leading clinical ecologists demonstrated conclusively that magnesium injections were beneficial for ME sufferers, confirming what clinical ecologists have been saying for years.

Also see zinc (112)

67. Malabsorption

Malabsorption is a term referring to a condition in which the bowel does not perform its digestive and absorption tasks satisfactorily. The classic disease in which this occurs is coeliac disease (*sprue*). The intestinal lining becomes damaged by gluten allergy, the tiny 'hairs' (*villi*) lining the gut wall are stripped off and absorption of digestive products is limited. This means that, even eating normally, a patient can waste away due to starvation. About 1 in 2,000 Europeans are affected, although in Western Ireland this figure rises to 1 in 300.

The cure, once the cause became known, was really very simple: the patient avoids all foods containing gluten. This allows the bowel lining to recover and the patient begins to gain weight dramatically. Unfortunately, few doctors seem to ask the obvious question: could the intestinal lining become damaged by other foods or food ingredients? Empirical investigations show that it most certainly does and that, in addition, malabsorption can occur as a result of any condition leading to inflammation of the bowel mucosa (lining), such as **Candida (16)** and **parasites (83)**.

What allergy and nutrition doctors are finding is that mild degrees of malabsorption are quite common. Variability in weight is one of the characteristics of food allergy, but being *under*weight is by far the most common. Even on an adequate diet, many allergics cannot seem to put on weight. On a typical, sparse diet due to rigid limitation of foods, this problem becomes even more pronounced.

In addition, as a result of the lack of adequate digestive secretions from the pancreas (a prime allergy **target organ (104)**), the characteristics of the stools change. Typical bowel motions in these patients are bulky, loose and offensive. They often float and may stick to the side of the toilet pan. This property is due to lack of adequate splitting of fats, which are lighter than water and also sticky. Motions may also be much paler than normal because of inadequate splitting of bile salts, which give faeces their typical brown colour.

Doctors dealing with patients with a dietary disorder should have a high degree of suspicion of malabsorption and not confine this diagnosis merely to known gluten allergics. If the condition is suspected, laboratory investigations may be helpful. The accepted test is to have the patient swallow a biopsy capsule which then takes a small sample of bowel mucosa for examination. The test is only helpful if the patient has a structural abnormality, which means a rather severe degree of pathological change. Unfortunately, the typical 'expert' makes no allowance for minor degrees of *functional* change and so will often pronounce the patient normal even though he or she is manifestly ill.

Estimating faecal fats and pancreatic enzyme function is rather technical and would need a hospital facility. Many practitioners, in an outpatient situation, will be confined to simpler tests, such as bowel transit time and the Hydrocheck test.

Simple Tests and Treatment

Transit time can be estimated by instructing the patient to swallow a number of charcoal tablets and report how long before the first signs appear in the faeces and how long until the last traces disappear. I have seen this down to one and a half hours in a patient who had no structural abnormality of the bowel. The longest lapse was three weeks.

The Hydrocheck test consists of the patient swallowing a small capsule of blue dye. The capsule's coating is acid sensitive and will break down if hydrochloric acid is present in the patient's system in adequate amounts. If the capsule breaks down the dye is released, colouring the urine. If no change in urine colour is noted (a negative result) the patient has achlorhydria (lack of acid) and (very likely) some degree of pancreatic insufficiency, by association. A partial result means the urine goes pale green.

Treatment of malabsorption is of course most successful if the proper cause is sought and found. Investigating the possibility of food allergy and eradicating Candida can lead to rapid recovery and weight gain. In the meantime, the patient may need some kind of pancreatic extract supplementation and betaine hydrochloride tablets. Some preparations, such as Muripsin, combine the two.

Chronic malnutrition or perhaps dysnutrition is quite common in Western societies, largely due to undetected and untreated malabsorption.

Also see **enzyme supplementation (37)** and **leaky gut syndrome (64)**

68. Mental Retardation

ALLERGY AND THE MENTALLY DISADVANTAGED CHILD

If you have a child who suffers from brain-damage, is mentally handicapped or in some way retarded in development, that is bad enough. But the situation can be made even worse when what you are being told is not the truth, or at least not the whole truth. Yet, there are a great many children imprisoned in the diagnosis of 'retarded' who need not be.

The fact is that a lot of children, when properly investigated with EEG and brain scans, show no obvious physical abnormality to explain their lack of development. The reason for the child's failure to learn to speak and progress normally in motor skills remains a mystery – 'just one of those things', the parents are told.

Over the years I have seen a great many of these children and, while I do not claim miracle results, I have seen many worthwhile and sometimes dramatic improvements in cases that were supposed to be hopeless. One 18-year-old handicapped girl, within three weeks of dietary treatment, learned to speak for the first time in her life. A 38-year-old woman who was written off as 'brain damaged' suddenly came to life and, even at that late age, learned to read, write, count and handle money, just because wheat was cut from her diet. Dyslexia may be switched on and off in some patients just by their eating the wrong foods.

Mild and intermediate stages of recovery, though less dramatic, may still be meaningful for the victim and his or her family. An improvement in psychological performance of even 10 or 15 per cent may not sound very much, but it could mean the difference between the child being able to live at home or having to be institutionalized.

Probably in these cases that do improve there is some degree of treatable brain dysfunction caused by food and other allergies superimposed on a permanent brain damage (see **brain allergy (12)**).

In addition, there is a category of performance we call *minimal brain dysfunction*. Modern allergy and environmentally-aware doctors recognize that many reactions to foods and chemicals result in minor degrees of mental and physical disability. Sometimes these reactions are so subtle as to be hardly noticeable, unless one looks for them. Often such behavioural and attitude changes are put down to 'normal' patterns. Certainly they are common, a lot of people experience the effects, but that doesn't make them normal.

Children are particularly badly dealt with in this respect. Often, when feeling sick or aggravated due to an allergic reaction, a youngster's behaviour changes for the worse. He or she may become naughty, destructive, whining or uncooperative and may be punished unjustly for what is, after all, a medical condition. The clue is that this behaviour is often out of character. If your child is normally placid and easy going but occasionally becomes a monster, probably some trigger is at work causing brain allergy. You can do yourself and your child a favour by trying to find out what the trigger is. Chances are it will be some everyday food, such as milk, that is to blame.

Also see **endorphins (33)**, **hyperactivity and minimal brain dysfunction (52)** and **phenolic testing (86)**

69. Mercury Toxicity

Mercury (also known as quicksilver) was named after the fleet-footed messenger of the gods. It is one of the most toxic substances known to humanity, particularly when combined with other atoms and molecules, such as the chloride or methyl forms. These have far greater biological penetration. Brain tissue is especially at risk. Most people know that the expression 'mad as a hatter' comes from the twitching and dementia once common among hatters, who used to dip felt in mercuric nitrate to soften it.

Despite its poisonous qualities, industrial applications of mercury have grown and grown until extraction has now reached in excess of 10,000 tons annually, worldwide. This might not seem a lot compared to iron and steel tonnages, but weighed against its toxicity, gram for gram the mercury load that we are bringing into our environment is probably the worst of all pollution going on today.

TOXICITY

The first major mercury health scare of modern times came with the discovery in the 1960s that children dying of pink disease were in fact being poisoned by mercury in 'teething powders'.

Then, in 1953, inhabitants of the Japanese fishing port of Minamata began to fall ill with a mysterious illness causing twitching, mental confusion, difficulty speaking and, ultimately, paralysis. Autopsies all showed the same thing: reduction and damage of nerve tissue and loss of brain cells.

Eventually, the cause was found to be mercury poisoning from a nearby factory which pumped its effluvia into Minamata bay, contaminating fish stocks. The problem had become especially severe when the factory switched to the production of vinyl chloride: the waste from this process was predominantly methyl mercury, which is quite deadly, and a massive human tragedy soon occurred.

A similar pollution crisis occurred in Sweden when farmers used methyl mercury as a crop dusting and fed treated seeds to animals. Swedish food produce became heavily contaminated. The government responded quickly and, to this day, Sweden leads the world in concern about the issues surrounding mercury.

The tuna fishing industry was especially hard hit with several of these scares in the 1960s. Even today, with strict guidelines as to allowed mercury levels in food, confidence hasn't fully returned. The limit set by the American Food and Drug Administration is 0.5 parts per million: the truth is, we just don't know what safe levels are.

DENTAL AMALGAM

The principal concern about mercury toxicity today centres around whether or not it is safe to use in dental amalgams (so-called 'silver' fillings). It is worth noting that dentists who are at pains to reassure us that there is no danger are themselves advised to treat mercury as a *highly toxic* substance.

Written recommendations include not touching it by hand, performing all operations involving mercury over areas that have impervious and suitably lipped surfaces so as to confine and facilitate the recovery of spilled mercury or amalgam, storing amalgam under water, working only in well-ventilated spaces and alerting all personnel, especially during their training or indoctrination period, of the potential hazard of mercury vapour and the necessity for observing good mercury hygiene practices.

All this led some wit to comment, 'The only safe place for mercury is in the patient's mouth!'

Politics of Poison

The offensive part of the debate is the very real attempts by the American Dental Association and similar bodies to cover up the truth and suppress open discussion. In the United States a dentist can lose his or her licence for questioning the toxicity of mercury amalgam fillings. The stated position is that 'the removal of amalgam restorations from non-allergic patients for the alleged purpose of removing toxic substances from the body, when such treatment is performed solely at the recommendation or suggestion of the dentist, is improper and unethical.'

This is politics at work, not science. A layman might be justly suspicious that the official attitude to the risk has more to do with protecting the dentist than the patient.

THREE TYPES OF PROBLEM

There are really three issues where mercury is concerned. The first is the tendency of mercury to concentrate electrical fields. This is an ordinary biophysical effect and explains why people with too many dental fillings cannot work in areas where large field currents are developed.

The second is **hypersensitivity (53)**. This is really more or less an allergic reaction to mercury and various estimates place this as applying to between 1 and 15 per cent of the population. Anyone in prolonged contact with mercury tends to develop a sensitivity – thus dental students show a sharp increase in the percentage of positive patch tests for mercury sensitivity as they progress through their studies.

In passing, it should be noted that similar sensitivities can occur with other metals, notably nickel, chromium, cobalt and gold, though these are rare.

The third and most important effect has been talked about already: that is, toxicity. We inhale mercury vapour from our amalgam and swallow its compounds. This loss of mercury is increased by chewing hot or salty foods.

Unfortunately, mercury from the teeth has an especially great affinity for brain tissue but it also lodges in other body organs. It can have a disastrous effect on the immune system.

ORAL GALVANISM

Another surprise reason for the release of the metal in its natural state, entirely unthought of until the last few years, is electrolysis – that is, the electrical dissolving of metal. Amalgam-filled teeth can actually act as tiny batteries and give off a current. Examination of the inside of such teeth shows oxidation (scorch) marks where the current has flowed over many years. So, far from being safe, having dental fillings is rather akin to sucking a mercury lozenge continuously!

THE SYMPTOMS

The symptoms of mercury toxicity can be many and varied. In fact the range of effects covers all **target organs (104)**. It seems to contribute to allergy problems, probably by increasing the **body load (11)**, so any allergy symptom can be prolonged or made worse by it. Suppression of the immune system

may coincidentally lead to Candida overgrowth and it may be difficult to eradicate this organism without first attending to the possibility of mercury poisoning.

Mercury toxicity should be considered in any allergy case not responding to proper treatment. This is especially important in degenerative and auto-immune diseases such as multiple sclerosis, lupus erythematosis, rheumatoid arthritis, colitis and even, it is said, arteriosclerosis (hardening of the arteries). Also any vague mental symptoms not responding to other treatment, such as lethargy, depression, loss of memory, etc. might well begin to recover after removal of toxic mercury.

TESTING AND TREATMENT

We have been bedevilled for years by the lack of a good, objective test to show whether or not the patient is reacting to mercury. The only standardized 'scientific' test for mercury allergy is patch testing. This is very unreliable and, although positive results may be helpful, negative ones do not exclude the presence of significant reactions. In any case, it may be possible to demonstrate a sensitivity to mercury while still having no way of being sure that it is what's making a person sick.

At present, a top expert would proceed as follows:

1. Check all teeth for galvanic currents, noting the most negatively charged teeth. Anything up to about 100 mV is 'acceptable', though hardly normal. Over that should give cause for concern.
2. Test for mercury sensitivity. If indicated then it is vital to test for safe replacements. Alternative filling substances such as Occlusion, P30 and Herculite also contain heavy metals and may not be safe. Gold fillings are best but should contain 80 per cent gold and no toxic metals. Naturally, this is an expensive alternative.
3. It may be suggested that the patient go on nutritional supplements to leech out mercury and other heavy metals (chelation). The simplest supplement is sodium alginate, found in seaweed – kelp

is a quite satisfactory source. Apple pectin is also efficient. A chelating vitamin and mineral formula is currently available from Lambert's (see Useful Addresses). It is called *Ultra-detoxi* and reflects the best knowledge we have to date.

4. Where the allergist is not the dentist it is necessary to write to the patient's dental practitioner at this point. He or she must be advised of several safety precautions.

Most important: If fillings are to be removed, they must be removed in the right sequence, otherwise the patient could get much worse. It is essential to start with the most negatively-charged tooth and then work gradually towards the positively-charged ones.

The dentist must use a rubber dam around the tooth and provide efficient air extraction to prevent the patient swallowing mercury vapour. It is also a good idea for the patient to take charcoal tablets before and after amalgam extraction, to adsorb any stray mercury.

For sicker patients, it may be a good idea to go on a hypoallergenic diet and take vitamin and mineral supplements through this period, starting a few days before the first visit to the dentist.

It needs to be understood that the alternative materials cannot be expected to be as durable as the mercury amalgam. Patients are advised to go to a dentist who has had a lot of practice with these alternative types of filling.

THE ROLE OF DRUGS IN TREATING MERCURY TOXICITY

Two new drugs are coming in to use to chelate mercury. Research in several countries has shown them to be generally safe and effective.

The first, meso-dimercapto-succinic acid (DMSA) is taken orally and has been shown effective in removing mercury from all organs, except the kidneys.

The second drug, 2,3,dimercapto 1, propanesulphonic acid (DMPS) has to be administered by intra-muscular injection. DMPS is better at removing elemental mercury, which is the kind chiefly encountered when the toxicity comes from dental amalgam. However, it should not be used where brain toxicity is suspected since it cannot itself be removed but is instead bound into brain tissues, with its mercury load. DMSA does not bind to neurological tissue and is the drug of choice in such cases.

Treatment with either drug is made more successful with proper preparation: the patient should go on an oligo-antigenic diet, avoid chemicals and other toxins and follow a supplement detoxification program, as outlined above.

Finally, at the time of writing there is an attempt being made to establish a test for mercury overload. The important thing, though, is that chronic low-level toxicity may not be measurable yet may still quite seriously damage body tissues.

SCIENTIFIC PROOF

Scientific proof that amalgam toxicity exists still falls far below standards accepted by medical science. To say otherwise is less than honest. However, this picture is changing rapidly.

One of the most exciting studies to date was carried out in 1989 in Calgary, Canada by a research team headed by Drs Hahn and Vimy. Initial results were presented at the 32nd Annual Meeting of the Canadian Federation of Biological Research.

They placed dental amalgam fillings containing radioactive tagged mercury 203 into 12 molar teeth of five pregnant sheep on the 112th day of pregnancy (sheep gestate for a total of 145 days). The foetuses received catheter implants to allow foetal blood to be drawn along with maternal blood, for comparisons to be made.

Briefly, the results found that as early as three days after the placement of amalgam fillings radioactive mercury had accumulated in maternal and foetal blood, amniotic fluid and maternal urine and faeces.

By 16 days levels were highest in the kidneys, gastrointestinal tract and thyroid gland of the mother sheep. In the foetus levels were highest in the pituitary gland, liver, kidney and parts of the placenta.

After 33 days (birth) the foetal tissues had

higher mercury levels than those of the mother, especially in the bone marrow, blood and brain.

Levels continued to rise in the mother. There was eight times the blood level found in the milk.

The researchers concluded that mercury vapour released from dental amalgam fillings is readily absorbed in the lungs, gastrointestinal tract and jaw bone and accumulates progressively in tissues.

The irony is that the UK's National Health Service offers free dental treatment to pregnant women, to encourage them to have fillings placed at precisely the time when it is most dangerous and potentially harmful to the unborn child.

The pro-amalgam lobby's response to the Hahn and Vimy experiment was swift and predictable: they denounced the whole study. John E. Dodes of the New York chapter of the National Council Against Health Fraud said 'The antimercury lobby has persistently failed to tie any disease to the release of mercury from silver fillings'.

The ADA's stance remains that ' . . .the continued use of dental amalgam as a restorative material does not pose a health hazard to the non-allergic patient.'

It can only be a matter of time before common sense prevails over vested interests.

Also see **hair analysis for minerals (47)**, **lead (63)** and **metal allergy (70)**

70. Metal Allergies

Some people are plagued by reactions to metals with which they come in contact. It can mean they are unable to wear certain types of jewellery, or may find themselves unable to handle money.

These are usually Type IV **hypersensitivity (53)** reactions, especially nickel and chromate allergy. Delayed dermal hypersensitivity testing (patch tests) can generally pinpoint this kind of allergy. Sensitivity, once established, is lifelong.

ALUMINIUM

Our bodies slowly accumulate a toxic load of aluminium from food, water and medicines. Aluminium may well be a major cause of premature senile dementia (Alzheimer's disease), now epidemic in Britain. Certainly kidney dialysis patients can experience irreversible brain damage if they accumulate too much aluminium. The facts so far suggest that aluminium accelerates the ageing process in normal men and women by the very fact that it accumulates slowly over decades rather than acting as an acute (immediate) poison.

European 'safe' limits have been set at 200 microgrammes of aluminium per litre of drinking water. This limit is not based on any scientific facts; it is entirely arbitrary. Significantly, water in many areas of Britain exceeds even this limit, some water having over 300 microgrammes per litre at times.

Aluminium compounds generally are added to beer to improve its clarity and to cheese during processing. Aluminium is an ingredient in baking powders used to make biscuits, cakes and breads. Aluminium compounds are also added to such foods as frozen strawberries, maraschino cherries and pickles – primarily to improve their appearance.

In the United Kingdom about 16,000 tons of aluminium sulphate are added to water supplies every year as a clarifying agent. Aluminium in tap water can be increased by ten or a hundred times by boiling the water in an aluminium saucepan, and can reach twenty times the European safe limit or more if the water is acidified with vinegar or the natural acids of fruit or vegetables.

Avoid aluminium cooking utensils.

NICKEL

One in every ten women is allergic to nickel. Almost all cases are women who have had their ears pierced. The problem may begin on the earlobes but soon spreads elsewhere, wherever the skin comes in contact with watches, buckles, clips, etc.

Nickel is widespread throughout the environment and it is almost impossible to avoid contact with it completely. Table 70.1 gives a guide to some of the more common sources of nickel:

Sources of Nickel Contact

- Jewellery: Earrings or clasps, necklaces or chains, bracelets, rings, watchbands and buckles
- Metal fasteners on clothing: Suspenders, hooks and eyes, snap fasteners, zips, buckles, eyelets on shoes, safety pins, buttons, (some of these can be replaced by nylon or rubber equivalents)
- Personal articles: Keys, lighters, pocket knives, lipstick holders, eyelash curlers, hairpins, curlers, hair slides, spectacle frames, umbrella handles, handbag fasteners
- Around the home: Needles, pins, thimbles, scissors, paper clips, pens, door handles, cutlery, vacuum cleaners, sewing machines, telephone dials, metal chains, nails and screws, screwdrivers, prams, metallic hair dyes. Some detergents contain small amounts of nickel
- Money: 'Silver' coins
- At work: metal alloys used in manufacturing, electronics parts and circuits, insecticides and fungicides, storage batteries, nickel catalysts, mordants (used in textile dyeing), hair dyes, electroplating, inks, spark plugs, duplicating fluids, ceramics

If contact with an object is unavoidable it can be painted with clear varnish or covered with tape. Ear-ring clasps may be painted temporarily with nail varnish for limited use. Generally, the effects of perspiration make reactions worse, therefore nickel allergy is worse in summer.

OTHER METALS

Stainless steel is usually non-allergic. It may contain nickel, but it is so strongly bound that even sweat fails to dissolve it.

Gold is far less apt to cause allergy than other decorative metals, but even 'pure' (24-carat) gold may be contaminated with traces of nickel or other metals. Sulphur and other chemicals in smog can tarnish gold, which may then cause a reaction.

Also see **lead (63)** and **mercury toxicity (69)**

71. Microwaves and the Electromagnetic Spectrum

Most people overlook the fact that radio waves and microwaves are part of the electromagnetic spectrum. Because they are so useful for communication these waves are somehow assumed to be 'friendly'. But just because the carrier waves, among other uses, transmit cheerful and entertaining TV programmes, this does not mean they are necessarily safe. In fact, new and disturbing evidence suggests that they are not.

We are exposed to levels of radiation that are (at a conservative estimate) over a million times the 'background' doses. There is no part of the globe unaffected and our bodies are exposed continuously. Radiation comes from many sources, including VDUs, microwave ovens and satellites in space. These satellite transmissions find out every nook and cranny in the remotest corners of the Earth, from the Arctic to Antarctica, meaning there is nowhere safe and nowhere to run.

The question no longer seems to be, 'Is it safe?' but 'Just how great is the danger?' We know that other parts of the electromagnetic spectrum (gamma rays, X-rays, ultraviolet light, etc.) can be harmful. It may be true that short-term bursts of energetic radiation do little measurable harm. But the concern is that continuous long-term exposure, such as we are now all subjected to, might indeed have serious consequences. This would parallel the known effects of chemical pollution, where it is clear that carcinogenic (cancer-causing) effects and other health hazards only build up slowly.

Experiments show that exposure to microwaves is capable of causing a rise in body temperature; this is called the 'thermal effect'. It has been assumed that if exposure does not cause a rise in temperature it is doing no harm. Yet this safety 'standard' adhered to in the UK and US was chosen by working out at what level the thermal effect occurs and reducing the dose by a factor of ten (a resulting supposedly 'safe level' of 10 milliwatts/m). Remember this ignores biological variation, which says that some individuals will feel the effect at far lower than average levels.

Now attention is being focused on non-thermal effects, that is, on biological changes that might take place in the absence of any rise in body temperature. Tests on animals have shown that T-cell function can be harmed by microwaves and can therefore lose their ability to recognize cancer cells and other foreign invaders. Readers will be aware of the connection between poor immune functioning and allergies.

Tests at the College of Pharmacy in Illinois have shown that lymphoid organs subjected to magnetic resonance go into a leukaemia-like state (a drop in white cells but no effect on red corpuscles) that is reversible. Similar work at the School of Aerospace Medicine in Houston, Texas showed that radio frequencies alter the immune system. Has this anything to do with the fact that amateur radio enthusiasts have triple the normal incidence of myeloid leukaemia? The disturbing thing about these tests is that the exposures were only around 0.01 to 0.1 V/m – well within the current permitted exposure levels that might be found in any home.

Other tests on animals demonstrated that exposure to microwaves reduces resistance to other forms of environmental stress. Additionally, those animals already stressed (in this case recovering from an X-ray dose) deteriorated measurably under the microwave load, a result that wasn't noted in the unstressed animals.

The exact effects of microwaves thus would seem to depend on a number of factors, including the timing of the dose, its duration, how fatigued the patient is, existing stress, etc. There is much here of concern to all of us.

The point is that our bodies, as with all other organisms, rely on what are called 'coherent' electromagnetic fields with which to organize internal messages. It is even possible that our physical shape is outlined by transmissions from the DNA molecule (which is formed in a perfect radio-transmitter shape) and that this is how our cells grow to give us the correct outward appearance. This fascinating theory has been given the name *cerebral morpho-genetic radiation* by Roger Coghill. If this were so, we could expect trouble from interfering electromagnetic radiation. There might be more birth malformations (which is true) and more cancer (also true). It is only a theory, but it is scientifically proven that the DNA molecule does absorb more electromagnetic radiation than the surrounding fluid.

DETECTION

With growing concern, you might want to test your environment for dosage levels. A number of so-called 'field meters' have now sprung up that detect electromagnetic pollution. The one I use is the *Kombitest* from Bio-Physik Mersmann marketed by Environmental Diagnostics Ltd and priced around £150. Roger Coghill produces a simpler model at around £40. It is available from Coghill Research Laboratories. (See the Useful Addresses section for both addresses.)

If general surveys you can do yourself give rise to concern, then call in an expert. Private practitioners can undertake this work. The National Radiological Protection Board are usually willing to become involved, if the situation is of some gravity (such as inexplicable infant deaths, leukaemia, etc.) and where high exposure levels can be demonstrated – but there may be a fee.

In the meantime, what should you do?

1. If you use a VDU, try to have the screen as far away from your seat as possible. If you double the distance, it reduces the radiation *four*-fold (not just by half).

   Turn the set off when it is not in use, or at least turn off the monitor. Take frequent breaks of at least ten minutes. Leave the vicinity of the VDU during these breaks: don't simply look away. Invest in a radiation protective screen.

   If you have the option, liquid crystal display (LCD) screens are much safer.

2. Make sure you are not indirectly exposed if you work near but not at a VDU. Don't use old sets, they leak far more. See they are properly earthed. Advice about earthing yourself (see **electrical fields and allergies (32)**) is also valid here.

3. Insist on a radiation screen. Don't be fooled into buying one that only reduces glare (they are much cheaper, of course). Ideally it should be earthed. It is also possible to buy material to cover the sides

and back of the monitor, to prevent sideways leaks.

4. It is said that the cactus *Cereus peruvianus* placed near a VDU will dampen radiation by absorbing some of it. Try it if you are prepared to believe this.

5. Avoid precautionary or 'routine' medical and dental X-rays just for check-up purposes. Women of childbearing years should have X-rays only in the 10 days following menstruation. Though this is now somewhat in dispute it is better to play safe. Allow no X-rays if you are trying to conceive. Children should not have X-rays except in a genuine medical emergency.

Try to obtain details of the dose you receive and keep a record that you can continue to update throughout your life of the total radiation received.

6. *Do not* attempt to screen your house or any other building with a metal plates or wires. You may inadvertently intensify a field and make it dangerous. A true 'Faradic cage' will screen out most or all radiation, but these are expensive and technically difficult. You are unlikely to come up with the right structure as a do-it-yourself enthusiast.

Also see **irradiation of foods (61)**

72. Migraine and Headaches

Headaches and migraine are frequently encountered symptoms in an allergy practitioner's work. Migraine has been studied more extensively, since it is a more serious – at times disabling – complaint. But almost all of what is said here about the causes of migraine can be applied to headaches as well.

The word migraine comes from a French expression meaning 'half a head'. This denotes the fact that a 'classic' migraine, as first described, was characterized by one-sided headaches. Typically there were warning signs of the onset such as flashing lights and other visual disturbances.

Nowadays several types of migraine are recognized. This is almost certainly due to different areas of the brain being affected, not a result of different causative agents. Similarly, treatment is the same for virtually all types. The possible exception is hemiplegic migraine, which may come about in a different way.

Less dramatic but still alarming to some patients is a partial (but reversible) paralysis that accompanies their headache. Others get no head pain but severe abdominal cramps ('abdominal migraine'). The headaches may come in attacks, with clear periods in between ('cluster headaches'). Migraine is said to strike especially in association with stress but usually just after the stress has abated (at weekends, for example, if the patient's job is stressful).

The incidence of migraine varies considerably and has been reported to be as high as 23 per cent in women and 15 per cent in men. It also appears to run in families.

The exact mechanism of migraine is not known. Perhaps it is best regarded as a neurovascular syndrome, that is, an arterial spasm or instability affecting primarily the blood vessels of the head and brain, brought on by factors operating on the central nervous system. These factors include emotions, food, exertion, upper respiratory tract infections, **hypoglycaemia (55)**, **lactose intolerance (62)**, irregular sleep, travel and bright lights.

Formerly, tyramine was mooted as the probable 'cause' of migraine. Nowadays we recognize there are several mediating chemicals such as serotonin, **histamine (50)**, **prostaglandins (92)** and catecholamines (adrenalin and noradrenalin), but all are likely to be secondary (i.e., not the primary cause).

As distinct from these 'triggers' are the real causes of migraine. Dentists have taught us that certain abnormalities of the temporomandibular joint (in the jaw) can cause headaches. But recent research has shown the overwhelmingly common cause of migraine is food allergy or intolerance. One study on children carried out at the Great Ormond Street Hospital for Sick Children in 1983 showed that no less than 93 per cent of cases had a complete remission when their diets were corrected.

All environmental allergens, as described in this book, are relevant causative factors in migraine. The **body load (11)** principle is fully valid: the more the patient can reduce his or her burden of bad foods, chemicals, hidden infection, hormone abnormalities, etc., the more likely a lasting and satisfactory cure.

Elimination and challenge dieting often yields dramatic and permanent results. Many people have heard of the 'Five Cs' for migraine: these are the food triggers chocolate, coffee, citrus, cheese and claret (meaning any red wine). In my experience, these are not as often the culprits as are other foods such as milk, wheat and egg. The fact is, any food can be to blame.

Also see **diets (27)** and **phenolic testing (86)**

73. Milk

Milk enjoys very favourable propaganda. This is probably related to past perceptions, when the introduction of free milk for school children earlier this century did much to ensure youngsters were better nourished. The virtual elimination of rickets in our society is probably due almost entirely to this provision.

It seems odd, therefore, to be condemning milk. But facts are facts: I see so much disease and misery *caused* by milk allergy and milk intolerance that I have no hesitation in denouncing it as unhealthy. It is implicated in a vast range of conditions such as arthritis, learning difficulties, **hyperactivity (52)** in children, **migraine (72)**, colitis, eczema and asthma – to name just a few.

Milk is frequently associated with catarrh. This is a very common experience, but few people ever take this observation further and realize that milk is unsuitable for them or indeed the majority of people.

The trouble is that despite all the propaganda to the contrary, milk is *not* a natural food. It doesn't belong in our diets. Nowhere else in the animal kingdom do beasts need to feed their young with milk from another species, nor do they continue to do so after merest infancy. The idea that we have to have it, or that our health is threatened without it, is patent nonsense. The people of Oriental nations, whose diets are virtually dairy-free, do not suffer with rickets (unless as part of general malnutrition) or osteoporosis in older women. Neither milk nor calcium has any preventive effect in osteoporosis.

The secret to milk being a 'cure' for rickets is that milk contains vitamin D. But this vitamin can easily be obtained elsewhere (from fish oils, for example). Iodine is also important but, again, milk isn't the only source.

So why bother with milk at all? We don't need it and it can have harmful repercussions. In fact some clinical ecologists have more than a suspicion that calcium in the blood may be *depleted* by milk. If the milk induces a degree of **malabsorption (67)** this would not only be possible but highly likely. Some of us have seen calcium levels rise in the blood after a patient gives up dairy produce.

DAIRY PRODUCTS AND ALLERGIES

Purely from my practice experience I find that cream is the least well-tolerated dairy product. Yoghourt, which seems to be different chemically, may be OK; also butter, surprisingly. There are quite a few dairy-free margarines now available. Don't forget that buttermilk is fermented and therefore not suitable on an anti-yeast programme.

The usual allergen in milk is in the phospholipid fraction, which means that skimmed milk may be OK. But for those patients allergic to the protein this would be the worst choice (true also of patients with a **lactose intolerance (62)**).

Many milk-allergics can take evaporated milk. Presumably the process of heating it kills off its allergenicity. You can experiment with using evaporated milk if you want.

Don't forget that beef comes from the same animal. It may be OK, but be suspicious.

Finally, if you have to give up milk and are worried about calcium, take a supplement. This is advisable especially for children. This way you cannot be criticized for neglecting your or your child's diet – but remember also my remarks about vitamin D above.

Goat's Milk

Goat's milk is often cited as a substitute for milk. It is supposed to be 'beneficial'. All the good it ever does is probably by getting allergics off cow's milk; not as a result of any positive properties it has.

In fact goat's milk is something of a health hazard in its own right. It is not subject to the same vigorous health controls that cow's milk is. Thus the risk of **brucellosis (14)**, TB and other infections is very real.

Furthermore, at least half the patients who react to cow's milk also react to goat's milk. So even for the allergic patient, it isn't a totally safe bet.

Nevertheless, it can provide the kind of nutrition that cow's milk is noted for but, in many cases, without the allergic drawbacks.

Soya Substitutes

Soya milk is another accepted substitute for cow's milk. People often naively assume it cannot be allergenic.

The truth is that soya allergy is getting steadily more common. There are also other potential drawbacks to soya milk. It may contain **antinutrients (7)**, particularly those that influence protein absorption. This may be sufficient to interfere with growth and could be an important consideration with children.

Sesame Milk Substitute

This recipe I learned from a nurse, Ann Lindstrom in Sweden. The plain taste is rather unappealing, but used in cooking or with the addition of summer fruits or other flavouring for drinking it is a pleasant addition to the dairy-free armoury:

Half a deci-litre of dark sesame seeds

Half a deci-litre of light sesame seeds

Process these in a blender or food processor until mushy. Add half a litre of water, in stages, blending between each stage. To flavour add honey, berries or half a banana.

If you find this too much effort, use halva instead:

Honey Halva Milk

Method: liquidize a block of honey halva with a half pint of water. Stir well before use. Halva is rich in calcium and this gets rid of one worry for dairy-free patients.

Also see **diets (27)**

74. Miller's Method

This way of testing for allergies is also known as provocation-neutralization (PN), or serial end-point skin titration.

It was first developed by Carleton Lee of Missouri in the late 1950s. Herbert Rinkel and others went on to improve it and promote its more widespread use, and the first definitive book explaining the technique in detail was written by Joseph B. Miller (*Food Allergy: Provocative Testing and Injection Therapy*); hence Miller's method.

THE METHOD

A reagent (food, dust or chemical) is injected superficially into the skin (intracutaneously), making a deliberate wheal. If this grows compared to a control (blank) over, say, 10 minutes, this suggests an allergy. Sometimes a symptom is produced (provocation) and this is much more conclusive. Remember these substances are tested one at a time, so there is usually no doubt which caused the symptom.

If a reaction occurs, the patient is then given a series of weaker and weaker injections of the substance at 10-minute intervals until the wheal ceases to grow and the symptom, if there is one, disappears completely.

This 'switch-off' dilution is called the neutralizing dose; it works as a kind of antidote. The procedure is illustrated in Figure 74.1.

Usually the patient can then be given a cocktail of these neutralizing doses. One drop of this cocktail under the tongue just before meals and he or she can then often eat

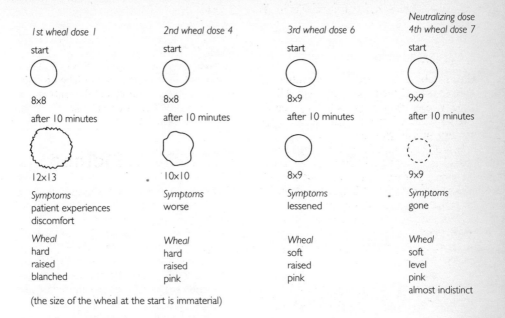

1st wheal dose 1	2nd wheal dose 4	3rd wheal dose 6	Neutralizing dose 4th wheal dose 7
start	start	start	start
8×8	8×8	8×9	9×9
after 10 minutes	after 10 minutes	after 10 minutes	after 10 minutes
12×13	10×10	8×9	9×9
Symptoms patient experiences discomfort	*Symptoms* worse	*Symptoms* lessened	*Symptoms* gone
Wheal hard raised blanched	*Wheal* hard raised pink	*Wheal* soft raised pink	*Wheal* soft level pink almost indistinct

(the size of the wheal at the start is immaterial)

Figure 74.1: Wheal responses in Miller's Method

the foods that would normally cause an allergic reaction. A percentage of patients, however, obtain relief only if they inject the neutralizing mixture subcutaneously – once or twice a week is usually sufficient.

The method's accuracy can be increased by asking the patient to undertake simple tasks, such as a handwriting demonstration and noting how these change under testing. At the neutralization point the patient's performance should return to normal (see Figure 74.2). More objective determinations can include measuring the patient's pulse rate and blood-pressure.

Before   After

Figure 74.2: Example of handwriting deterioration while testing mould

One important advantage to this method is that the symptom provoked gives the patient a vivid subjective demonstration of each allergen, which helps to fix it in his or her mind. This is far more meaningful than the abstract results of a blood test or some other laboratory report. But remember, not all allergens provoke symptoms.

Another advantage is that a patient with multiple allergies need not be restricted to a very meagre diet; allergenic foods can be eaten in moderation, under the umbrella of the 'drops'. Only foods that cause a severe reaction are banned – and the patient may even become desensitized to these by taking the drops and avoiding the food for several months.

PROBLEMS

When it works, the method works very well. A number of difficulties may occur, however. About 10 per cent of cases are plagued with shifting end-points. Repeat testing becomes necessary and this is troublesome and may be expensive. These shifts can occur very rapidly, so that by the time the patient is supplied with his or her prescription, it is ineffective. In these cases, even retesting won't help. However, this only applies to less than 5 per cent of those tested.

Unfortunately, the people who need this kind of treatment most, the very sick, 'unstable' patients, are the ones most likely to be troubled by this shifting end-point phenomenon.

Even if the antidotes are not effective, however, the method is still good for diagnosis. It can pinpoint rapidly the worst allergens for a patient. This will help reduce his or her **body load (11)**. The method is also very safe. Reactions are common but rarely severe, and in any event can be relieved rapidly by the corresponding neutralizing dose. Nevertheless, it would seem prudent to avoid injecting anything into an individual who has experienced a dangerous anaphylactic reaction.

An outstanding feature of this neutralizing technique is that it is usually effective against environmental chemical triggers – *no other method* is. This makes it superior in my view to **enzyme potentiated desensitization (36)**.

HORMONES

An important special application of Miller's method is in neutralizing hormones. Women tested with oestrogens and progesterone often experience reactions, particularly to progesterone in cases where the woman deteriorates badly health-wise at around her period time. We can hypothesize that these women are allergic to their own hormones (see **hormones and allergy (51)**).

In fact there are two phenomena we encounter. If the reaction is straightforward and neutralizes easily, this probably represents a true 'allergic' reaction by the woman to her own hormones. But sometimes it can be very difficult or impossible to neutralize a symptom once provoked. We take this to be evidence that the real problem is a hormone imbalance – hormone replacement therapy (HRT) can be considered as a possibility in management.

SUBLINGUAL PROVOCATION AND NEUTRALIZATION

A modification of the Miller-Lee technique is to test substances under the tongue (sublingually). A food or other concentrate is placed under the tongue and the reactions noted. If the patient experiences a symptom, this is neutralized, as before, by serial dilutions. The dilution that switches off the symptom completely is taken as the end-point.

There is no essential difference between this approach and using an injection, although naturally there are fewer parameters by which to judge reactions or the lack of them. Instead of being able to view a wheal, its size and characteristics, the clinician has only the patient's subjective symptoms to rely upon, plus what he or she can observe objectively. Yet with practice it is possible to become quite adept at spotting subtle shifts in the patient's mood or attitude, skin colour, etc. The neutralizing dose would be that which leads the patient to declare his or her symptoms 'switched off' and the clinician to note that whatever manifestations arose have disappeared again.

Obviously, subtle reactions may be missed. Well-masked allergens may not react at all. But the technique is especially suitable for children, many of whom don't like injections and would not willingly sit for several hours having intracutaneous needles every 10 minutes.

A paper on sublingual testing by the late Lawrence Dickey, former surgeon and latterly clinical ecologist and editor of the journal *Clinical Ecology*, is available as a useful booklet for practitioners from Action Against Allergy (see the Useful Addresses section).

DERMAL APPLICATION TESTING

A further modification of this technique, developed by Drs Jean Munro and Ray Choy, is to test substances directly on the skin. This method arose from an observation that probably all clinical ecologists have made from time to time: that an extremely sensitive individual sometimes feels unwell just *being in the presence of allergens*. Such patients may have to be relocated away from the storage and display areas where test solutions are kept in order that they can be tested.

Munro and Choy were finding that some patients were reacting quite severely to the usual technique and decided to test these patients by simply having them hold a phial of the solution. Even this was too much for some; and so dermal application was resorted to. It was found quite workable.

By placing a dilution of the extract on the skin of, say, the back of the hand, biological and subjective reactions could be provoked and then neutralized by further dermal applications. Sometimes these dilutions may reach 'homoeopathic' levels (i.e., they are *very* dilute) but still seem to work.

The important safety measure is that if a strong reaction develops, the test solution can be wiped off swiftly.

CONTROVERSY

No technique of clinical ecology has been more heavily criticized than Miller's method. Nevertheless, most of us who use it do so because we are aware of its capabilities and accept its scientific validity. More and more papers are being published that show its effectiveness. Yet the controversy won't go away.

Over the years a number of studies have been cited to show that Miller's method is a fake. Almost without exception these have been improperly reported, evidence for key statements has been missing and data has been altered (or withheld) or the protocol so bad that it was obviously designed to invite failure.

In 1973 the Food Allergy Committee of the American College of Allergists, using sublingual provocation testing (see below),

carried out a study that showed that the neutralization basis of Miller's method was quite effective. Did they publish their findings? No, they *repeated* the whole test again in 1974 and this time found that the statistics were not as good. The second study was therefore termed 'The Final Report' while the first positive study was simply cast aside.

The 'Jewett trial' carried out in 1981–83 was appallingly defective. The results remained unpublished for seven years, so clinical ecologists world-wide were deeply shocked when it was suddenly published in August 1990 in the *New England Journal of Medicine*. This, the world's second most prestigious medical journal, even went to the extraordinary length of issuing a press release announcing that at last the clinical ecologists were going to be sunk. I won't say such spite is without precedent in medicine, but it certainly has no place in a scientific periodical.

To my mind, Miller's method is an outstanding contribution to medicine. Like all medical techniques, it requires skill if it is to be performed correctly.

Also see **challenge testing (18)**

75. Moulds

Moulds are a serious health problem. More food crops worldwide are lost to mould than any other single cause. Yet we need moulds to rot away rubbish and dead matter. Along with certain bacteria, moulds clean up organic waste and stop the planet becoming a gigantic garbage heap. Thus we live in an uneasy relationship with them.

Fungi include mushrooms, moulds and yeasts. They may invade human tissues – causing, for example, skin infections or Candidiasis of the bowel – and also cause direct or indirect toxic effects via secreted poisons called **mycotoxins (76)**. These substances are often powerful immuno-suppressants and thus further reduce the individual's resistance, not only to mould infections but also to bacteria and viruses.

A number of clinical conditions are caused by mould infections, apart from the more obvious athlete's foot and ringworm.

These include farmer's lung (caused by mouldy hay), cheesewasher's lung (from a strain of penicillin) and bagassosis, a condition that affects those working with sugar cane infected with moulds (bagasse is the remains of the treated cane plant, after sugar extraction).

We are all exposed to mould spores in the atmosphere, which are freely breathed, much like all-year-round pollen. These spores are only absent on cold, frosty days and when snow lies on the ground. At different times of the year, different fungi dominate.

There are some 4,000 indoor moulds that flourish in our homes. Even an apparently dry house is subject to moisture from cooking, perspiration of the occupants and moisture exhaled in breathing. Measurements show that an average family may give off up to 20 litres of moisture daily. Particularly bad areas for mould are rooms where the moisture is at its highest, such as the kitchen and bathroom.

Of course, not all houses are structurally dry. Older property especially tends to be damp; also low-lying dwellings and those near rivers, lakes and marshes. Some homes are particularly bad for mould content and, indeed, it may be evident as green or black patches growing on the walls. Familiar 'dry rot' is a mould – *Merulius lacrymans* – despite its name, dry rot needs moisture to grow. Even when not visible, mould may be hidden in fabrics, carpets and furniture, especially if these are damp, old or have food particles embedded in them.

FOOD CONTAMINATION

There are moulds in our diet, too. Not just in cheese and mushrooms – unwanted moulds. Bread is a shocking and surprising avenue of exposure. In 1980 the following fungi were found in flour milled in the UK: *Penicillium, Cladosporium, Aspergillus candidus, Aspergillus flavus, Mucor, Aspergillus terreus, Alternaria, Aspergillus versicolor, Absida, Aspergillus fumigatus, Verticullium* and *Paecilomyces* (Food Surveillance Paper, HMSO, no 4, 1980).

Mould contamination of animal feeds can lead to further exposure. Both moulds and toxins (along with antibiotics, hormones and sedatives) pass into dairy produce, meat, eggs, bacon and poultry.

As the moulds' main port of entry is the mouth, the digestive tract tends to be the most affected. Darkness and moisture within the gut suit these organisms very well. Add to that the fact that our immune systems seem to be already under siege and, not surprisingly, we have a formula for trouble of epidemic proportions. **Malabsorption (67)** syndrome develops due to intestinal inflammation together with an inability to eliminate cellular waste. As my friend Dr Nancy Dunne in Dublin is inclined to put it, 'Pseudo-coeliac disease with negative alpha-gliadin antibody titres and normal jejunal biopsy but full symptomatology is now as rife as the common cold.'

THE MOULDY PATIENT

It is possible, indeed probable, that many symptoms supposed to be mould allergy are actually the poisoning effects of traces of mycotoxins. Ergot mould contains LSD; 'magic mushrooms' contain a hallucinogen called psilocybin. It isn't hard to imagine that there may be many more such chemical compounds, as yet undiscovered, lurking in moulds.

I call the true mould allergic the 'mouldy patient'. There seems to be a syndrome of reacting to dietary mould, damp weather, old musty buildings, etc.; the patient often has intestinal Candidiasis; cravings for sweets seem to be a major feature and tolerance of alcohol (yeast) is poor. Athlete's foot and skin infections with mould (ringworm or Tinea) may be present, suggesting the patient is somehow a breeding ground for moulds.

For some reason I am unable to explain, but it is extremely common, mould-allergic patients become highly sensitive to ambient chemicals in the environment. Possibly moulds are suppressing the enzymes of **detoxification (26)** pathways in much the same way as they are capable of causing immune suppression.

Symptoms Suggesting Mould Sensitivity

- Worse on damp days
- Worse in musty old buildings, with old fabrics and papers
- Cravings for sweet foods
- Cravings for bread and yeast foods
- Chemical hypersensitivity
- Poor tolerance of alcohol, craving for alcohol
- Skin infections with mould, e.g. troublesome athlete's foot
- Known Candidiasis
- Vaginal thrush
- Fatigue
- Mood disorder, spacey 'unreal' feeling

GETTING RID OF MOULD

The most important preliminary is to eradicate damp where it exists. If there are structural problems to the building you must engage a qualified builder who can advise you what to do. Rising damp, leaking gutters or faulty plumbing can all be fixed and need tackling definitively.

A dehumidifier may help dry out the indoor atmosphere. There are several models around now aimed at the domestic market, but be careful: make sure that the moisture they collect doesn't become a focus for growth of mould and other pathogens.

Remove any obvious sources of mould contamination, such as old damp fabrics, lumber and other household waste. You may need to increase the efficiency of garbage disposal. House plants, too, are sources of mould. Parting with them may be necessary in very severe cases. There are some very good artificial plants. If, like me, you love the sight of green foliage, even fakes are better than nothing.

National Safety Associates (UK) Ltd produce personal environment air systems. These are a great boon to allergics: they ensure a clean local environment and they are very effective against airborne mould spores indoors.

Also see **Candida (16)**, **environmental allergies (34)** and **intestinal fermentation (59)**

76. Mycotoxins

Mycotoxins are a group of poisonous and often cancer-causing chemicals produced by a number of **moulds (75)**. LSD is an example and comes from the cereal mould *ergot*.

Most mycotoxins are present in insignificant quantities and many appear to pose no toxic threat to humans. But a few are deadly. Most people have heard of the potent liver poison and carcinogen aflatoxin B1, secreted by the common mould *Aspergillus flavus* that grows on wheat, maize, peanuts and other crops. Many environmentalists regard aflatoxin B1 as the most powerful carcinogen known. Most mycotoxins survive cooking, so even this way of potentially neutralizing them is no good.

Sale of aflatoxin-contaminated food for human consumption is illegal under the UK Food and Drug Act of 1955. One of the problems, however, is that mycotoxins in animal feeds may turn up in our food when we eat the flesh of these animals.

Nor is aflatoxin the only culprit. It appears there are plenty. Some species of Penicillium produce ochratoxin-A on wet grains which may go on to contaminate offal meat. Ochratoxin-A can cause kidney damage.

A Fusarium toxin, deoxynibalenol (DON) has been linked indirectly to disorders of the immune system. DON is also known as vomitoxin because it causes pigs that eat it to vomit. It may also be implicated in oesophageal cancer.

OESTROGENIC EFFECT

Zearalenone, another toxin from Fusarium, has been identified as a cause of abortion. Zearalenone and its derivatives mimic female sex hormones by binding to the same cellular receptors as do oestrogenic hormones. This gives rise to similar physiological and pathological effects.

The chief concern regarding human health is the possibility of such mycotoxins inducing hormone-dependent cancers such as cancer of the uterus. In addition to cancer, all these oestrogen-like agents can produce foetal abnormalities (see **preconceptual health (89)**).

We are already exposed to significant hormone levels in our food supplies, from treated livestock. Many women also take the Pill. It isn't unreasonable to suppose that the recent increase in the incidence of cervical, uterine and breast tumours among young women and of testicular abnormalities among young men could be related to abnormal amounts of oestrogenic substances.

Also see **candida (16)**, **environmental allergies (34)**, **intestinal fermentation (59)** and **plant toxins (87)**

77. Natural Gas

Natural household gas from underground deposits is now used instead of town gas (from the coking of coal), as used to be the case. Most of the UK's gas supply comes from beneath the North Sea. The gas pumped into our homes typically contains about 88 per cent methane, 5 per cent ethane, up to 7 per cent nitrogen, 1 per cent propane, 0.5 per cent carbon dioxide, 0.05 per cent butane and 0.03 per cent of longer chain relatives (C5 and upwards). The gas board also adds an odourant – around 10 parts per million – to alert the user to possible gas leaks.

When it is burnt, gas gives rise to carbon dioxide, water, some oxides of nitrogen and small traces of oxides of sulphur and aldehydes. The latter are intense irritants and account for many of the unpleasant symptoms experienced if a person comes in contact with gas combustion fumes.

Little wonder, then, that many allergic patients react to gas. We pipe into our homes one of the most serious ecological pollutants. There should be far more public awareness of what the potential hazards are. I have seen a tremendous diversity of illness caused by exposure to *ordinary ambient domestic levels* of natural gas: patients with joint pains, asthma, peculiar rashes, deranged thinking, blindness and countless other symptoms. One teenager had been on tranquillizers for years before I discovered she was highly sensitive to gas. Once the supply was shut off, she recovered completely.

It is wrong to call these reactions 'allergy'. Really, they are the result of a kind of low-grade poisoning, one which seems to affect some individuals more than others. Natural gas is quite toxic and will make anyone ill in sufficient quantity; sensitive patients react at levels *far below* those that would trouble the rest of us. Often these patients have an acute sense of smell and may be able to detect gas when no one else can.

LEAKS

It is not possible to avoid small leaks of gas in the home. If you can smell gas, call in the gas board. You may need to be persistent: often the engineer or inspector will pronounce that there is 'no leak' even though you can still smell gas. This is because a keen human nose is far more sensitive than detector equipment. If you continue to smell gas, keep pestering the gas company until they get it fixed.

Sometimes rotted piping *outside* can be the source of a leak, since by its nature gas tends to seep along pipes and can travel a long way through the soil and up into buildings. Two of my patients even reacted to a leak in the house next door!

Also see **chemical cleanup (19)**, **electrical fields and allergies (32)** and **formaldehyde (42)**

78. Nitrates

Nitrate from agricultural fertilizers finds its way into ground waters, rivers, lakes and seas. It is highly probable that too much nitrate in drinking water is a health hazard and that excessive amounts in both fresh and salt water can disrupt ecology. Nitrate has given rise to heavy algae overgrowth in the Adriatic Sea, threatening bathing in sensitive resorts like Venice. This algae 'bloom' is called *eutrophication* (from the Greek *eutrophos*, rich food)

Some researchers believe that nitrates may be the cause of cancer of the stomach and windpipe in adults, but studies are conflicting. A more definite connection exists regarding Blue Baby Syndrome (methaemoglobinaemia), a serious and potentially fatal blood disease affecting infants (see below).

Unfortunately, the usage of nitrates is still on the increase. In 1950 the average tonnage throughout the world was 14 million. By 1985 that figure had risen to 125 million. Plants without adequate nitrogen are thin, pale and weak; replenishing their nitrogen levels by adding nitrates to the soil causes them to resume normal growth. Even healthy plants seems to become bigger and stronger (up to a point) with the addition of nitrates to the soil.

However, this problem of nitrate 'pollution' isn't quite as simple as ecologists like to believe. Researchers have shown that only about 7 per cent of applied nitrogen is actually leached from the soil into water supplies. Furthermore, there is an alarmingly high nitrogen content in the run-off even from unfertilized arable land, enough to cause problems. It seems that agriculture of any kind results in the release of precious nitrogen from the soil.

SAFETY LIMITS

In certain parts of Europe water supplies already exceed the EEC safe limit (50 mg per litre) and it is likely that, as time passes, more and more areas will fail to meet these moderate standards.

Hard hit zones in Britain are mainly in the arable farming areas such as East Anglia, Norfolk, Cambridgeshire, Lincolnshire and Hereford.

The concern is that even if farmers change their habits at once (admittedly very unlikely) there may be enough contamination of the soil filtering through to our water supplies to pollute the water table for decades to come.

BLUE BABY SYNDROME

Too much nitrate in drinking water can cause Blue Baby Syndrome, a serious blood disorder in babies under three months. Bacteria in the child's gut convert nitrate into nitrite, which is taken up by haemoglobin in preference to oxygen. The result is *methaemoglobinaemia* and the baby suffers severe respiratory failure. Its lips and body may take on a markedly blue hue, due to the lack of oxygen.

The World Health Organization reported 2000 cases of this disease between 1945 and 1986; 160 of these babies died. So great is the concern about the problem in the UK that in summer, when evaporation from reservoirs concentrates water contaminants, at least one British Water Authority supplies bottled water to households with small infants.

Also see **algae (3)** and **water (110)**

79. Nitrous Oxide

Nitrogen dioxide, or nitrous oxide (laughing gas) is a product of combustion, emitted from sources burning organic fuels at high temperatures. It is often found at elevated levels indoors, together with **carbon monoxide (17)**. It is an irritant gas affecting the mucous membranes of the respiratory tract and eyes; it may cause allergic-type symptoms. It is also a powerful neurological toxin and can produce low-grade dissociation of the thinking processes – this makes it of interest to clinical ecologists, who often see vague undifferentiated symptoms with obscure environmental causes.

Hundreds of animal studies have been performed with nitrogen dioxide. Chiefly these have been to do with lung function. The results of most of these toxicological studies give rise to concern that chronic exposure of humans to nitrogen dioxide could result in chronic irreversible lung disease. It may also be implicated in decreased immune defenses, leading to increased susceptibility to infectious disease and, of course, unwanted allergic or intolerance reactions.

There are difficulties extrapolating the effects of nitrogen dioxide on animals to what might occur if humans were exposed to it. Controlled human studies have produced conflicting evidence. It may potentiate decreased lung function when administered with broncho-constricting agents (but not alone).

So far as the evidence goes, the US Environmental Protection Agency's Office of Air Quality Planning and Standards (OAQPS) considers the main people at risk are children, chronic bronchitics, asthmatics, individuals with emphysema and anyone with impaired and/or sensitive respiratory or nasopharyngeal systems (such as hayfever sufferers).

DOSAGES

Probably the concentration of nitrogen oxide a person is exposed to is more telling than the length of exposure. This is important because the pattern of exposure to appliances such as gas stoves and kerosene heaters is episodic and more likely to lead to short-term, high-level concentrations than continued low-level doses. Homes with gas appliances or kerosene heaters were shown to have four or five times the ambient levels of nitrogen dioxide found in homes with neither.

Also see **atmospheric pollution (10)** and **formaldehyde (42)**

80. Noise

We are all subject to an environmental stress that is often under-rated or even missed: sound. The sounds around us can cause very unpleasant effects: headaches, tiredness, an inability to concentrate and, if too loud or going on for too long, actual physical damage – deafness.

The British Acoustical Society warn us that low-frequency vibrations (10 to 20 cycles per second) may disturb the brain, in the way that flashing lights are known to bring on fits in susceptible individuals. These 'infrasonics' from vehicle engines may be responsible for a number of accidents in which car drivers behave in strange and inexplicable ways. The vibration effects of machinery and even air-conditioning may be an undetected factor in **sick-building syndrome (98)**, causing nausea and disorientation.

Very low-frequency sound waves have surprisingly destructive qualities and have even been said to be responsible for deaths. Early experiments in France killed one engineer horribly when he was subject to a high-intensity 'sound' blast of these low frequencies. A subsequent test, though carefully controlled, managed to shatter all the windows for a half-mile around the test site. It is now said that two low-frequency generators can create a 'directional' sound that can be aimed to destroy a building many miles away.

Probably most people are aware that certain sounds ('white noise') are capable of being used as torture. This alone should give pause for thought. Clearly, sound waves can be very harmful indeed and it is not unreasonable to warn that if levels go on steadily escalating, we may all be in for trouble of an as yet unsuspected kind.

NOISE MEASUREMENT

Noise is measured in bels, each progressive level being 10 times the sound pressure of the previous level. It is customary to sub-divide these units into tenths, hence deci-bels (dB). The lowest detectable pressure, only just above absolute silence (zero), is taken as 1 dB. Normal conversation (60 dB) is thus 1,000,000 times more intense than this first faint sound. In fact, instruments for measuring sound are weighted electrically, to approximate what the ear actually perceives.

Loud sounds, as opposed to merely low-frequency noises, are a recent phenomenon. Up to the age of the Industrial Revolution, apart from the rare sound of gunpowder explosions and thunder, the loudest sounds would be very infrequent and caused by something falling with a crash (80–90 decibels). The general background noise was probably as low as 30–40 decibels.

In the twentieth century we have noises produced by jet aircraft and rock bands that reach levels of 120 to 140 decibels, billions of times greater than a whisper. It is no wonder then that at 140 decibels we experience pain. See Table 80.1.

Part of the problem with loud sound is that the ears cannot be selective in the way that the eyes can. If a light is too bright or a view repulsive, you need only close your eyes to be rid of it, whereas with a sound you cannot prevent yourself receiving its shockwaves whether they are welcome, painful or not.

Noise Levels

Decibels

140	Jet engine at 300 ft/100 m. Threshold of pain
130	Rock band
120	Loud thunder, jet aircraft at 500 ft/170 m
110	Pneumatic drill, many discotheques
100	Loud street noise
90	Loud office or factory machinery
80	Noisy office, interior of a car
70	Average radio and TV, vacuum cleaner
60	Average conversation
50	Typical home or quiet street
40	Private office, quiet conversation
30	Watch ticking, rustle of paper
20	Quiet countryside
10	Leaves rustling
0	Threshold of hearing

Remember: each 3-decibel increase means approximately double the sound intensity.

It is very important from the point of view of well-being for people to avoid as much sound stress as possible. Double glazing keeps out traffic noises. Try to get into the habit of having the TV and radio turned down as low as you can (though not so low that you have to strain to hear what's being said).

If there are sound hazards in your work it is vital that you follow recommended safety procedures and wear ear protection. Don't be tempted to ignore this precaution: 20 or 30 years from now, when you experience noise-induced deafness, you'll regret it.

Finally, there *are* 'good' sounds. Music is the most obvious and, for all the derision heaped upon 'musak', it can have relaxing and calming properties. The main problem with it is its repetitive nature and the fact that, if you can't switch it off, it can become 'pollution'. Nevertheless, gentle, easy music can have enormous de-stressing potential – experiment for yourself to find which music soothes you most.

Much more research could be done into the subject of aesthetics from a medical point of view. Good art and good music, well-designed homes and pleasant, harmonious surroundings, not to mention relaxing sounds, good food and pleasing company, can all have a positive effect on well-being which *must* have incidental benefits to the organism. The converse must also be true: that those of us who live in depressing, squalid and ugly surroundings become imbued with a mean emotional response that we know can have an adverse impact on the immune system, not to mention other aspects of health and integrity.

Also see **seasonal affective disorder (97)**

81. Nutrition and Allergies

Allergics need extra good nutrition for two reasons:

1. Vitamins and minerals can help strengthen the immune system and so fight allergies.
2. Long-term food allergies cause underperformance of the gut and poor digestion, leading to chronic deficits of major and minor nutrients. Some allergics are noticeably skinny and underweight due to **malabsorption (67)** of macronutrients (protein, carbohydrate and fats). But for the vast majority, malnutrition is at the micro-nutrient level.

THE MYTH OF THE BALANCED DIET

There is a grave misconception in the field of dietetics and nutrition, which is that if one eats a 'balanced diet' there is no need to be concerned about nutrition – one will have a sufficiency of every known nutrient. Yet what is usually recommended only means a balance of the wrong ingredients, often junk, much of it stale and having lost its nutrients due to storage, processing or cooking techniques.

Antinutrient (7) factors are ignored. Yet food combinations, by their interaction, sometimes interfere with one another. It isn't much use adding up the total ingredients of somebody's diet if these are blocking each other and so preventing full bio-availability.

Probably the biggest (and lamest) sacred cow of conventional dietetics – one that needs putting to sleep once and for all – is the notion of recommended dietary allowances (RDAs).

RDAs were formulated years ago on very inadequate data and are entirely misleading. They were based on the levels of vitamins needed to avoid getting a frank deficiency disease such as scurvy or beri-beri. It is absurd to consider this to be the same as the *optimum* dose of a vitamin. Just scraping by without losing your skin, hair and teeth isn't my idea of health. Yet RDAs continue to be the classic ideal of what personal nutritional requirements should be.

Even if these were adequate recommendations, a UK nutrition survey carried out in 1986–87 (*The Dietary and Nutrition Survey of British Adults*, HMSO, 1991) reveals that the British are borderline on most nutrients – and these are average levels, which implies that some individuals are way below RDA levels. Thus, for B_6 (RDA = 2 mg per day), the overall intake is reported as 2.02 mg a day. But breaking this average down, we find that men get 2.48 mg and women only 1.57 mg, some even less than that.

Two other instances should suffice: folic acid has an RDA of 300 mcg, yet at the lowest end of the scale over 2 per cent of women were getting under 100 mcg daily; vitamin C has an RDA of 30 mg, yet a significant number of women in the age range 25–35 were getting only a third of this amount. But, 'on average', we all meet the RDAs.

There are other serious flaws with the whole concept of RDAs. For one thing, an individual's requirements vary according to his or her levels of stress, illness and other factors. It is also faulty to assume that whatever is in food is being absorbed by an individual. Many people, we know, simply don't absorb nutrients efficiently.

Finally, and most importantly, food itself is variable. Tables listing what is *supposed* to be in fresh fruit, etc. may not be applicable to modern commercial supplies, which have often been stored for long periods in unsatisfactory conditions. Tests on fresh fruit have shown that sometimes there is no vitamin C whatever present. The idea that an 'apple a day' or drinking fresh orange juice will supply full daily requirements is therefore nonsense.

Agriculture is no longer what it was a half-century ago. Crops raised by today's farming techniques have often been forced artificially and have had insufficient time to gather necessary nutrients.

VITAMINS

The word vitamin comes from 'vital amine'. It was found that these substances were essential for health yet our bodies could not manufacture them. If they are not present in our food, we suffer disease. For example, a lack of adequate vitamin B_1 causes the condition beri-beri.

Some vitamins have names. B_1 is thiamine and B_2 is riboflavin. A system of letter coding started off all right, with vitamins A, B, C, D and E, but the next few were later found not to be vitamins and so there are gaps in the sequence. The only other one that now remains is K. Possibly others will come to light.

In addition, vitamin B was found to be a complicated mixture of substances and so was subdivided; B_1, B_2, etc. B_4 is missing, so are 7 to 11, but we have a B_{12}.

You will hear many other vitamin names bandied about. We've reached B_{17}, according to some enthusiasts. These designations are not official and should be discontinued until it is proved that a substance truly is a vitamin – that is, essential to life, not just contributory.

Other substances important for health, and apparently working in conjunction with vitamins, we call co-factors. Some are vitamin-like, others are simply minerals (these are discussed below). Co-factors include folic acid, biotin, inositol and choline, all reckoned as part of the B complex.

MINERALS

A number of elemental substances are vital for health. For example, it has long been known that lack of iron leads to anaemia, and that iodine deficiency gives rise to retarded growth and cretinism (in children), goitre and loss of thyroid function in adults.

In fact, in recent years there has been a huge expansion in our understanding of minerals and the part they play in our metabolism.

Probably the most important element to be studied in recent years is **zinc (112)** (see below).

Other key minerals, called 'trace elements' include selenium (see below) and chromium (important in carbohydrate metabolism; lack of it may predispose a person to diabetes).

ESSENTIAL FATTY ACIDS (EFAs)

Almost accorded the status of vitamins are certain **essential fatty acids (38)** (EFAs). The body cannot make them but they are vital for optimum health.

Probably most people would benefit from extra EFAs. Modern processed diets are very deficient in it. But certain conditions are sometimes especially helped: eczema, **hyperactivity (52)**, arthritis, **PMT (90)** and obesity.

DOSAGES

It might seem odd suggesting doses after what I've said about biological variations and requirements. Nevertheless, some guidance must be given.

Nutrients *interact* and are *interdependent*. Thus the effect of taking vitamin B_6 is minimal without adequate E, C, zinc and **magnesium (66)**. Even more important, substances can sometimes *compete*, so that, for example, too much zinc can displace magnesium or copper.

One method of supplementation is to take large doses, to make sure there is more than enough (few vitamins are toxic). This is called *megavitamin therapy*; I don't recommend it. It is wasteful and not certain to be safe.

A better approach is to try and work out what you need; this is known as the *orthomolecular* approach. The idea is to take increasing doses of each vitamin until you get as much improvement as seems possible. This isn't easy to judge, because the effects are both subtle and long term. In general, the doses chosen are moderate, but much higher than RDAs (10 to 100 times higher).

Undoubtedly, the easiest way of taking vitamin and mineral supplements is in a well-formulated multi-preparation. You can always add extra individual vitamins or minerals, if that seems to suit you better. Suggested ingredients for a good daily multi-formula are given in Table 81.1.

Suggestions for a Daily Multiformula

This is not intended to be a prescription and should not be construed as such.

C: 500 mg
B_1: 25 mg
B_2: 25 mg
Niacin: 50 g
B_6: 50 mg
B_{12}: 20 mcg
Pantothenic acid: 100 mg
A: 4500 units
E: 200 units
D: 200 units
Choline: 500 mg
Inositol: 200 mg
Biotin: 200 mcg
Folic acid: 300 mcg
Magnesium: 400 mg
Zinc: 15 mg
Oil of Evening Primrose: 1 g
Chromium: 200 mcg
Iron: 50 mg
Selenium: 200 mcg
Manganese: 5 mg

Do remember that it is possible to react to vitamins. Don't be puzzled if this happens: after all, B vitamins are synthesized from yeast; vitamin E usually comes from wheatgerm; vitamin C from corn, and so on.

Always get *hypo-allergenic* supplies. Those free of unnecessary starches, sugars, colours, etc. are best. However, there is no such thing as a non-allergenic vitamin preparation.

Initial supplementation should be continued for 3 to 12 months depending on the patient's general state of health. Unfortunately, the body's uptake and restoration of depleted stocks is very slow, even when deficiencies are quite pronounced, so it is a long-term strategy. After that, a more convenient maintenance dose can be used.

With improved digestion and a good diet it isn't necessary to take vitamins for life. However it's something which most people need to do repeatedly for optimum health, bearing in mind what was said above about the balanced diet.

NUTRIENTS AND THE IMMUNE SYSTEM

Since Linus Pauling first made history by showing the importance of vitamin C in combating ordinary viral infections, such as the 'common cold', we have learned a great deal about nutrients and the immune system. How important this is can be seen historically from the fact that as a result of better nutrition we have seen the virtual demise of major terminal diseases such as tuberculosis in Western society.

Malnutrition or poor nutrition is usually thought of as affecting starving communities of the Third World. We call this protein-energy malnutrition (PEM) or protein-calorie malnutrition (PCM). It may come as a surprise to some to learn that PEM is the most frequent cause of acquired immune deficiency in humans (AIDS is still a long way behind). But the important point is that we see this phenomenon to a surprising degree in Western society, not just among aged or impoverished individuals but those who eat too much manufactured food. The impact on immune function can be highly significant, especially for allergics, many of whom are eating self-imposed diets which are, in fact, of only PEM standard.

Some Nutrients Individually Considered

Apart from the generalized nutritional aspect of immunity, there are several individual nutrients of particular concern in relation to the proper functioning of the immune system. It should be pointed out that, in clinical terms, human malnutrition generally involves multiple nutrient deficiencies. This makes causal relationships harder to investigate. Also, whereas any single nutrient deficiency (vitamin, mineral, protein, carbohydrate or lipid) may cause immune aberrations, such isolated deficiencies rarely exist in Nature.

ZINC

Zinc is probably the most important trace element. It is essential for normal T-cell function, thymus function and overall cell-mediated immunity. Zinc deficiency can lead to decreased cellular and humoral immunity. Unfortunately, excess zinc seems to lower the ability of phagocytes and macrophages to engulf foreigners, so it needs intelligent supplementation – megadoses are *out*.

Zinc has also been found to be important in preventing dwarfism, infertility, hair loss, poor skin, diarrhoea, bad wound healing and anorexia nervosa.

Orthomolecular levels: 10 to 15 mg daily.

VITAMIN B₆ (PYRIDOXINE)

Pyridoxine is similar to zinc in its effects on the immune system. It is not surprising, therefore, that vitamin B₆ and zinc seem to potentiate (encourage) each other's effects. Isolated pyridoxine deficiencies cause more profound effects on immune system functions than deficiencies of any other B vitamin.

It is popularly accepted (though with little scientific footing), that the way to establish how much B₆ you need is to go on taking increased doses until you begin to recall your dreams vividly (this is called the *dream recall dose*). This does not necessarily mean nightmares, but that your dreams don't vanish on waking, as is usually the case – you can recall their content clearly.

Start with around 50 mg daily and increase by 50-mg steps until this dream phenomenon occurs. Then take just *less* than this amount; if 250 mg gives you the dream effect, limit yourself from then on to 200 mg a day.

The liability of this method is that not everyone dreams. If nothing is happening by the time you reach 300 to 400 mg, then stop. Go back to a maximum of 200 mg daily. Too much B₆ can be toxic and cause bizarre mental disturbances. It also interferes with blood clotting – so if you are contemplating surgery or have had a stroke you should only take it under the advice of your doctor.

The exception to this is the people who cannot function mentally without very high doses of zinc and B_6 (see **brain allergy (12)**).

Orthomolecular levels: 100 to 200 mg daily.

VITAMIN B_3 (NIACIN OR NICOTINIC ACID)

Lack of niacin leads to pellegra – red, scaly dermatitis, diarrhoea and dementia – scourge of the American south (corn, the staple dietary starch, does not make its B_3 bio-available). Factually, pellegra-like states are not rare in the Western world, even in the UK. Psychiatric wards are probably rife with examples.

B_3 is a vital precursor in certain **detoxification (26)** pathways. Its use as a means of detoxifying and removing pollutants from the body is discussed in the relevant section of this book.

Note: You may also encounter nicotinamide (nicotinic acid amide). This is not a direct metabolic substitute and you should not mix the two. Nicotinamide does not have the troublesome side-effect of flushing of the skin that B_3 may cause, but neither is it as effective.

Orthomolecular levels: 50 to 500 mg (can cause unpleasant flushing at these levels).

VITAMIN A

The presence of vitamin A is essential in non-adaptive immunity, being required for the production of lysozymes in tears, saliva and sweat. It also plays a part in both cell-mediated and humoral immunity.

Vitamin A is an important scavenger for oxidation radicals. It is believed that vitamin A can revert the immunosuppression usually caused by corticosteroid hormones. This would make it very valuable at times of stress, when immunity is often sharply reduced.

There has been some concern over the safety of high levels of vitamin A. However, it should be pointed out that some studies show it is surprisingly safe even at mega-doses. Short-term levels as high as 50,000 to 100,000 international units (IU) have been used in conjunction with vitamin C with good effect against acute infections. More permanent doses should not exceed 20,000

IU daily, except under the supervision of a doctor. Note that alcohol increases the toxicity of vitamin A.

I repeat here the official warning that vitamin A supplements may be teratogenic (causing damage to a foetus during its development) but this is based on the worst kind of data processing. Ironically, vitamin A is vital for a healthy foetus and successful pregnancy (see **preconceptual health (89)**).

Orthomolecular levels: around 5,000 IU daily (maximum 20,000 without supervision).

VITAMIN E (ALPHA-TOCOPHEROL)

Vitamin E is an important **anti-oxidant (8)**. It is believed to protect membranes against lipid **peroxidation (84)** by chemical free radicals. This may be the key to its role in protecting against heart attacks.

Its most important role, however, is its part in immunity. Numerous animal studies have confirmed that vitamin E enhances humoral antibody response.

Orthomolecular levels: 100 to 200 IU daily.

VITAMIN D

In the past few years the biological role of vitamin D has been expanded beyond its effects on calcium metabolism. Vitamin D receptors have been found in the hypothalamus of the brain, with the suggestion that this vitamin may play a role in hormonal regulation by the pituitary gland.

Vitamin D is steroidal in structure and could thus act as an immunosuppressant. Excess doses are toxic.

Orthomolecular levels: 100 to 200 IU.

VITAMIN C (ASCORBIC ACID)

Vitamin C is probably unique among nutrients in that it has a beneficial effect even in tiny amounts yet is not toxic or detrimental in very large quantities.

Tests show that vitamin C is vital for the immune system. A deficiency leads to loss of cell-mediated immunity, with diminished T-cell function (see **immune system (56)**).

Interestingly, antibody levels remain unchanged, even in severe vitamin C depletion.

Vitamin C is also a powerful anti-oxidant and vital, along with A, E and selenium.

Orthomolecular levels: 100 to 500 mg – but see 'Your Own Ascorbic Acid Dose', below.

YOUR OWN ASCORBIC ACID DOSE

Because of its properties in assisting immunity, allergics might benefit from substantial doses of vitamin C. Over and above its vitamin properties it does seem to have a detoxification function when taken in larger doses and is valuable for those who find themselves reacting to ambient chemicals.

Patients are encouraged to work out their own dose of vitamin C, using the 'fill and flush' approach. This is done by taking incremental doses (increasing by half a teaspoon each time) until side-effects are noticed. Usually, excess vitamin C causes diarrhoea. Take just less than this amount, if you need to. Say four teaspoons cause diarrhoea – your dose is three and a half teaspoons.

But, by going on, the body can get to tolerate larger amounts and this is often where the real magic lies. Some doctors insist that there is no real therapeutic bite until the diarrhoea stage has been reached and passed. Experiment yourself and see.

Unless on the advice of a physician, it is probably not desirable to take large amounts of Vitamin C continuously, only when needed. The body seems to get used to the higher dose and signs of scurvy may appear on dropping the dose significantly, even to what would be easily anti-scorbutic levels previously.

If you can't tolerate vitamin C this may be because you are sensitive to corn. Most supplies are derived from this source. Palm is an alternative. Others may appear on the market.

VITAMIN B₁₂ AND FOLIC ACID

Both of these nutrients are required in the prodigious output from the bone marrow (approximately 10,000 million leucocytes alone, daily). Deficiency leads to a less-than-optimum performance of the red and white blood cell-forming tissues. The result is anaemia and/or too many immature white cells that can't do their job.

Advice is *not* to supplement folic acid without B_{12}, otherwise peripheral nerve damage may result.

Orthomolecular levels: Folate, 5 mg daily (will need a prescription in the UK, due to concern about B_{12} interference).

B_{12}, 200 to 1,000 mcg. By far the best way to supplement is to get a doctor to prescribe injections. B_{12} is stored for up to two years in the liver.

IRON

Iron deficiency is commonplace in menstruating women and in malnourished children throughout the world. It is one of the few likely forms of single-nutrient deficiency.

Both a deficiency and excess of iron can cause immune dysfunctions. A deficiency would lead to a reduction in haemoglobin and decrease in the delivery of oxygen to the tissues (anaemia). Cells of the immune system, with their rapid turnover and therefore relatively high oxygen demand, would be hit especially hard.

Microbes, too, need iron to reproduce and grow. Because of this it is recognized that there are dangers in providing iron supplements to malnourished individuals, who may be immune compromised. It renders them very liable to serious infections because the iron will give a temporary advantage to potential pathogens before the rest of the immune system has had a chance to recover.

It is better to raise the level of general nutrition first – especially of protein, in order to raise the serum iron-binding capacity – before providing large amounts of supplemented iron.

Orthomolecular levels: 10 to 50 mg.

MAGNESIUM

Care may be needed in supplementing magnesium. It can lead to diarrhoea and a worsening in magnesium status, due to loss of electrolytes from the colon.

Orthomolecular levels: 200 to 400 mg daily.

SELENIUM

In laboratory animals, sodium selenite administration raises the antibody responsiveness to a variety of antigen challenges. The combined use of selenite and vitamin E provides an important synergistic effect in aiding the immune system and as antioxidants. This is probably central to selenium's role against cancer: it has been observed that high levels of dietary selenium are associated with lowered incidence of cancer deaths.

Selenium is also important for the elasticity of tissues/helping to prevent ageing.

If taking a supplement, try to get an organic form. L-selenomethionine, especially if combined with zinc, is the best.

Orthomolecular levels: 100 to 200 mcg daily.

Also see **hair analysis for minerals (47)**

82. Osteoporosis

Nearly a third of all American women will during their lifetime develop osteoporosis sufficiently severe to cause a fracture. At least 1.2 million fractures are said to occur each year as a direct result of this condition. The medical and social costs of this condition are estimated to be from $6 billion to upwards of $10 billion annually. It affects 15 to 20 million Americans (mostly women) annually. There are 200,000 hip fractures alone every year. It should not be forgotten also that the complications of a hip fracture are fatal to many of these patients. In fact more women die every year of hip fracture than all those who die of cancer of the breast, cervix or uterus combined.

The UK picture is equally gloomy.

Formerly known as senile osteoporosis, it is now obvious that in women the bone mass begins to decline even before the menopause, at around 35 years of age, and then accelerates rapidly for some eight to ten years. Thereafter it continues at a slower rate.

It is a disease of Western women. Chinese female octogenarians, for example, show almost no osteoporosis or fractures of the femur. This leads to the speculation that osteoporosis is an environmental condition, caused mainly by diet.

HORMONE THERAPY

The current therapy focuses mainly on oestrogen, supposedly to retard the advance of the menopause, and calcium supplementation, since osteoporosis is seen largely as a loss of calcium tissue in the bones. However, it is probably not really as simple as this.

Oestrogen therapy really only defers the inevitable and therefore its 'success' as a treatment is debatable. Moreover, some doctors would see the risk of hormone replacement therapy as wholly unacceptable when used for this purely prophylactic reason.

Calcium supplements (around 800 to 1500 mg a day) are usually recommended but it must be said that studies on how effective this is are confused and contradictory. Calcium supplementation will not restore lost bone tissue. The likelihood is that calcium supplementation is of little value on its own. The paradox is that it is known that calcium deposition is a factor in hardening of the arteries, arthritis, kidney stones, gall stones and cataracts, so for some patients it may be a question of ageing one way or decaying another.

BONE DENSITOMETRY

Probably the single biggest factor in whether a woman will develop osteoporosis is her bone density at the age of 35. Those with dense bones are unlikely to reach severe osteoporotic levels even during the seventh and eight decade. Those whose bones are thin even before menopause are likely to end up with difficulties, no matter what treatment is attempted. It is to be hoped that routine bone densitometry screening will be available to all menopausal women.

The truth is that osteoporosis is probably

a holistic condition and needs treating holistically. It is doubtful if single nutrient supplements, even such obvious ones as calcium and vitamin D, would be effective in the absence of good whole-body nutrition.

Bone, remember, is more than just a collection of calcium crystals. It is an active living tissue, constantly remodelling itself through deposition and absorption and continually participating in a wide range of biochemical reactions – reactions that will be compromised by any degree of under-nutrition.

NUTRITIONAL FACTORS

Vitamin K is known to be important primarily for its effects on blood clotting. However, it is also required for synthesizing osteocalcin, a protein found uniquely in bone and on which the calcium crystallizes. It is usually assumed that vitamin K deficiency is rare, but in one study (of only 16 patients) with osteoporosis their mean serum vitamin K levels were only 35 per cent of those of age-matched controls.

Vitamin D is required for intestinal calcium absorption. Reduced vitamin D levels are common in elderly patients, especially women. Studies have failed to show conclusively that vitamin D supplements help, yet it would be logical to ensure that D status is adequate.

Magnesium (66) is probably far more important than calcium, but scientific proof is lacking. The critical bone enzyme *alkaline phosphatase* (involved in forming new calcium crystals) is activated by magnesium. Its relative lack, therefore, could be expected to block the deposition of new bone tissue. Whole-body concentrations of magnesium were found to be below normal in 16 out of 19 osteoporotic women.

Manganese is also required for bone mineralization. Rats fed on manganese-deficient diets had smaller and less dense bones. In one study of osteoporotic women, blood manganese levels were found to be only 25 per cent of those of controls! About 5 mg daily is accepted generally as a suitable supplement.

Folic Acid

The interest in this vitamin co-factor stems from the fact that homocystine metabolism seems to be at least partially folic acid-dependent and patients with a genetic failure in the metabolism of homocystine are known to develop severe osteoporosis at an early age. Folic acid deficiency is relatively common, particularly in those who do not follow a hunter-gatherer type diet. Supplementation would therefore seem to be prudent.

Boron

Previously thought to be important only for plants, it is possible now that boron plays a role in human nutrition, particularly in relation to bone health. Supplementing the diet with boron (3 mg daily) was shown to reduce urinary calcium excretion by 44 per cent. Also, interestingly, it increased the serum concentration of the hormone 17-beta-oestradiol, which may be the most biologically active form of naturally occurring human oestrogen. Dietary requirements are not known; supplementation is suggested at 2 to 3 mg per day.

Attention has also been focused on a number of other nutrients including strontium, silicon, vitamin B_6, zinc, copper and vitamin C. In other words, we are working towards the conclusion that any important nutrient could lead to as yet undiscovered deficiencies in bone metabolism; good holistic nutrition is vital.

NON-NUTRITIONAL FACTORS

● Exercise has been shown to have a positive effect on bone density; thus those who lead sedentary lives are more likely to develop osteoporosis. Animal studies show that lack of use leads to rapid bone reabsorption (breakdown by cells). It is likely therefore that regular gentle exercise will benefit all women at or beyond the menopausal years.

● Some drugs accelerate bone loss. Particularly important are steroids such as prednisolone, though it appears that the type of osteoporosis this can lead to is quite different biochemically from post-menopausal osteoporosis. Certain anti-convulsants (phenytoin, for example) may also lead to increased bone re-absorption.

● Smoking is said to hasten the menopause by about five years and reduces oestrogen levels thereafter. Other evidence suggests that smoking may alter osteoblast function (osteoblasts are the cells that 'build' bone).

● There are also racial and genetic factors.

A number of disease states need to be considered in any clinical evaluation of osteoporosis. All are rightly the preserve of a qualified physician and are not for self-medication. They include: anorexia nervosa, testicular failure, thyrotoxicosis, bone cancer disease and immobilization after surgery.

Also see **nutrition and allergies (81)**

83. Parasites

New work has called the attention of clinical ecologists to the phenomenon of bowel parasites and the problems they may cause.

These problems aren't nearly as rare as might be supposed. Despite the British standard of hygiene and well-known phobia for exotic travel and anything 'foreign', Britons carry quite a lot of unwelcome passengers around in their bodies. Those that do not harm us are called *commensals* (living together) but the ones that 'live off' us, as opposed to living *in* us, we consider to be parasites.

It is now realized that as many as 15 per cent of us may be carrying *Giardia lamblia*, a minute flagellated protozoan that causes severe fatigue and bowel disturbance. That's 1 in 6 of the population. Perhaps 10 to 12 per cent carry Cryptosporidia infestation: a mild enough companion if you are healthy but, for those with compromised immunity (such as AIDS victims), it can result in a fatal overwhelming disease. One of the reasons that the incidence of these parasites has been underestimated for so long is simply that detection techniques have been so bad.

Parasites may produce illness in several ways. They can undoubtedly produce immune suppression, which will hinder the body's attempts to get rid of them.

Secondly, parasites compete for nutrients. Whatever the host organism eats, they take their share. In some cases, if the infestation is severe, frank malnutrition will result (as for example with a tape worm). If not protein energy malnutrition (PEM, see **nutrition and allergies (81)**), the result may be a micro-nutrient deficiency. Diphyllobothrium latum, a worm found in freshwater fish in Scandinavia and North America, is capable of inducing a B_{12} deficiency severe enough to cause anaemia.

Finally, the host can become sensitized to the parasitic organism within and experience allergic reactions to it: they are, after all, foreign protein.

Many people have an asymptomatic parasitic infection and remain unaware that they are harbouring an unwanted guest until some incidental occurrence tips the balance in favour of the invader. This could be the arrival of a second parasite infection (many people have two or more) or some other increase in **body load (11)** that will reduce host resistance. Thus allergy patients are especially at risk.

Probably the majority of patients simply get vague grumbling symptoms that come and go, never quite adding up to a 'disease' or something the doctor would wish to have fully investigated. Most of the symptoms are especially referenced to the bowel, where mild symptoms of the 'irritable bowel'-type are quite common. However, systemic symptoms can be caused too, particularly fatigue and lack of energy, muscle weakness, headache, sore throats, enlarged lymph glands, night sweats and occasional fever.

GIARDIASIS

Giardia lamblia is a flagellated protozoan which is found world-wide. Prevalence is high throughout the tropics; modern travel has spread it to more temperate zones. The very high incidence in the general population has been referred to above. It is an important cause of traveller's diarrhoea and chronic fatigue states. Patients with irritable bowel or 'food allergy' can often date the onset of their symptoms to an episode of tummy upset on a holiday abroad.

Person-to-person spread is more common in day nurseries, residential institutions and between male homosexuals. It exists in a free swimming form and as a cyst, the latter being the form in which it is transmitted. Symptom-free carrier states are common. These individuals may pass on the infection while being unaware that they are carrying it.

Severe **malabsorption (67)** may occur, not unlike the changes of coeliac disease, from mild to total atrophy of the gut lining. Typical symptoms include nausea, anorexia, abdominal discomfort and distension. Stools may be bulky, float and stick to the pan (steatorrhoea). If the illness is prolonged, weight loss can be quite pronounced.

It is common for patients with Giardiasis to have secondary deficiency of the enzyme lactase and they may also fail to absorb folic acid and vitamin B_{12}, leading to anaemia.

Diagnosis

Diagnosing giardiasis is very difficult. Most labs do not have the requisite detection skills. The 'gold standard' for giardia is jejunal biopsy, where a capsule is passed through the stomach and a small specimen of mucous epithelium is sampled. The parasite is visible with microscopy. Unfortunately this test is rarely carried out.

Routine hospital screening of faeces for the presence of cysts misses the diagnosis 98 per cent of the time. A newer and probably better method, described by the researchers Bueno and Parrish in the US, consists of a superficial biopsy of rectal mucosa taken by means of a small cotton bud swab pressed firmly into the mucosal lining. The specimen is centrifuged and examined immediately under a microscope or, if this is not possible, it is held in an incubator at 98.6°F/37°C until ready. A positive result would include visualization of the protozoa, which are actively mobile for up to 24 hours. Cysts may also be present and can be recognized by their form.

Treatment

Originally mepacrine, an anti-malarial drug, was used. Co-trimoxazole (a combination of sulphonamide and trimethoprim, also known as *Septrin*) and metronidazole (*Flagyl*) have been the most widely used drugs to date. Unfortunately the relapse rate is very high and treatment may need to be repeated, showing that the organism was not eradicated properly in the first place.

A new drug, tinidazole (*Fasigyn*) has become available and appears to be effective. It may cause short-lived abdominal discomfort and drowsiness. The usual dose is 2 g as 4 tablets taken on a single occasion. Treatment should be avoided if the patient is pregnant or breastfeeding; patients may feel ill if they consume alcohol concurrently with the treatment.

TOXOPLASMOSIS

Toxoplasmosis is an infection caused by *Toxoplasma gondii*, an intracellular protozoan which requires for its life cycle a definitive host such as a cat, sheep or pig and an intermediate host, e.g., a human. Infection of humans occurs either congenitally (passed on from the mother) or by ingestion of foods contaminated by infected cat, lamb or pork faeces, or by eating lamb or pork contaminated with *T. gondii* cysts.

Toxoplasmosis is rare in the UK but not in the southern US. Five major clinical forms are recognized:

1. A mild asymptomatic form with only swollen lymph glands which is occasionally found by chance.
2. A more severe disturbance with swelling of lymph nodes and a mild fever. This is the form that can mimic ME or infectious mononucleosis (Epstein-Barr virus) but the Paul-Bunnell test for the latter will be negative and remain negative.
3. Neurological abnormalities which include neck stiffness and headache, sore throat and rashes. The cerebral spinal fluid has a raised pressure and its protein level is elevated.
4. An acute febrile illness with widespread rash, swollen liver and spleen. The complications of this form include inflammations of the eye, the myocardium

and the liver. The latter two forms are more common in those with a poor immune system, such as AIDS sufferers.
5. Congenital toxoplasmosis, which often leads to mental retardation, epilepsy and even spasticity or paralysis.

Diagnosis

Diagnosis is made chiefly from serological tests for IgG antibodies to *T. gondii*. Other antibody tests include indirect fluorescence or haemagglutination. Raised antibody levels are not rare in the general population, and only an increasing level is suggestive of active toxoplasmosis.

Treatment

Most patients require no therapy as the disease is mild. For those with the more severe form, pyrimethamine (25 to 50 mg three times a day) and sulphadiazine (4 to 5 g daily) are used in combination. Therapy needs to be continued for at least one month. Since pyrimethamine causes foetal abnormalities it should not be used during pregnancy or if a woman might be pregnant. Steroids are occasionally used to dampen down any inflammation in the eye.

Prevention is better than cure. Domestic cats that kill mice and birds are the chief source of infection and strict codes of hygiene should always be observed around pets.

CRYPTOSPORIDIA

In the last decade, *Cryptosporidium* species have become recognized as one of the most frequent causes of acute gastroenteritis caused by a parasite. It is common in farm workers but affects the population generally. Usually it gives rise to a mild self-limiting attack which lasts no more than a few weeks. But it is particularly disastrous for AIDS victims who cannot fight it off and suffer a severe life-threatening diarrhoea with dehydration.

Six species are known which infect mammals, birds, reptiles, fish and humans. *C. parvum* is the major species responsible for clinical disease in humans and domestic animals. Transmission is direct transfer (faecal-oral route). That is to say, cysts are excreted in the faeces and, due to inadequate hygiene, eventually find their way into the mouths of uninfected hosts.

Secondary symptoms include fatigue, headache, joint pains and general debility. The antibody response to Cryptosporidia may interfere with treatments being attempted such as **enzyme potentiated desensitization (36)** or **Miller's method (74)**.

Treatment

To date, there is no really successful treatment for Cryptosporidium infections. *Flagyl* can be tried and a number of herbal preparations (listed below) may succeed in keeping it in check.

ENTAMOEBA HISTOLYTICA

This well-known tropical protozoan infection is surprisingly widespread in temperate zones (as high as 5 per cent of the population in the US). People are largely 'symptom-free' because they are healthy and well-nourished – once again, it is probably responsible for a lot of chronic mild complaints. 'Carriers' may exceed 50 per cent of the population in poorly sanitized areas.

E. histolytica probably only attains its killer dysentery form in a compromised host. There seem to be some strains more virulent than others. Except in these special cases the dangerous spread to the liver and brain, causing amoebic abscesses, is very rare.

Diagnosis

Stools are characteristic and may show specks of blood. The organism or its cysts can be found on microscopy. Serological tests are almost always positive when the disease is present, but since antibody levels stay high long after infection this isn't a good guide to current disease.

Immunofluorescent techniques are better (see **conventional allergy tests (22)**).

OTHER SUSPECTS

There are many other such organisms and the list is growing constantly. *Blastocystis hominis* is an example. This organism was formerly considered to be a yeast but is now re-classified as a protozoan. Its frequent pleomorphic forms (odd, changing shapes) make diagnosis exasperatingly difficult.

Endonylax nana is another type of amoeba. Formerly thought to be non-pathogenic, it is now realized that it may be, given a weakened host. It is often present with other organisms. It may be associated with inflammatory arthritis.

NON-SPECIFIC AND HERBAL TREATMENTS

For many of these organisms, the imidazoles such as metronidazole (*Flagyl*) and tinidazole (*Fasigyn*) are the treatment of choice. Therapy may need to be kept up for several weeks. Even if apparently successful, relapses are common. These are probably due to incomplete eradication, rather than re-infection.

Herbal treatment can be strikingly effective. Dr Damien Downing speculates that many traditional 'bowel remedies' gained their reputation from the fact that they were effective against organisms of this type. We have had parasites with us since long before the dawn of history and centuries of trial and error may have led to the cure.

Particularly effective are plants from the genus *Artemesia*. These are the worts such as wormwood (*Artemesia absinthium*) and mugwort (*Artemesia vulgaris*), etc. Moxa, used in moxybustion by acupuncturists, is from this group of plants.

Best known as an antiparasitic is *Artemesia annua*. It is currently under study by the World Health Organization as a possible treatment for chloroquine-resistant malaria. It is available as a bowel preparation (take 1 g three times a day for 60 to 90 days). Better results may come from combining it with some other herbs. Grapefruit-seed extract, known under several brand names such as *DF100*, *Parcan* and *Citrocidal* (100 mg three times a day) has a similar range of activity. The two combine very well. If a short-term course of *Flagyl*

is added, this makes up just about the best ammunition we have got.

Even then, there is no guaranteed cure. Relapses may occur and life-long maintenance therapy may have to be considered.

A final problem with these parasites is that they spread very quickly through a family. It is important to examine and treat other family members, despite lack of symptoms, otherwise they may be a source of re-infestation.

In Britain, rectal swabs and the Bueno-Parrish method can be done at the London Clinic (see Useful Addresses)

Also see **candida (16)**, **gut flora (46)** and **intestinal fermentation (59)**

84. Peroxidation

A group of AIDS patients have been trying the effect of hydrogen peroxide (H_2O_2) on themselves. The theory is that, since active oxygen generated from this substance is the same as that used by the body's white cells to attack cancer cells, viruses and other micro-organisms, it must have a therapeutic effect. Claims from the 'peroxide lobby' have grown steadily, until now even cancer is said to be treated successfully by this method. Some clinical ecologists claim to have obtained good results against **Candida (16)**. The data is given here because you may hear about it and (as patients who are desperate sometimes regrettably do), try it for yourself.

What is true is that 'excited' oxygen, the super-oxide radical, is harmful to life. It will kill microbes – but will also harm body tissues as well. Scavenging white cells in the body are able to generate this active form of oxygen on the spot, but they are provided with an enzyme – peroxidase – which breaks the excited oxygen down quickly before it does any harm.

It seems doubtful that artificially supplied peroxide is adequately covered by this safety mechanism. Remember that we now advocate the health-giving benefits of certain vitamins known as **anti-oxidants (8)**. It makes little sense to intervene with a method which does, in effect, contradict this treatment.

DOSAGE

Try it if you must. Start with 1 oz of 0.5 per cent (dilute 1/200), taken with water. Some will find they need to start with less. Nausea is the main side-effect. Reduce the quantities even more if this occurs.

Otherwise, increase by 1 oz daily for five days (5 oz daily). After one week go to 5 oz three times daily for a week (or until the disease is no longer present). Then the dosage can be tapered back down over a five-week period.

Use food-grade peroxide if you can get it, since the common 3 per cent H_2O_2 contains small amounts of chemical stabilizers and other impurities. Cleaning-grade (35 per cent) is dangerous unless diluted. It can be used, but take care. Take 3 drops of 35 per cent H_2O_2 in a glass of water, three times a day, increasing by one drop each dose, to a maximum of 25 drops *per dose*.

If the bleachy taste is unpleasant, wash your mouth out with water afterwards or have a fruit juice 'chaser'.

Adding seven drops of 35 per cent H_2O_2 to a gallon of drinking water and shaking well purifies it and gives it a pleasant fresh-from-the-waterfall flavour.

If the oral route is not well tolerated, take a bath in peroxide. Anywhere from 1 to 8 pints of 3 per cent H_2O_2 in a standard size bathtub, half full of water.

H_2O_2 may be administered intravenously but only under the supervision of a qualified physician (250 cc of .075 per cent to .15 per cent, or roughly 1/1300 to 1/650).

ADDITIONAL COMMENT

Perhaps the greatest potential benefit of 'oxywater' might turn out to be the reversal of the slight brain damage caused by long-term oxygen depletion, which can be observed in the average human and is sometimes not all that slight. This is part of the ageing process and is due to arteriosclerosis blocking off bloodflow to the brain. It is better not to get arteriosclerosis – and the evidence is that a good diet and lifestyle will prevent it – but once it is there, any extra source of oxygenation is necessarily beneficial.

It could be more than a coincidence that proponents of oxywater therapy claim it banishes tiredness, depression, irritability and poor judgement and that it improves alertness, reflexes, memory and apparently intelligence, and may offer the elderly a new weapon against senility and related disorders.

Also see **chronic viral infections (20), hyperventilation (54)** and **the immune system (56)**

85. Pesticides and Health

Most people today are concerned about the widespread use – some might say abuse – of pesticides. It is not even a question of whether pesticides are safe or not but actually of whether we need them at all. Their use seems to be geared largely to agribusiness profits rather than to general human benefit, and certainly in the Western world, where most pesticides are used, we are already grossly overproducing foodstuffs to the point where there seems little sense in polluting the environment to grow yet more.

It is debatable whether pesticides actually do any good. Over the 30 years leading up to 1974, while insecticide usage increased 10-fold, crop losses actually rose from 7 per cent to 13 per cent. Even with pesticide warfare on today's grand scale at least 30 per cent of the world's potential crop production is lost each year due to pests.

Some pesticides are used to combat, not loss of yield, but the disagreeable appearance of produce caused by attack from pests (such as apple scab). In this case their use is really only a 'cosmetic' one.

One of the worrying aspects of the pesticide toxicity debate is the vexed one of end-usage. Even given that manufacturers may have carried out proper toxicity studies and made clear recommendations for their application, there are at present no regulatory mechanisms to make sure that these instructions are actually followed. Farmers may misunderstand explanatory leaflets or deliberately choose to ignore them. There simply can be *no* safety while proper controls of end-usage do not exist.

HOW TOXIC?

We are constantly reassured that pesticides are 'safe' – meaning they won't kill you if you are careful with them. Unfortunately the attitude seems to persist that we, the public, have to prove that a product is a menace, rather than the manufacturers paying for and carrying out adequate research into safety.

The usual stance when challenged on safety issues is 'there is no scientific proof of a threat to health'. The fact is, lack of evidence may simply mean that nobody has been looking for any, not that proof has been sought and found wanting. It seems unlikely that evidence of risk will be sought vigorously while research is left to the chemical companies themselves.

Difficulties in determining toxicity centre round the possible cumulative effect of long-term exposures, even at low levels. This may turn out to be far more serious than the toxicity of acute episodes, even though an 'accidental event' is more dangerous for the individual. Probably, pesticide residues accumulate in our body and may ultimately reach dangerous levels. We know from ecological disasters that have already occurred that poisons can become more and more concentrated as they advance along the food chain. Humans, of course, are at the end of many food chains.

There is also the additional phenomenon of potentiation, where two substances may interact and produce a dramatically greater effect than either on its own. With so many complex chemicals present in our environment it is intellectual folly to maintain these interactive summations are unimportant. Indeed, it is possible to predict with some certainty that they *do* take place. We just don't know enough about what is happening.

ALLERGIES AND IMMUNITY

As well as the purely toxic effect, there is also growing alarm over the possibility that pesticides may suppress the immune system. Temik (*Aldicarb*) is known to produce AIDS-like symptoms. If this and other pesticides have an adverse effect on the immune system, it can be predicted that allergy and intolerance, as well as infections and possibly cancer, will be a consequence. It has even been suggested by knowledgeable clinical ecologists that ME could be due to chronic pesticide poisoning. Certainly, this illness only emerged in the second half of the twentieth century, as did the use of synthetic chemical toxins on a massive scale.

A related problem is the possibility of an individual becoming sensitized to a pesticide. This is of special concern to farm workers who are in contact with large amounts, but again the cumulative problem may be at work and building up trouble for us all. Already a number of pesticides are known allergens or sensitizing irritants.

THREE CATEGORIES

Pesticides fall conveniently into three main categories: insecticides, herbicides and fungicides. Dr Jean Monro points out that the word itself is a trick. There is no such thing as a pesticide, only *biocides* (meaning: life-killing). All these agents have deleterious effects on human beings and other animals, not just on 'pests'. Numerous fish kills, bird fatalities and livestock disasters testify to this.

Insecticides

The most toxic and dangerous by far are the insecticides. Most of these are equivalent to the nerve gas used in human warfare. Insecticides can be subdivided into organo-chlorides, organophosphates, carbamates and pyrethroids. Organophosphates and carbamates suppress the breakdown of acetylcholine in the body. Since this is an essential neurotransmitter, this leads to a variety of malfunctions of the nervous system and, in sufficient quantity, certain death.

Organochlorides include the notorious polychlorinated biphenyls (PCBs), which are no longer manufactured in Britain or the US. These are stable environmentally, however, and are still around.

ORGANOCHLORIDES

Organochlorides are neurotoxic although the precise mechanisms are not yet fully understood. DDT is the best known example, also BHC (*Lindane*) and Aldrin.

They are remarkably well tolerated by humans, as shown by a classic series of tests done in 1956 in which brave volunteers swallowed massive amounts of DDT (220 times the average US daily intake over 18 months). They suffered no immediate ill effects and monitoring since that time has shown no apparent long-term hazard.

The chief concern is the way organochlorides accumulate in the environment, since they are not biodegradable. People may be safe but many other animals in the food chain are not. Fish are highly susceptible (their bones become deformed) and birds cannot make hard egg cases, so are unable to reproduce. Residues of DDT are now found all over the world, even in the most remote and inaccessible lakes.

ORGANOPHOSPHOROUS COMPOUNDS

These are relatives of the very lethal nerve gases developed for potential use in the Second World War. They interfere with the enzyme acetylcholinesterase which regulates the neurotransmitter, acetylcholine. The result is a violent discharge of all nerve tissue, resulting in uncontrolled spasms followed by death due to paralysis. A horrible end not to be contemplated lightly.

Malathion is a typical example. But here we should not get carried away. Malathion itself is relatively harmless. It is only when it undergoes biotransformation by hydrolysis into malaoxon that it becomes deadly. Insects have the necessary enzyme but humans don't and so are (more or less) spared the consequences.

CARBAMATES

These have an action similar to the organophosphorous compounds. However, they are twice as expensive and only regarded for use when other methods have failed.

PYRETHROIDS

Pyrethrum has long been known as an insect repellent. Natural pyrethroids are produced from the dried flowers of *Chrysanthemum cinerariaefuram*. They have a fast knockdown effect for flying insects, which suggests some kind of neurological toxicity. Unfortunately they are not selective and also kill helpful insects such as bees and other pollinators.

Herbicides

Herbicides have a number of modes of action, some of them hormonal (forcing the plant to overgrow until it dies). A concern about this effect on the growth of the human foetus would thus seem logical and justified. Some herbicides are specifically toxic to plants and not to animals; others affect humans in unwanted ways, the most notorious example being 2,4,5-T.

Agent Orange, so much used in the Vietnam War, was a mix of 2,4,5-T and 2,4-D, but also contained a much more deadly substance, dioxin. Publicity of the birth defects after women had been directly sprayed with Agent Orange led to 2,4-D being banned in the US. It is not banned in Britain, however.

Paraquat is an example of a selective plant toxin. Nevertheless, overdoses to humans are hazardous and cause respiratory failure and death. Its metabolism is discussed briefly in the section on **anti-oxidants (8)**.

Fungicides

Fungicides are a different matter. Over a quarter of the world's total crops are lost each year to fungus attack. Trying to eradicate this economic blight with chemicals is obviously tempting. The problem is that we then eat the foodstuffs that have been treated. We know very little about the cumulative effect of fungicides.

Eliminating established fungus is much more difficult than preventing it in the first place. Continuous applications are therefore needed. This is where the danger lies: we end up consuming the accumulated substances with the crop.

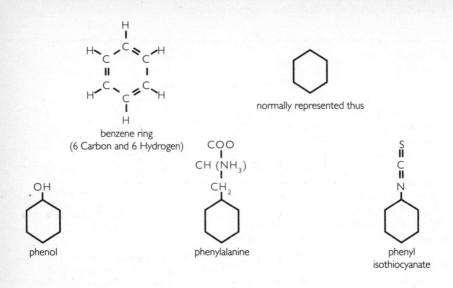

Figure 86.1: Derivation of phenolic compounds

Also see **detoxification (26)** and **thermal chamber depuration (106)**

86. Phenolic Testing

The neutralizing technique led to an interesting new development: the subject of phenols in foods. In a sense we have discovered 'molecular allergy'. This is a true allergic reaction; thus intradermal testing with chlorogenic acid, a phenol found in green coffee, castor bean and orange, gives a wheal and flare reaction in sensitized individuals that is characteristic of Type I **hypersensitivity (53)**.

There are many such compounds found in food, based on the phenol (carbolic acid) molecule (see Figure 86.1).

Caffeine is an example and is, of course, a poison. In fact most phenolic substances are toxic. How are we able to tolerate them? The answer is, evidently, some people don't!

Phenolic compounds colour and flavour foods. Their toxicity may protect the natural plants against micro-organisms. They also help in the dispersal and germination of seeds and attract flower pollinators because of their scent.

Some individual phenolic compounds have been correlated with specific disorders. Tyramine and nicotine, for example, are implicated in migraine and headaches. A little experience with phenol 'families' leads to new diagnostic skills in allergy. For example, a patient sensitive to cheese, beef, banana and potato might really be sensitive to nicotine.

Individual phenols can be tested and neutralized using **Miller's method (74)**. Avoidance is another option, where the range of related foods is not extensive.

Note: Many substances are now included in phenolic testing that are not really phenol-based, such as dopamine and adrenalin. But the term 'phenolic' persists as an overall generic name for the *test procedure*.

HISTORY AND BACKGROUND

In 1979, Dr Robert Gardner, Ph.D., professor of Animal Science at Brigham Young University, began to speculate that his own allergies might be caused by a sensitivity to some aromatic compounds found naturally in all plant foods and pollens. He acquired some of these pure compounds, made serial dilutions and

Phenolic Compounds in Some Common Foods

	Capsaicin	Cinnamic acid	Coumarin	Eugenol	Gallic acid	Malvin	Menadione	Nicotine	Phenyl isothiocyanate	Phlorizin or phloridzin	Piperine	Piperonal	Rutin (quercetin)	Vanillylamine	Apiol
Almond				•	•							•		•	•
Apple		•	•	•	•	•				•			•	•	
Banana		•	•												
Beef				•	•				•	•	•	•	•	•	•
Beet sugar		•			•					•	•	•			
Cabbage				•	•				•			•			
Cane sugar				•	•								•		
Carrot				•	•	•	•						•		•
Celery		•	•	•	•	•	•						•		•
Cheese		•	•	•	•					•	•		•	•	•
Chicken			•			•			•		•		•		
Egg			•		•	•	•		•	•			•		
Grape		•			•	•	•			•	•		•	•	
Lamb			•			•			•	•	•	•	•	•	
Lettuce		•	•		•	•				•			•		•
Milk (cow)	•	•		•	•	•			•	•			•		•
Onion	•	•		•	•	•				•		•	•		
Orange			•	•	•					•			•	•	•
Pea		•	•	•	•				•		•		•		•
Potato	•		•		•			•			•		•	•	
Rice			•										•		
Soya bean			•	•		•			•	•	•		•	•	•
Tomato	•	•	•	•	•	•		•	•		•	•	•	•	•
Wheat				•	•								•		
Yeast			•					•		•	•	•	•	•	

Adapted from Robert Gardner, Brigham Young University.

started sublingual tests, monitoring changes in his own pulse rate.

He experienced reactions to various extracts and neutralizing doses were found for each compound. Gardner found that neutralizing doses of these compounds would kill his allergic reactions to specific foods. After several months he had succeeded in neutralizing many of his own dietary allergies and he was able to eat most foods without reactions. He experienced a major improvement in his health.

A colleague began to hunt for phenolic compounds in foods and found, for example, that cow's milk contains 13, tomato 14, and soya 9. Table 86.1 shows the phenolic content of some common food substances.

Practitioners claim that neutralizing treatment has been particularly successful with infants and children, giving excellent results in cases of autism, **mental retardation (68)**, **hyperactivity (52)**, dyslexia, insomnia, enuresis, respiratory allergies, headaches, abdominal pains and asthma.

In adults, remissions have been achieved in many chronic problems including **migraine (72)**, fatigue, depression, asthma, arthritis, colitis, hypertension, menstrual disorders, dermatological problems, chronic constipation and cardiac arrythmias.

METHOD

Those who use the phenolic approach rely diagnostically on the **Vega machine (109)** or 'Dermatron'. It is quick, non-invasive and consequently cheap for the individual. It is possible to test over 20 items in a matter of minutes.

On the down side, this instrument isn't easy to use and many cannot make it perform at all. It is also difficult to 'sell' it to members of the medical establishment, who view such equipment with undue caution.

The standard 1:5 dilutions of test reagent are used, exactly as for Miller's method. Neutralizing dilutions tend to run high, up to and exceeding the fortieth dilution (which is virtually unheard of in intradermal testing). In fact it is now advocated that 1:5 series is used only up to about the tenth dilution and a 1:10 from there on, to speed

up matters. Children are mostly found to neutralize on lower dilutions, usually between one and twenty.

Patients return on a monthly basis and receive a 10 cc dropper bottle containing their neutralizing doses and are instructed to take two drops sublingually, three times a day *after* meals. Upon return, the patient is retested and a new neutralizing dilution is administered, which is almost always lower than the previous one. The aim is to get down to a 'No. 1' dilution, meaning the patient has become tolerant to that particular phenolic.

The patient is then instructed to take one dose three times a week in order to prevent a recurrence of the original symptoms.

RAST TEST NOTE

Interestingly, perhaps remarkably, the RAST test (see **conventional allergy tests (22)**) supports the phenolic hypothesis. Cross-reactions on this test sometimes seem to occur between allergens, not of the same botanical family, but of a common phenol group.

Finally, there is the possibility that phenolics *may* protect us in some way. Many foods contain **lectins (65)**, which should have a severely damaging effect on our gut and indeed the body as a whole – we ought to suffer more than, in practice, we do. Perhaps phenolics are shielding us? And one experiment has shown that the phenolic rutin (quercitin) has a protective effect against mast cell disintegration (mast cells in the body trigger allergic reactions to substances). Maybe these phenols work like drugs, too!

The door is open to many exciting discoveries.

Also see **plant toxins (87)**

87. Plant Toxins

Nature has seen fit to endow a number of plants with the capacity to synthesize substances that are toxic to humans and other animals. Humans are probably only able to tolerate the majority of foods because of the discovery of fire, which cooks away toxins (although several plant toxins are heat-stable).

Farmers and veterinarians, who are more advanced in clinical ecology than many doctors, have known for years that animals become sick if they graze on certain types of plant (for example, bulls become enraged if they eat loco weed – 'loco' being Spanish for crazy). Many plant substances are toxic to humans in quite small quantities, including deadly nightshade, acorns and hemlock. Ricin, the toxic principle in castor seeds (*Ricinus communis*), is one of the most poisonous substances known: a minute drop on the tip of a needle was used in an infamous political assassination on the streets of London in 1978.

The fact is that all plants, including edible ones, contain quantities of poisons. Carrots, for example, contain a nerve toxin: *caratotoxin*. And someone once pointed out that if cabbage had to undergo the tests that drugs are now subjected to before being pronounced fit for humans, it wouldn't pass. Obviously, most often the amounts of poison in foods are tolerable. Toxicity is a matter of degree.

Ironically, some of the 'best' (most nutritious) foods are the most toxic, such as grains, nuts and legumes. It seems as if we face either cumulative poisoning from plants, cancer and heart disease from animal products, or starvation!

TOXINS IN EDIBLE PLANTS

It is possible to classify the toxic elements in plant foodstuffs:

Lectins

Lectins (65) are large protein molecules; they are toxic and also mimic allergies.

Lectins are widespread and may be up to 20 per cent of the protein content of plants, especially of seeds and pulses. They have the curious property of imitating antigen-antibody reactions without actually sensitizing the immune system.

Anti-enzymes

These interfere with body enzymes such as trypsin (a protein digestive enzyme). In experimental animals this interference has been shown to cause retarding of growth, abnormal hypertrophy (enlargement) of the pancreas and, in the case of prolonged feeding, even the formation of cancer of the pancreas. Soya-bean protein derivatives have been shown to retain some of this effect, leading to concern that infants fed on soya milk might suffer growth retardation.

Goitrogens

Goitrogens are substances causing goitre or thyroid enlargement. Soya-bean extract is in this category and goitres have been seen in human infants fed with soya milk. Iodine appears to counteract this effect, so infant soya milks are fortified with iodide as a precautionary measure.

Goitrogens are a common constituent of plants belonging to the Crucifer family (cabbage, turnip, swede, broccoli, cauliflower, kale, brussel sprout, rape and mustard seed). An epidemic goitre seen in Tasmania is probably due to milk from cows fed on kale and turnips.

Oestrogens

There are naturally occurring oestrogenic compounds in many plants. These heat-stable compounds are capable of eliciting an oestrogenic response (feminization) in experimental animals.

Nerve Toxins

Also known as cholinesterase inhibitors, these affect chiefly animals, causing paralysis and sometimes death, though humans are occasionally afflicted.

Lathyrism, a condition associated with high intake of lathyrus bean (chickpea), is a kind of paralysis.

Carcinogens

A well-known example is *aflatoxin*, from **mould (75)** on nuts. There are probably many more waiting to be discovered.

Poisons

These include prussic acid and its

precursors, nicotine, solanin, atropine and a host of others.

Antinutrients

Antinutrients (7) are substances that interfere directly with the absorption of vitamins, minerals and other nutrients.

Phytate occurs in several plant groups, particularly grains and also the pulses. These are known to chelate, that is, combine with and remove, valuable minerals such as calcium and magnesium and trace elements such as zinc, copper and iron, which are vital for health.

Flatulence Factors

The pulses (peas and beans) are especially noted for this effect. The cause is low molecular weight oligosaccharides (simple sugars), namely raffinose and stachyose. Flatulence is generally attributed to the fact that humans do not possess the enzyme alpha 1,6-galacto-sidase necessary for breaking down these sugars.

PSYCHOGENICS

There is growing interest in drug-like substances in plants. Well-known are the psychedelic substances such as those in marijuana and peyote cactus; the coca plant gives rise to cocaine and the opium poppy is notorious for its forbidden juices. But there have been opium-like alkaloids called exorphins, and many other pharmacologically active substances, found in plants. These may have beneficial effects as well as unwanted ones.

Alkaloids

These are small organic molecules, usually comprising several carbon rings with side chains, one or more of the carbon atoms being replaced by a nitrogen (which confers the alkalinity). About 7 to 10 per cent of all plants contain alkaloids, of which several thousand are now known.

Famous alkaloids include nicotine, quinine, strychnine, ergotamine and atropine. The less toxic ones, such as caffeine, are used for pleasant social effects or as hallucinogens (cannabis, LSD and mescaline).

The well-known food allergy effect of addiction, where withdrawal from the food causes unpleasant symptoms, may be due at least in part to the addictive properties of alkaloids present in the food.

The action of alkaloids on the nervous system is generally to disrupt electro-chemical transmission at nerve junctions (synapses), either preventing transmission (as in the case of the plant curare) or enhancing it inappropriately (as, for example, physostigmine). Locoism, referred to above, is of this latter class.

Outbreaks of food poisoning due to solanine (from potatoes), tomatine (tomatoes) and dioscorine (yams) have all been reliably observed in either humans or domestic animals. Death due to alkaloid overdose is fortunately uncommon in humans; in Socrates' case (hemlock) it was deliberate murder by the state. But subclinical alkaloid intoxication occurs all the time. The 'edible' nightshades (potatoes, tomatoes, capsicums, peppers) are especially rich sources, but cabbage, peppercorns and many other foodstuffs are not far behind.

Exorphins

These are morphine-like peptides derived from partially digested grain, milk and legume proteins. Pharmacologically they behave, when tested on isolated tissues, very much like **endorphins (33)** (hence the name). It is reasonable to propose that in people whose intestinal digestion of these foodstuffs is incomplete, exorphins are absorbed and have the effect of a small dose of an opiate drug – for example, patients who take wheat bran and find their constipation gets worse.

Milk Sickness

A disease known as milk sickness, characterized by weakness, nausea and collapse, has occasionally reached epidemic proportions in certain parts of the US. It probably caused the death of Abraham

Lincoln's mother. The name derives from the fact that the disease is brought on by drinking milk from cows made ill with a disease known as the trembles. This was eventually tracked down to the consumption, by cattle, of a plant known as snake root (*Eupatorium rugosum*), containing the chemical tremetone.

Along the same lines, lupin alkaloids have been known to be transferred to human beings via goat's milk. Birth abnormalities have been reported and, significantly, lupin alkaloids have the same effect on goat offspring.

Caffeine Family (Methylxanthines)

It is commonly forgotten that caffeine and theobromine (which occur in tea and coffee) are toxic substances. Taken in sufficient quantities they can cause cerebral oedema (so-called 'water on the brain'), convulsions and even death, though no one has ever been able to establish tissue damage caused by chronic ingestion at normal levels.

Salicylates

Salicylates (96) are aspirin-like chemicals that occur in many fruits and vegetables. They tend to cause pharmacological rather than allergic reactions. Adverse reactions are dose-related and only occur in sensitive individuals who have a constitutional predisposition.

Hypertensive Substances

These are aromatic amino compounds such as serotonin and noradrenalin, which constrict blood vessels and thereby elevate the blood-pressure. Such substances occur in chocolate, pineapple juice, avocado, alcohol and cheese.

Also see **phenolic testing (86)**

88. Post Viral Fatigue Syndrome

This unfortunate condition has been known by many names over the years including Myalgic Encephalomyelitis (ME), Epidemic Neuromyasthenia, Tapanui Flu, Iceland Disease, Royal Free Disease and Chronic Epstein Barr Virus (CEBV).

There is currently a fervour to find '*the* virus' that causes this condition. I don't believe any one virus is guilty. In fact, PVFS may not be a disease caused by a virus at all but rather a disease of the immune system (a 'flat' or underperforming immune system). Nobody seems to have asked whether the patients might not have contracted a virus *because* they have PVFS, instead of the other way round. Many patients, when asked, are quite simply unable to give any clear history of viral illness.

In fact there seems to be a spectrum of illnesses – including **Candida (16)**, multiple allergy, chronic chemical toxicity and post viral fatigue – that all mimic each other; indeed they overlap considerably. The final result (or perhaps the starting point?) is that all of them compromise the immune system. Is it a coincidence that our modern world, with all its toxicity, has seen the emergence of PVFS on a massive scale and a possible pandemic of AIDS? We must ask ourselves what we are doing to our immune systems, and whether we want to go on doing it. Doctors should know that this condition has now been recognized by the WHO as an organic brain disease.

CHARACTERISTICS OF PVFS

Two symptoms dominate the presentation of PVFS: fatigue and depression. Moods are often black and, indeed, suicides occur. Fatigue can be limiting to the point of crippling an individual's life. The psychological impact of this can be appalling and is enough to cause mental distress, so that a careless or unsympathetic doctor could easily imagine it to be a 'psychogenic' illness.

The limitation on physical activity has a peculiar and distinctive characteristic. It is as if the exercise itself brings on symptoms, just like an allergy.

Not appreciating this important point, many doctors make the mistake of telling the patient to 'do something'. There is the false belief that if he or she could only be made to run about and get fit, the patient would somehow recover. However frustratingly tempting this idea is, it is *false*. Individuals soon learn what their limitations are and learn to keep within these boundaries, for fear of the consequences. This gives the appearance that they are lazy, because friends and relatives see them looking fine but seemingly unwilling to do the things they once did with ease.

THE MYTHS

Two myths seem to have become entrenched in the PVFS story. Both are false but doctors cling to them avidly and patients, in ignorance, begin to believe these untruths themselves. The first is that PVFS will get better in time. The second is that it can't be treated.

Factually, none but the mildest cases will recover spontaneously. Waiting for something to happen is to court failure and unhappiness. The longer the condition persists, the more the patient will come to believe that he or she is special and 'can never be cured'.

PVFS is actually not difficult to treat. The basic condition (whatever it turns out to be) can be helped by the general application of the principles outlined in this book. Thus an improved diet works; detecting and getting rid of food allergies is often *dramatically* successful. Most sufferers, as I have remarked above, have Candida; many respond to a cleaner chemical environment, and good nutrition strengthens an ailing immune system.

None of this is necessarily going to 'cure' PVFS but it certainly can eliminate a host of symptoms and return a despairing sufferer to an active and useful life. Even a modest 20 per cent improvement may mean no longer having to lie in bed, but perhaps being able to return to work or studies. Many cases have a far greater degree of improvement – often 90 per cent or more.

The one thing that doesn't seem to respond too well to treatment is the limit to the amount of exercise a sufferer can take. It may improve a lot but it is often the last thing to improve and it rarely ever reverts 100 per cent to what the patient could do before the illness.

Antidepressants do *not* help. Giving gamma-globulin injections is 'playing at doctors and nurses' and not getting down to real issues.

TESTS FOR PVFS

There are claims made for a test for PVFS. Since we do not know the cause, this is entirely misleading and symptomatic of the medical profession's obsessive desire to have something to measure in the lab. What concerns me is that somehow, by default, a supposed culprit will be elected and those who haven't got the 'real' illness will once again be ignored.

Of course, other physical parameters may change in PVFS. Dr Behan in Glasgow has done a great deal to show that PVFS cases exhibit measurable physical changes, in neurological, muscle and immune tissue. It is *not* a psychosomatic disorder.

I am fond of drawing attention to the fact that lymphocyte changes in chronic PVFS are remarkably similar to those in AIDS. The only exception is that natural killer cells are not lost in PVFS (see Figure 88.1). Is this telling us something?

Treating PVFS

- Find and eliminate food allergies
- Desensitize (**enzyme potentiated desensitization (36)** or **Miller's method (74)**)
- Ensure an adequate and nutritious eating programme (maybe a **rotation diet (95)** for the time being)
- Clean up Candida
- Do chemical testing and unburden (see **body load (11)**) where necessary
- Try nutritional supplements: vitamins, minerals, **Co-enzyme Q10 (21)**
- Check: are **detoxification (26)** pathways normal? Consider **zinc (112)**, **magnesium (66)** and glutathione, etc.
- **Parasites (83)**: clean-up?
- Is **mercury toxicity (69)** an added problem?
- **Electrical fields (32)** or **geopathic stress (45)**?
- Adequate rest, harmony at home, outside interests or hobbies and a positive view of the future?

IN THE LONG TERM

It is vital for patients to maintain a positive attitude. It is all too easy to avoid the

	Total lymphocytes	Suppressor lymphocytes	Helper lymphocytes	Ratio	Natural killer cells
Acute PVFS	↓	↓	normal	↓	normal
Chronic PVFS	↓	normal	↓	↓	normal
AIDS	↓	normal at last	↓	↓	↓

Figure 88.1: Lymphocyte changes in PVFS, compared with AIDS

company of others who may not understand the illness. Once established, this kind of psychological deficit becomes very difficult to break, even when treatment should be signalling success. It will also alienate others, who then assume the patient doesn't want to get well.

The support of relatives and friends is needed. Yet all too often this is lacking, aided and abetted by medical practitioners who make pronouncements that are at best misguided and, at worst, downright destructive. The last thing a patient needs, when in the grips of a nightmare illness, is scorn and disbelief from those who are nearest and dearest.

Also see **chronic viral infections (20)**

89. Preconceptual Health Care

Despite sophisticated modern medical technology, around one in ten children born in the UK are deformed or handicapped in some way. Instead of decreasing, the incidence has been rising steadily. In Britain we hold the world record for cases of spina bifida; *ten times* that of our nearest rival (Canada) if we include Eire in the figures. The fact that geography seems implicated strongly argues an environmental cause. Yet this is one of the most under-researched areas in all of medicine. Table 89.1 summarizes some of the influencing factors known to date.

Factors Contributing to Foetal Malformation
- Alcohol
- Smoking
- Oral contraceptives
- Medical drugs (e.g. Thalidomide)
- Street drugs
- X-rays
- Maternal diseases (e.g. rubella, jaundice)
- Gross malnutrition (lack of protein and low food intake)
- Vitamin deficiencies (especially A, B_2, B_6)
- Vitamin excess (too much vitamin A, for example, causes neural tube defects)
- Folic acid deficiency
- Deficiency of trace elements, e.g. zinc
- Exposure to toxic elements (lead, mercury, cadmium)
- Exposure to other environmental pollutants (e.g. PCBs, 2,4,5-T and mycotoxins)

THE FORESIGHT ASSOCIATION

Veterinarians have known for years that it makes no sense to try to breed healthy offspring from malnourished, substandard stock. Yet we do it all the time with humans. Most couples pay no attention to their lifestyle or state of nutrition, blissfully assuming that all this has nothing to do with healthy babies. At the very best, they assume that proper antenatal care will deal with any potential problems. We now know this is not true. Stillbirths and congenital malformations in babies can be influenced markedly by what would-be parents do *before* they even try to conceive. By the time pregnancy has been established it may be *too late*; the damage may already have been done.

The Foresight Association, under the capable care of Mrs Peter Barnes, has for years been accumulating and codifying scientific evidence and doing their best to spread their findings to doctors, midwives and other health care workers. Some of their cases are quite remarkable: women who have had a succession of disastrous pregnancies have suddenly been able to go comfortably to term and produce a healthy, *normal* child! Even more remarkably, to date, no damaged child has been born to a couple who have gone through the Foresight programme properly.

Advice on improving your chances of a healthy pregnancy and baby is best sought from a physician practising Foresight counselling. A list of these doctors may be obtained direct from Foresight (see Useful Addresses). All couples could probably benefit from this care, but those who have had more than one unsuccessful pregnancy are especially advised to seek help. The man is as important in this as the woman: both members of a couple are counselled for best results.

THE SOCIAL POISONS

Three areas are of particular concern here. Smoking, alcohol and many drugs (including barbiturates and street drugs, such as marijuana and morphine) depress gonadotrophin secretion in both men and women (the gonadotrophic hormones make the sex cells productive). High doses of these toxins in women inhibit luteinizing hormone (LH) and so prevent ovulation. Lower doses simply postpone ovulation; this delay is well known to be associated with an increased frequency of pathological outcomes to pregnancy: either miscarriage or congenital malformations.

Based on animal studies and epidemiological surveys, the danger period seems to be from the beginning of ovulatory maturation until after fertilization, before the first division of the zygote. In other words, a matter of days only, around the time of conception. However, in men the risk of sperm abnormality seems to extend backwards several weeks, in fact some three or four months before conception. This is logical, since average spermatazoa take about three months to reach maturity.

A heavy intake of alcohol may result in the complete suppression of gonadotrophic hormones. The effect of more moderate doses is unclear, but it has been suggested that as little as two glasses of wine a week can affect the reproductive integrity of sensitive individuals.

Smoking is also a major risk, not just for the child in utero but preconceptually. Again this applies to both sexes. In women, the known vascular effects of nicotine would adversely affect the mucosal lining of the uterus. In males, abnormal sperm are produced. Cannabis has the same effect.

The link between smoking, drinking and pregnancy was illustrated by a study on 2,800 women in New York. Basically, those who smoked 20 a day and who drank daily had over four times the incidence of miscarriage risk than non-smokers and non-drinkers; non-smokers who drank daily had two and a half times the risk; and women who smoked but didn't drink were down to just over one and a half times the risk.

CHEMICAL POLLUTANTS

What about other so-called xenobiotics (foreign substances)? In view of the known risk of teratogenesis (malformation) associated with certain notorious chemicals such as 2,4,5-T, this is an important concern.

Thalidomide, although a drug, was also a xenobiotic chemical. The fact is that we are probably unaware of many chemicals that act on a pregnancy; there could be very many.

Heavy metal toxins (mercury, aluminium, lead and cadmium) can play their part. Many of the children born to mothers in Minamata in Japan, scene of the worst mercury poisoning incident ever recorded, were stillborn or malformed.

The connection between **lead (63)** and sterility, abortion and irregular menstruation has been known for over a hundred years. Now we can go further: there is conclusive evidence that if *either* parent is significantly exposed to lead, there is an increased risk of birth defects, mental retardation or behavioural disorder in the first year.

The term *behavioural teratogenesis* has been coined to cover those cases where the resulting effects may not be as severe as a malformed limb or spina bifida but where there is significant neurological impairment after birth. In other words the child grows up behaviourally disturbed, mentally retarded or in some other way disadvantaged. In view of the fact that these problems are now so prominent in our society and that contemporary levels of the toxins discussed above are so high, the connection seems clear.

NUTRITIONAL FACTORS

Many nutritional factors can affect fertility and the viability of a pregnancy: not only are gross nutrients such as protein (starvation and malnutrition) important, but also micronutrients. Work by Professor John Dickerson at Surrey University suggests that the disastrous effects of Thalidomide were due to that drug's effect in blocking B_2 utilization. In other words, it induced a serious vitamin deficiency and this was sufficient to produce the abnormal limb growths that so shocked the world.

The importance of **zinc (112)** is also particularly well documented; almost equally so is that of pyridoxine (vitamin B_6), **magnesium (66)** and folic acid. There are minerals and trace elements that have yet to be fully assessed.

Some of our evidence comes from animal studies, but the message is too clear to be considered inapplicable to humans and is at any rate confirmed by data gathered in Europe in times of food shortage, such as the Dutch famine winter of 1944–45 and Dresden following the defeat of the German army and Russian occupation (1944–45). It has been shown clearly that maternal malnutrition around the time of conception is much more damaging to the outcome of pregnancy than malnutrition during the later months. Once again, this is telling us that by the time pregnancy is established most of the critical factors have already come into play. By the time of the first antenatal visit, damage may have already been done (this should not be taken to mean that nutrition later in pregnancy is not important: it is).

In case you are wondering, this applies to the men also. Male fertility is partly controlled by the same pituitary hormones that control female fertility. Some nutrient deficiencies act directly on the male gonads and prevent spermatogenesis (development of sperm), which cannot be restored with pituitary hormones. Tests show four such nutrients are probably essential for spermatogenesis in rats, independently of hormone status: linoleic acid, vitamin A, vitamin E and zinc.

Adults appear to recover completely from periods of malnutrition lasting many months and severe enough to cause infertility. However, in the long term, poor reproductive performance associated with poor nutrition is highly correlated with age-specific death-rates of women and their husbands. In other words, poor breeders die younger.

Iodine is often overlooked, since we have it supplemented in our table salt and at other sources. However, deficiencies can lead to infertility. South American Indians living in the high mountains had a long tradition of feeding their womenfolk fish eggs (that are rich in iodine) lest they become infertile. They didn't know about iodine but they certainly knew about nutrition and fertility.

THE PILL

Dr Ellen Grant points out that the physiological changes in a woman caused by the contraceptive pill are very similar to those caused by smoking. There is a significantly greater risk to the health of a pregnant woman and that of her unborn offspring if she has taken the Pill for any length of time.

One study for the Family Planning Association showed that women who had never taken the Pill had a low incidence of abnormalities (0.4 per cent), compared to 3.8 per cent in those who had used the Pill, or almost 10 times as great a risk, though this did apply only to the first baby.

We know that age increases the incidence of chromosomal abnormality in mothers. Down's syndrome (mongolism) is one of the conditions caused by chromosomal abnormalities. It has been shown that there are increased rates of abnormal chromosomes among women taking 'low-dose' Pills.

We also know that young women on the Pill have a high level of glutathione peroxidase and that this leads to a lowering of B_2 and thus an increased risk of foetal abnormality (see remarks under the section on Nutritional Factors, above).

The advice, therefore, if you have been taking or are taking the Pill and you want to get pregnant, is to wait a full six months after stopping the Pill before trying to conceive.

Also see **nutrition and allergies (81)**

90. Premenstrual Tension (PMT)

Also known as pre-menstrual syndrome (PMS), this condition causes many women to feel dreadful at or about the time of their period. This has always been attributed to 'being a woman' and most doctors are unsympathetic on the assumption that these unpleasant symptoms are somehow supposed to happen. Hormones were blamed and women who 'complained too much' were viewed as weak-minded or hypochondriacal.

Recently, however, there has been a shift in opinion. We now recognize that a real illness exists when a woman feels unwell because of her monthly cycle. Symptoms are usually at their worst leading up to the menses and, to some extent, abate as soon as the flow starts. Hence the term *pre*menstrual tension (PMT), the 'tension' part referring to the fact that women tend to be extremely anxious and irritable either as a primary symptom or in consequence of other accompanying ones. It should be pointed out, however, that some women suffer 'premenstrually' almost all the time.

It is reckoned that 80 per cent of women now get PMT at some time in their lives and for 10 per cent it can be disabling. Even women who have had a hysterectomy and who, therefore, no longer have a period can get PMT.

THE SYMPTOMS

Symptoms can be severe. PMT may wreck lives and ruin relationships. Sometimes there is a strong temptation to violence that can only be kept in check by an effort of will. Some women fear they will harm their children; others act irrationally, taking their feelings out on their partner or friends. Afterwards they feel embarrassed and guilty, which only adds to their distress.

There are several different but related aspects of PMT. It is important to realize, however, that there is plenty of overlap and that few women suffer just one category of symptoms. Also, the pattern may change at different times in a woman's life.

Psychiatric Symptoms

Women can experience a tremendous and at times baffling array of moods and thoughts, experiencing anything from tension, irritability, vivid dreams and low mood to extreme anxiety and savage emotions – there have been famous cases of PMT leading to murder. Often fatigue is an important additional symptom. Most common are irritability, weepiness and anxiety.

DEPRESSION

Some women become profoundly low and filled with black gloom just before their period. Suicide in women is highest at this time. An easy diagnosis for the doctor is 'depression'. True, the woman *is* depressed, but the real cause is PMT.

Often a woman has nothing to be depressed about. She may have a loving partner, warm friends, a good job and a comfortable home. But when PMT strikes there is nothing she can do to ward off the misery.

Accompanying symptoms are weeping, forgetfulness and confusion (sometimes christened 'brain-fag').

Physical Symptoms

WATER RETENTION

Some women experience symptoms related to premenstrual fluid retention. This leads to weight gain, swelling of the breasts and possibly swelling of the abdomen and ankles.

CRAVINGS AND BINGEING

A curious symptom associated with PMT is that of craving certain foods, especially sweet things. The desire may become uncontrollable and the woman gorges herself until she is sick. This leads inevitably to weight gain and feelings of guilt. Too much sweet food can also aggravate psychiatric symptoms.

There may be concomitant **hypoglycaemia (55)**, associated with headaches, weakness, dizzy attacks, extreme fatigue and even fainting.

TREATMENT

Treatment is along sound clinical ecology practice lines. The patient should be helped to alleviate stress as much as possible and eat a varied, balanced and nutritious diet, *avoiding* certain obvious food triggers for several days before the anticipated onset of PMT.

These danger foods are principally white flour, white sugar, tea, coffee and alcohol. But all manufactured foods are best avoided, since these usually have a high sodium content and little nutritional worth. Other individual sensitivities may be known; these too should be given a wide berth. If other aspects of the treatment suggested here are

not working, the patient should try more vigorous exclusion dieting. Many allergic patients can eat a number of foods safely only at times when menstruation is not imminent.

Nutritional supplementation need not be aggressive but should be applied intelligently:

First, a good general multi-vitamin formula taken for several months will help with basic nutrition. In addition there must be no lack of **magnesium (66)**, B_6, **zinc (112)** or gamma-linolenic acid. Oil of Evening Primrose (500 to 1,000 mg, three times a day) or some other supply of linolenic acid should be maintained throughout the cycle, as too the multivitamin. Extra B_6, zinc and magnesium should be added, commencing about 10 days before the menses, concurrent with the start of dietary restrictions, if any.

Suitable doses are zinc citrate, 15 mg daily, magnesium chelate or orotate, 200 to 400 mg daily and B_6 to personal levels (B_6 levels can be established according to the regime outlined on page 150 of **nutrition and allergies (81)**. No more than 200 mg daily should be taken without advice from a physician).

An anti-hypoglycaemia diet and chromium (glucose factor) may help with the cravings and hypoglycaemia, as too might clearing up Candida, if present.

Finally, bloating and pain, if severe, may need medication. A diuretic or aspirin should be tried, if all else fails.

Hormone replacement therapy (HRT) is the counsel of desperation. Some women are helped; some made much worse.

Also see **hormones and allergy (51)**

91. Probiotics

One of the worst examples of excess in modern medicine is the over-prescription of antibiotics. These admittedly remarkable drugs come with a price-tag few doctors take into their reckoning or even seem aware of: for every unfriendly bacterium killed there are also friendly ones destroyed. This can have far-reaching and unpleasant consequences for the host organism.

We *need* the bacteria that live in our intestines. They protect us from unwanted pathogenic micro-organisms that would otherwise take over and make us very sick. An analogy would be weeds and flowers in the garden: if the beds are crowded with healthy plants, these will choke off weeds before they can become established. In fact, we now understand precisely how important normal bowel 'flora' is: if it is disrupted with antibiotics, what might be called *dysbiosis* sometimes is the result (dysbiosis = abnormal bowel flora, especially pathogens).

Symptoms of dysbiosis usually include bloating, flatulence, abdominal distress and diarrhoea or constipation. Fatigue, feeling unwell and numerous non-specific symptoms may also be part of the picture. Dysbiosis can lead directly or indirectly to poor nutrition. Inflammation of the intestinal wall will result in poor digestive and absorptive performance. Dysbiosis may also be a key factor in **'leaky gut' syndrome (64)**.

The main friendly bacteria to be found in the intestine are anaerobic (don't need oxygen): Bifidum and bacteroides bacteria. *Lactobacillus acidophilus* is more widely known but not present in such numbers. There are of course many other organisms, some of which cause disease if they leave the - intestine and travel, for instance, into the bladder. Probably as much as a third of faeces consists of the solid particulate matter of these dead bacteria, particularly Bifido and bacteroides bacteria.

The best-known offending pathogen to take over during dysbiosis is Candida albicans, although it is becoming clear that it may not be the only culprit (see **Candida (16)**). It now seems quite probable that other fermenting mould-type pathogens proliferate as well, yet they simply have not been assessed fully to date. Candida gets all the blame, and the condition is labelled 'Candidiasis'.

TREATMENT

The main point of treatment is, so far as possible, to remove the cause. If the patient has been subjected to a regular barrage of antibiotics, this should be discontinued. By definition, repeated courses are simply not solving the *real* problem but only treating the end result – the infections.

Return to normal flora can be assisted by taking oral supplements containing suitable live bacteria. These are called *probiotics*. *Lactobacillus acidophilus* is a suitable example, but *Lactobacillus bulgaricus* is equally effective. Both are found in live yoghourt, which may be a satisfactory supply for those not troubled with dairy allergy.

It makes more sense to top up with Bifido bacteria and bacteroides. The best preparations therefore include large amounts of Bifidobacteria, as well as 'acidophilus'. A recent refinement has been to select Lactobacillus strains from human sources. Logic says that these are antigenically more suitable for the human host environment and therefore more likely to flourish. Dairy-free brands are readily available.

Eat a diet that avoids refined carbohydrate in the form of white flour and sugar, as found in most commercial food supplies.

Also see **moulds (75)**

92. Prostaglandins

This important group of active body substances was first discovered in the early 1930s by a Swedish doctor, Ulf von Euler. He found that semen caused experimental smooth muscle samples to contract. Because the active ingredient was thought to originate from the prostate gland, the generic term *prostaglandin* was coined.

In the 1940s another Swede, Dr Sune Bergstrom, took the research further and found that prostaglandins were derived from fatty acids. He identified two types, which he called PGE1 and PGE2. It was also found that there were prostaglandins in many tissues, not just semen.

In 1971 a UK research student, Jim Willis, showed that aspirin and similar non-steroidal anti-inflammatory drugs (NSAIDs) used in treating pain actually worked by blocking the synthesis of prostaglandins. In 1973 Dr David Horrobin injected himself with prolactin and developed symptoms not unlike those that women get when premenstrual: bloating, irritability and depression. He later showed that prostaglandin El opposed this unpleasant effect.

Since then, we have learned that prostaglandins are hormone-like substances involved in a great variety of body functions, some of which appear to cause inflammation, blood clotting and other tissue damage, some of which appear to be beneficial. Probably the two types interact, keeping each other in check; perhaps a correct balance is what is needed for perfect health.

We now have a nomenclature for prostaglandins similar to that for vitamins: E, F, A, C and D. More than 50 have been identified so far, with a range of differing activities. Understanding the diverse roles of prostaglandins has advanced rapidly as intensive research continues.

SYNTHESIS

Prostaglandins are derived from **essential fatty acids (38)**. Linoleic acid is converted to gamma-linolenic acid, this is then turned into dihomogamma-linolenic acid, a precursor of prostaglandin El. But dihomogamma-linolenic acid is also a precursor of arachidonic acid, which leads to the E2 chain of prostaglandins (see Figure 92.1). Both PGE1 and PGE2 are vital to optimum health – an imbalance or lack seems to have adverse effects on the skin and cardio-vascular, reproductive and immune systems. The last is of special importance to allergics.

PGE1 is an extremely active substance with a whole range of properties, including inhibiting inflammation, preventing platelets sticking together, vasodilatation (leading to lowering of raised blood-pressure), inhibiting cholesterol production, and stimulating underactive brown adipose tissue (the kind that burns off excess fat).

The 2-series prostaglandins (derived from arachidonic acid), on the other hand, produce a reddening of the skin and tissue swelling. They are important in the pain-producing properties of chemical mediators such as bradykinin and **histamine (50)**.

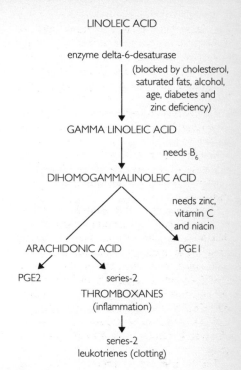

LINOLEIC ACID

enzyme delta-6-desaturase

(blocked by cholesterol, saturated fats, alcohol, age, diabetes and zinc deficiency)

GAMMA LINOLEIC ACID

needs B_6

DIHOMOGAMMALINOLEIC ACID

needs zinc, vitamin C and niacin

ARACHIDONIC ACID   PGE1

PGE2   series-2
THROMBOXANES
(inflammation)

series-2
leukotrienes (clotting)

Figure 92.1: Prostaglandin production

Arachidonic acid can also produce a group of substances called leukotrienes, which tend to promote inflammation or be converted to substances called thromboxanes. These have important blood-clotting effects which, although inconvenient in respect of myocardial infarction (heart attack brought on by a blood clot in the arteries of the heart) are nevertheless vital to the body. Without adequate blood clotting we would be at great risk (as haemophiliacs once were).

Together, the PGE1 and PGE2 play a part in regulating the immune system, controlling T-cell-mediated immunity (see **the immune system (56)**).

Also see **nutrition and allergies (81)**

93. Pulse Testing

Dr Arthur Coca, a leading American allergist, stated that his wife once reported that her pulse raced after eating certain foods. On this simple observation this great, pioneering doctor – who bridged the gap between clinical ecology and conventional immunologically-oriented allergy work comfortably – built a very interesting technique for detecting allergies, especially to foods.

Because Coca identified clearly a group of patients who had food allergies, ascertained that it ran in families and found no antibodies or other humoral agents to explain the reaction (nor yet have been), he called it familial non-reaginic food-allergy. A further characteristic of this type of allergic reaction is that it frequently raises the pulse rate. It is a very widespread phenomenon in the population: Coca put it as high as 90 per cent on circumstantial evidence.

He gave two important factors as the basis of his discovery, pointing out the dependability of the heart rate as a constant, if all other factors remain equal:

1. The daily pulse range (the difference between the slowest and fastest pulse rate of the day) is rarely greater than 16 beats per minute.
2. The daily maximum, remarkably, does not vary by more than two beats per minute.

Coca goes on to say that if the daily range of the pulse exceeds 20 and the daily maximal counts per minute vary by more than two beats, the patient is practically certainly affected with an allergy of the non-reaginic type. Furthermore, if the maximal count is 88 or higher, this is good corroborative evidence and the diagnosis can be upheld.

It must be pointed out that all this refers to a *resting* pulse rate and that there must be no other manifest clinical condition (such as a fever, heart disease, thyroid excess, anaemia, etc.) that would account for a high or variable pulse rate.

As Coca observed, a patient with allergies may present a completely normal pulse-record for several days on an unrestricted diet, though this is rare. We now know that if this occurs it is due to the 'masking' phenomenon (see **hidden allergy (49)**).

Coca's method has two aspects. First, he advocates a charted survey of the pulse over several days, the patient taking his or her pulse before getting out of bed in the morning, before each meal, twice after each meal (30 and 60 minutes afterwards) and then on retiring. This record may then be studied in the light of the above criteria. The chart we use in my own clinic is shown in Table 93.1. It is the chart of a 55-year-old woman with arthritis. It shows a range of 28 beats. Also you may note that each time she ate banana her pulse rate increased sharply, and she did indeed turn out to be allergic to banana. She was also allergic to tea, milk, egg and beef, but these caused no reaction on this survey, presumably due to the masking effect.

It is difficult to identify specific allergens by means of a chart such as this. It serves only as a general guide to the case. If by chance, however, it shows periods of normal pulse rate (such as on Day 1 and Day 6), the foods eaten before these periods may be selected as 'safe' and if the patient concentrates on those foods he or she may then have a steady baseline upon which to project individual feeding tests.

Coca carried out individual food tests on the basis of five small meals a day, consisting of one single food to be tested at each sitting. He recommended small portions so that the reaction, if there is one, clears more quickly. The resting pulse is used and must be counted for a full minute. It is recorded before ingesting the food and again 30, 60 and 90 minutes afterwards. Naturally the patient should avoid any provocative activities in the interim, otherwise confusion may occur, though it is not necessary to sit still for the entire one-and-a-half hours.

Safe foods may be used cumulatively. That is, foods that do not raise the pulse may be eaten along with the new food being tested. The time of day and also the sequence in which foods are tested is unimportant, Coca stated, though today we benefit by being able to suggest avoiding foods from the same family within the same two-day period, in case inadvertent cross-reaction and masking occurs.

Essentially this is a simple method and can easily be carried out by the individual on

One-Week Pulse Survey

	Day 1	Day 2	Day 3	Day 4	Day 5	Day 6	Day 7
pulse before breakfast	72	88	74	78	82	77	80
List food eaten for breakfast here	tea/milk, melon, egg	tea/milk, toast	tea/milk, bacon, egg, toast	tea/milk, apple, banana	tea/milk, smoked haddock, toast, egg	tea/milk bacon, egg, toast	tea/milk, apple, toast
30 mins after breakfast	74	86	78	93	80	83	76
60 mins after breakfast	80	80	82	85	81	76	76
pulse before lunch	76	70	76	81	74	80	68
List food eaten for lunch here	cheese, sandwich, chocolate biscuit, apple juice	ham, tomato, lettuce, banana, tea/milk	nut roast, tomato, lettuce, coleslaw, apple juice	cod in batter, potatoes, tea/milk	roast beef sandwich, orange, tea/milk	ham salad, tea/milk, biscuit	cheese sandwich, banana, ice cream, coffee/milk
pulse 30 mins after lunch	82	72	74	78	78	72	84
60 mins after lunch	72	84	68	84	83	74	82
pulse before dinner	78	76	72	80	74	71	76
List foods eaten for dinner here	steak, potato, broccoli, swede, gravy, cheesecake, coffee/cream	lamb chop, potatoes, cabbage, pear, cheese/biscuits, wine	spaghetti bolognese, date and walnut cake, coffee/cream	roast pork, roast potatoes, cabbage, swede, gravy, coffee/milk, cake	shepherd's pie, peas, carrots, gravy, tinned pears, cream, coffee	lamb casserole, with onions, carrot, potato, turnip, ice cream, cheese/biscuits, coffee	chilli con carne, salad, apple pie, cream, coffee
pulse 30 mins after dinner	80	76	74	76	78	65	80
60 mins after dinner	80	78	80	78	76	70	72

him- or herself. However there are one or two pitfalls. For example, cumulative reactions can occur. That is, a food that has little or no effect at first may, if eaten repeatedly as a 'safe' food, steadily increase the pulse rate. This problem can usually be sorted out by rotating safe foods.

Environmental factors may also confuse the issue. It may appear that a food is causing a reaction when in fact it is due to something in the room at the time of testing. It is important to keep conditions as consistent as possible, to avoid this difficulty.

Also see **applied kinesiology (9)**, **challenge testing (18)**, **cytotoxic tests (24)**, **Miller's method 74)** and **Vega machine (109)**

94. Radon

A build-up of the radioactive gas radon-222 within the home has only recently been perceived as an important environmental health hazard. The UK National Radiological Protection Board (NRPB) has recommended that levels of 20 milliSieverts be adopted as a desirable upper limit of domestic exposure for the time being and that this figure should be reduced to 5 mSv for homes built in future.

Radon is natural radioactive gas with a half-life (the time it takes for half the initial dose of radiation to fade and disappear altogether) of 3.8 days. It originates in the Earth's crust as a result of the decay of radium, which is itself a radioactive decay product from uranium and thorium. Because all soil contains uranium radon is widespread, but amounts vary from locality to locality.

High indoor levels of radon gas are now more prevalent, probably because of our energy-efficient, double-glazed and insulated buildings that trap air and keep it from circulating freely.

Granite rock areas are worst affected. In the US, high-risk localities are Maine, Pennsylvania, New Jersey and Florida. In Britain, danger zones are Cornwall and the Aberdeen area (Grampian). Sweden seems particularly hard hit and the government there has taken the matter very seriously.

The real concern is not radon gas itself, which is technically inert, but so-called 'radon daughters'. These are decay products – radioactive solids that can then attach themselves to airborne microscopic particles such as dust or cigarette smoke and lodge in the lungs. Here they will irradiate tissues and are known to add to the likelihood of lung cancer. Exposure to radon daughters by inhalation represents about half of the total dose of radiation humans get from all natural sources.

The American Environmental Protection Agency estimates that exposure to excessive radon levels may be responsible for as many as 10,000 to 30,000 lung cancer deaths each year. According to the National Radiological Protection Board 6 per cent – that is some 2,500 lung cancer deaths – may be the figure for the UK.

In areas considered 'high-risk' the NRPB will undertake a free survey of radon levels. For those who want to go it alone, there are devices on the market that measure radon levels in the home (contact Tech/Ops Landauer Inc. – see Useful Addresses).

Advice on reducing radon levels consists largely of improving the ventilation to house basements using extra-aeration bricks, assisted by fan extraction if the risk warrants it. Cracks in foundations should be sealed, as should openings at which pipes enter and leave the building.

Note: Radon exposure is not the same phenomenon as 'earth currents' or the radiation described under **geopathic stress (45)**.

Also see **irradiation of foods (61)**

95. Rotation Diets

This important subject for allergics has no relationship whatever to the rotation diet that was described for weight loss. The confusion of terminology is regrettable.

Those who have multiple allergies and are prone to rapid development of intolerances to new foods need to go on a rotation diet. Probably the combination of low-dose desensitization and a rotation diet is about as close as it is possible to get to an 'ideal' allergy programme. *Note:* the rotation principle is generally held to be counter-productive to the **enzyme potentiated desensitization (36)** approach.

It is very important not to remain on a long-term diet which is nutritionally inadequate. You will complicate your health problems considerably. If you find yourself reacting badly to a large number of substances, a rotation diet is a better answer.

It is rare indeed to have to avoid completely more than a handful of foods. The usual exceptions are the classical allergy reactions (Type 1 – see **hypersensitivity (53)**) that are very severe or even life-threatening. Usually it is possible to eat even poorly tolerated foods on an infrequent basis, provided your response isn't too severe and recovery is rapid. Keep a large repertoire of foods at all times and vary it constantly.

The minimum rotation period is four days. Less than that just isn't long enough to rest your system adequately. Some patients feel better rotating one day in five. Very sick patients sometimes can only allow themselves to eat one food per meal, and that food only once every seven days, but this is extreme.

You can construct your own rotation diet: a different meat for each day, a different fruit, a different drink and so on. The rules are quite simple. Any single food is allowed every four days. Members of the same food family can appear every second day (see Appendix A: Food Families).

A vexed question is whether you should eat a food more than once on the allowed day. The answer again depends on you: try it for yourself and see. Some people can get away with it, some can't.

Rotation dieting will often show up an allergy by unmasking it. If you start to react on a particular day, test the foods you ate that day again, individually (if you wake with the symptoms, of course, you will need to test the previous day's foods).

Basically, rotation diets are an onerous chore. Do not follow one unless there is a real need because of the seriousness of your illness or your tendency to develop new allergies.

An example of a rotation diet is given in Table 95.1, but you should modify it or make up your own.

Try to get organic foods if you can. Manufactured items are not permitted; many of these are adulterated. For example, a beefburger may contain not only beef, but soya, wheat (rusk), onion and several other items that cut right across the rotation plan. Similarly, complex foods such as cake, are not allowed. You must eat only simple, unprocessed items, bought fresh. This in itself makes for an improvement in health.

Once you have worked out a successful rotation diet on which you feel well it should continue to support you in good health, perhaps indefinitely, barring any adversity or stress. That means many of the foods you were formerly allergic to can be avoided for long periods; thus you may lose many food allergies by regaining your tolerance. Eventually, you should be able to enjoy, in moderation, many of your favourite indulgences. However, it must be stressed that these must only be returned to your diet on an occasional basis, otherwise you will soon be in trouble with them again. Remember: you may lose your individual allergies, but you are unlikely to lose the tendency to develop them.

EXTENDING THE ROTATION DIET

The diet is fairly simple and can be extended in a number of ways: for example, you may add a nut each day, a hot drink, a cold drink, and so on. The only practical limits to this are just how much complexity you can allow without getting confused and making mistakes; and how many safe foods you can find. Keep food families firmly in mind when making an addition, and don't cross these; in general, add similar foods on the same day or leave two days between foods of the same family.

MORE SEVERE CASES

Unfortunately, this straightforward approach may not be enough. Some people – again, usually the severe cases – need to follow a stricter set of rules in relation to rotating in order to be successful. This only applies to a minority of very sick patients who are temporarily overloaded, and on the advice of a physician.

The task is to work out a rotation diet based on the principle of 'one food, one

Expanded Four-Day Rotation Diet

Day	1.	2.	3.	4.
Meat	Pork	Beef	Lamb	Rabbit
Fowl	Chicken	Turkey	Pheasant	Duck
Fish	Cod	Salmon	Halibut	Mackerel
	Hake	Trout	Plaice	Tuna
Vegetables	Peas	Potato	Lentil	Tomato
	Broad bean	Peppers	Green bean	Lettuce
	Carrot	Leek	Parsnip	Onion
	Cabbage	Marrow	Broccoli	Courgettes
	Cauli	Artichoke	Celery	Asparagus
Fruit	Apple	Orange	Pear	Grapefruit
	Banana	Grape (raisin)	Pineapple	Sultanas
	Strawberry	Melon	Raspberry	Mango
	Kiwis	Peach	Papaya	Nectarine
Starch	Wheat	Buckwheat	Rice	Tapioca
	Corn	Sago	Oats	Quinoa
Drinks	Camomile tea	Fennel tea	Rooibosch Tea	Rosehip
	Apple juice	Grape juice	Pineapple juice	Grapefruit juice
Nuts	Brazil	Cashew	Walnut	Hazelnuts
Cooking Oil	Corn	Olive	Ground nut	Sunflower
Specials	Yams	Dates	Sweet potato	Figs
	Scallops	Shrimps	Venison	Lobster
	Soya milk	Milk	coffee	Goat's milk
	Chocolate	Honey	Carob	

Table 95.1

meal'. This may sound drastically restrictive – it is; but in almost all situations it is better than feeling ill. Of course, you would not need to stay on this regime permanently. It is wholly inadequate nutritionally. If you get your **body load (11)** down, you should be able to extend your food options in accordance with the seven-day diet plan given in Table 95.2, which was worked out by one of my patients.

PROBLEMS WITH THE ROTATION DIET

It is possible for your tolerance of a food to break down, even on a rotation diet. This could be caused by extra stress or an acute illness, or by exposure to some other type of allergen such as a gas leak. It is unfortunate if this happens but very important that you know how to deal with it. The key is forward planning. As soon as you succeed in making the rotation diet work for you – that is, as soon as your symptoms subside and stay away – at once begin testing to identify new and useful foods. Don't wait until the problem arrives before solving it: be ready.

After a week on the diet all other foods are now unmasked. You can then test one or two, following the usual procedure. Any that you find safe can be 'held in reserve' in case you need them. You don't need many, especially if you pick items from rare families that will fit more or less anywhere into the rotation without cutting across the scheme. Avoid

Seven Day Rotation Diet
Use fresh foods wherever possible – not tinned or frozen

	Sunday	Monday	Tuesday	Wednesday	Thursday	Friday	Saturday
Meat and Fish	Halibut Plaice Duck Deer	Chicken Eggs Pheasant Quail Turkey Anchovy	Beef Veal Milk Cream Cheese Yoghurt Rabbit Tuna Mackerel Skipjack	Pork Ham Bacon Sausage Lard	Cod Haddock Ling Hake Salmon Trout	Herring Pilchard Sardine	Lamb Mutton Goat Crab Lobster Prawn Shrimp
Vegetables	Peas Beans Liquorice	Cauliflower Swede Brussels Sprouts Broccoli	Onions Leek Garlic Chives Asparagus Mushrooms Chanterelle Yeast	Carrot Celery Parsley Parsnip	Potato Tomato Red, Green, Yellow Pepper Aubergine	Courgette Marrow Cucumber Pumpkin Spinach Olive Sesame	Cabbage Turnip Radish Chinese Leaves
Fruit	Cherry Plum Peach Apricot Prunes Lychee Loganberry Blackberry Strawberry Raspberry Grapefruit Chocolate	Pineapple Banana	Guava Kiwi Fruit	Grape Raisin Sultana Mango	Orange Lemon Lime Satsuma	Melon Apple Pear Quince	Rhubarb Buckwheat Currant Gooseberry Papaya Paw Paw
Nuts	Peanuts (Bean Family)	Pistachio (Mango Family)	Walnut Pecan	Cashew (Mango Family)	Brazil	Almond (Apple Family)	Hazelnut Coconut
Grain	Sugar Cane	Rye	Wheat	Oats	Millet Bamboo Barley	Rice	Corn
Juice/Drink	Grapefruit Juice	Pineapple Juice	Milk	Grape Juice	Orange Juice	Apple Juice	Blackcurrant Juice
Oil	Peanut Oil	Safflower Oil	Soya Oil	Grapeseed Oil	Sunflower Oil	Sesame Oil Olive Oil	Rapeseed Oil Corn Oil

spending too much time experimenting if it makes you ill; concentrate on maintaining your well-being instead. If a food does start to cause a reaction, you will then be able to find a substitute for it at once.

The following examples are foods which are, to all intents and purposes, separate families in their own right: eel, horsemeat, pigeon, carp, guava, brazil nut, papaya, kiwi fruit (Chinese gooseberry), sweet potato, quinoa, sesame and yam. Not all of them are easily available unless you happen to live in a large, cosmopolitan city, but the principle is important. By consulting the extensive list of food families given in Appendix A you should be able to choose items that are not related to the foods you were already accustomed to eating.

Also see **cyclical and fixed allergies (23)**, **diets (27)** and **dynamics of food (31)**

96. Salicylates

Aspirin is the commonly used name for the medicine *acetylsalicylic acid*. Allergy to this drug and its relatives remains high on the list of drug reactions. However, there are many similar substances throughout Nature, in plants, herbs, fruit and vegetables (indeed, aspirin properties were first discovered in the bark of the willow or *Cinchona*). These naturally-occurring salicylates also concern the allergist.

Aspirin allergy results primarily in skin rashes (hives), asthma and behavioural disturbance with children. However, any other **target organ (104)** can be affected, leading to colitis, headache, rhinitis (sneezing), etc.

Aspirin allergy does not necessarily occur in isolation. In one study, 75 per cent of people allergic to aspirin were also sensitive to inhalants (such as pollen and dust), 74 per cent were allergic to some sort of food and 43 per cent were allergic to other drugs. Also, cross-reactions to other analgesic drugs (painkillers) are quite common.

Dr Ben Feingold's original, now-famous diet to counteract **hyperactivity (52)** was based on the avoidance of aspirin and related compounds. It had limited success but was more successful when food colourings such as tartrazine were also removed, since these definitely cross-react. My experience with salicylate reactions, however, is that they are grossly overrated and often succeed incidentally (e.g. the patient is actually allergic to apple or a fruit and so gets better by chance on a 'salicylate-free' diet).

Foods Containing Salicylate
- Almonds
- Apples
- Apricots
- Blackberries
- Boysenberries
- Cherries
- Cucumbers and pickles
- Currants
- Dewberries
- Gooseberries
- Grapes and sultanas
- Nectarines
- Oranges
- Peaches
- Plums and prunes
- Raspberries
- Strawberries
- Tomatoes

Salicylate in Flavourings
- Antiseptics (e.g. ointments and mouthwashes)
- Bakery goods (except plain bread)
- Cake mixes
- Sausages/frankfurters
- Gum
- Ice-cream
- Jam and jelly
- Speciality meats (salami, bologna, etc.)
- Mint flavours
- Oil of wintergreen
- Margarine
- Sweets
- Toothpaste and toothpowder

Beverages
- Beer
- Cider and cider vinegars
- Diet drinks and supplements
- Gin and all distilled beverages (except vodka)
- Soft drinks (various)
- Tea
- Wine and wine vinegars

Plants

(Including the leaves, flowers, fruits, stems, bulbs, bark, and roots)

- Acacia
- Aspen
- Birch
- Calcanthus
- Camellia
- Hyacinth
- Marigold
- Milkwort
- Poplar
- Spiraea
- Teaberry
- Tulips
- Violets
- Willow

Suntan Lotions

Look for chemical names containing the words 'salicylate' or 'salicylic acid' (e.g. acetyl salicylic acid, ammonium salicylate, para amino-salicylic acid etc.)

- Arthropan Liquid
- Sal ethyl carbonate
- Salicylamide
- Santyl Ointment (santalyl salicylate)
- Stroncylate

Miscellaneous Contacts

- Methylene disalicylic acid (in lubricating oils)
- Perfumes and cosmetics
- Salicylanilide (antimildew)
- Soap (green, wintergreen fragrance)
- Sulphosalicylic acid (chemical)

DRUGS THAT MAY CROSS-REACT WITH ASPIRIN

A number of anti-inflammatory drugs cross-react with aspirin. The proprietary names are many and varied. Look for the proper (chemical) names fenoprofen, naproxen, ibuprofen, indomethacin, sulindac, tolmetin and phenylbutazone.

Note: Aspirin shows up in a variety of non-prescription remedies for headache, pain, menstrual discomfort, colds, fevers, etc. Aspirin allergics must exercise care. Dentists sometimes insert aspirin-containing wicks into tooth sockets during dental repair work.

Remember, also, tartrazine may be in many drug preparations, even laxatives, suppositories and vitamin preparations. Up-to-the-minute lists are difficult to maintain since they change constantly. Anyone who is allergic must therefore be vigilant on his or her own behalf.

Also see **chemical cleanup (19)**, **diets (27)** and **food additives (41)**

97. Seasonal Affective Disorder

Most of us feel happier, more cheerful and energetic during the warmer months. The long sunny days seem to bring out the best in us. The colder months are a time of greater ill-health and moody introversion.

In the past, this could be explained in part by the loss of vitamins and nutrients available from fresh food, which became more scarce with winter. We now get many of our foods fresh almost daily from distant, sunnier parts of the world, even in the depths of winter. Yet the problem hasn't gone away. This suggests another factor may be at work.

Many animals solve the problem of cold weather torpor in northern latitudes by going into hibernation. It has long been assumed that such seasonal biological variations do not affect humans – after all, we have fire. Yet some of us, is seems, are not quite free of winter malaise. The key to this condition is *light*.

A number of studies in recent years have shown that diminution in the surrounding light levels can result in a marked decline in mental activity. For most of us this might be hardly noticeable, but for some individuals, this change can bring on symptoms, such as depression. Because it is thought to be seasonal and the medical word for mood is *affect*, this postulated condition is called *seasonal affective disorder*, or SAD for short.

Estimates place sufferers at between 5 and 10 per cent of the population. Women experience it more than men by about 4:1. It is said to be associated with weak immunity and increased susceptibility to infections, so this is of interest to allergy doctors and patients. So too is the fact that patients tend to crave sweet foods, binge and put on weight, which sounds very like food intolerance. There may also be a loss of libido, and SAD can run in families.

RESEARCH

Links between health and light have been understood for a long time. For example, sunlight on the skin is known to be one of the sources of vitamin D. Rickets became very common in large cities, where smoky atmosphere cut off the sun, before the vitamin D connection was discovered and smoke-free regulations helped to solve the problem. Light also helps clear jaundice in the newborn child.

However, the realization that light is important to mood has been slow in coming. Now psychiatrists in the US and Britain have carried out studies that seem to prove the existence of SAD. Adults suffer primarily from symptoms of depression, lethargy and overeating. Children, it appears, tend more towards lack of sleep, irritability and withdrawal. The effect on school performance can be quite detrimental.

We are used to the idea of 'biological clocks'; they are such a nuisance when it comes to travel, causing jet lag. The menstrual cycle of women clearly originated aeons ago from phases of the moon. It seems quite logical, therefore, that the sun, so much more powerful and dominating, should also have regulating effects. In fact, researchers believe that solar radiation levels play a part in controlling, or at least influencing, endocrine function, immune responsiveness, stress, fatigue, control of viral infections and absorption of calcium and phosphorus, as well as those factors already mentioned.

Light Intensity

Artificial light is poor compared to natural lighting. Even on a dull day, outdoor light levels may be 200 times brighter than those indoors. The trouble is we now spend more time indoors than ever before; we have cut ourselves off almost completely from the sun.

The problem is made worse, it seems, by the wrong *quality* of light. Electric lamps produce a very distorted light, with an excess of red rays. Even fluorescent 'daylight' lighting, which is better, comes nowhere near the true composition of natural ambient light. It has far too much yellow and green (cool colours). Incidentally, do not confuse this term 'daylight' lighting with *full-spectrum lighting*, which is discussed below.

TREATMENT

Predictably, most doctors prescribe anti-depressants for this condition. Yet the best treatment for SAD sufferers is light! Obviously, real sunlight is best and one of the reasons that winter holidays abroad are becoming so popular among the British is the fact that they are undoubtedly healthful and invigorating, allowing for large doses of full-spectrum natural light just when it is most scarce at home.

For more lengthy treatments, some source of 'artificial sun' is required. It is vital to get units that deliver so-called *full-spectrum light*, which equates as nearly as possible the quality of sunlight. These are now available commercially at a reasonably economical price, though they are of course many times more costly than fluorescent so-called 'daylight' tubes. Details of a supplier in the UK are given in the Useful Addresses section of this book.

Medical workers in this field suggest several hours a day of exposure to full-spectrum light. The most practical way to achieve this is to work near a high-intensity source, but for many this isn't practical. It may be necessary to divide the 'dose' between two sessions, night and morning. This way, up to six hours a day might be taken to advantage.

If you suspect SAD in your own case, draw back the curtains and blinds, open the windows as often as the weather allows and make a point of frequent walks in the open air. Even the pale, wintry sun is many times brighter than any artificial light source! Try to arrange two weeks' holiday in the sun in the depths of winter, when experience tells you that you are at your lowest ebb. This should help you recharge psychologically until spring comes along.

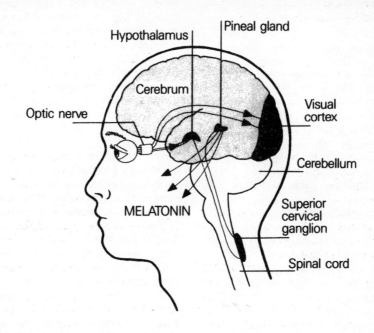

Figure 97.1: Optical pathways and the pineal gland

Incidentally, it is light to the eyes that matters – not, as in some medical conditions, light to the skin.

Finally, there is an association for those who want support for SAD, the Seasonal Affective Disorder Association (see Useful Addresses).

Also see **environmental allergies (34)**, **hormones and allergy (51)** and **noise (80)**

98. Sexual Hypersensitivities

Allergic reactions that interfere with sexual activity cause a particularly distressing condition that is not nearly as rare as is supposed. The effect on a woman of finding that she is allergic to her husband's semen can be devastating psychologically as well as physically.

The whole area of sex-related allergies is complex and is rendered even more difficult due to the natural reticence of most patients.

There are a number of true allergic reactions and also hypersensitivity reactions and straightforward irritation. Diagnosing the correct cause of trouble is crucial to managing it successfully. Even so, some cases are difficult to resolve.

With any kind of inflammatory reaction, both men and women can be affected. Women usually experience vulvo-vaginitis, that is, inflammation and irritation of the vulva and vaginal area. In males, inflammation of the tip of the penis (balanitis) occurs. The reaction can spread to other parts of the body. This is especially true of women, who have been known to have severe systemic (total body) allergic reactions following intercourse.

Sexual reaction can have a number of causes:

- Infective organisms
- The products of ejaculation
- Contraceptive substances and devices
- Cosmetics
- Incidental contact with unusual substances

MICROBIAL HYPERSENSITIVITY

A number of organisms in infective conditions can affect the genital area. 'Honeymoon' cystitis of course does not confine itself solely to the honeymoon period. Repeated attacks of painful urination and bladder irritation can frequently follow intercourse.

Bacterial vaginosis is more directly related to intercourse with an infected partner. A vaginal discharge is the usual accompaniment. Pathogens are mostly mixed, including *Gardnerella vaginalis* and various anaerobes (bacteria that live without oxygen). The characteristic foul smell of the discharge is produced by volatile amines such as methylamine, ethylamine and putrazine. These substances can be released by contact with seminal fluid, which is alkaline, and the sudden spread to the tissues can give rise to flushing, irritation and other symptoms that may lead the partners to assume (erroneously) that they are 'allergic to sex'.

Candidiasis

This may not show itself on repeated vaginal swabs but can be a cause of intense vulvo-vaginal irritation made worse by intercourse. In addition, patients may show a true allergic IgG-mediated type **hypersensitivity (53)** to Candida albicans.

Balanitis

De-epithelialization of the glans penis is a poorly documented condition that often affects men. Perhaps because the penile epithelium is unaccustomed to exposure, prolonged or forceful intercourse, especially if lubrication is poor, may occasionally rub and inflame it. This condition needs to be distinguished from a true inflammatory balanitis caused by hypersensitivity reactions to vaginal micro-organisms, spermicides, etc.

SEMEN

Allergy to semen was first described in 1967 by Halpern et al, who reported a case of a 29-year-old atopic woman who developed asthma after intercourse. In another case, reported in 1974, increasing hypersensitivity reactions culminated in an anaphylactic-type circulatory collapse. Since then, the condition has been widely described and this unusual diagnosis is now only missed when the attending physician is insufficiently attentive to the patient's reported history.

Diagnosis may be made by patch testing or, as is done at our clinic, with intradermal testing of the serial titration type. For moral and ethical reasons we prefer to use the husband's own semen, though the semen of most men appears to contain the same sensitizing agents. Apparently these agents come from the seminal vesicles.

Note: Women can also have allergic reactions to substances *via* their partners' semen. One of my patients reacted to her husband's medication. This was discovered by her having sex with and without condoms and with and without the medication; we were able to show that the allergy was not a semen allergy. Literature also contains a case of a woman who had an anaphylactic reaction to walnuts. She was highly allergic to them and, if her husband had been eating walnuts immediately prior to coitus, she would have a similarly severe reaction after intercourse. Walnut protein was demonstrated in the semen.

A woman may react to her partner's aftershave, topical ointments, etc. by direct contact. This may be very puzzling until the true cause is deduced. The usual culprit is propylene glycol, which is also widely used as a vehicle for cosmetics, body lotions, anti-perspirants and topical medicines.

CONTRACEPTIVES

Some men (and also women) experience a hypersensitivity reaction to the rubber of contraceptive sheaths. The usual culprits are additive reagents to the rubber itself, but reactions may also be due to the 'sensitizing' solutions used by the condom manufacturers for enhancement purposes. Allergic hypersensitivity to *K-Y Jelly* and other lubricants has also been reported.

COSMETICS

A number of local applications to the genital area may cause hypersensitivity reactions, which on occasion could be aggravated during sex and appear to be caused by sex. Such applications include perfumes, hygiene sprays, soaps, bubble baths and locally applied medications containing notorious sensitizers such as amino glycocides, tetracyclines, chlorohexadine, hexachlorophane and chloroxylenol. Some women wear self-adhesive pads to contain vaginal secretions, which may contain disinfectants and scents (acetyl acetonate and derivatives). Hypersensitivity to clotrimazole, a common anti-Candida treatment, may be the cause in a woman whose vaginal irritation worsens when she receives treatment for thrush.

Taking a detailed history is very important. This may bring to light unusual sexual practices – as in the case of the woman who had a severe inflammatory vulvo-vaginitis caused by her lover anointing his penis with a rubefacient cream, the idea being to cause both partners stimulation from the warm 'glow' that resulted.

INCIDENTAL ALLERGENS

Sometimes allergic reactions may occur at intercourse due to some non-obvious cause, for example, allergy to the duvet. Another reported case was allergic hypersensitivity to newsprint, which was transferred to the vulva via the husband's fingers. He was in the habit of reading the newspaper before retiring for the night and he carried with him sufficient chemicals to cause his wife to react.

TREATMENT

The most obvious treatment is avoidance where possible, for example no spermicides, cosmetics, douches, etc. Identification is clearly important. Patch tests are not reliable.

For semen allergy, desensitization may be tried with the Miller's low-dose technique, which is the only safe method. Antihistamine creams or tablets, such as diphenhydramine hydrochloride, may be tried.

The use of condoms, if acceptable, may be a way of avoiding semen hypersensitivity or a reaction to a partner's ingestants.

Genital infections need treating in the usual way and are seldom tackled vigorously enough. For example, it makes good prescribing sense to treat both partners at the same time, to prevent 'ping-pong infections' (backwards and forwards). Broad spectrum antibiotics such as tetracycline may be needed for chlamydia and anaerobes, metronidazole (*Flagyl*) is the recognized treatment for Trichomoniasis vaginalis and chlamydia.

ALLERGIES AND APHRODISIACS

Allergies play a part in arousal for many people, whether they know it or not. Reactions to food are often rather like intoxication, the effect on the brain being alterations in function very similar to those everyone is familiar with in connection with **alcohol (2)**. Many patients, especially women, are able to describe dramatic events of arousal following allergy **challenge testing (18)**.

Certain foods since time immemorial have been ascribed the power of increasing sexual desire (aphrodisiacs). You may be aware of the reputation of some of them. But as you will see from Table 98.1, any food may do it if the individual is maladapted to it and it produces a slightly enhanced reaction! Alcohol has always been the most potent of these foodstuffs, simply because by its nature it tends to provoke stimulatory reactions to the foods contained in the beverage. Those of you who know what 'brewer's droop' is will understand that it also impairs function. Thus Shakespeare was right when he had the porter in *Macbeth* declare that alcohol 'provokes the desire, but it takes away the performance' (II, iii).

In fact allergies can both stimulate and suppress, though usually depression follows too much stimulation (exactly as with alcohol). Dr Theron Randolph tabulated the main effects, and these are shown here. Compare this table with that given for general cerebral stimulation due to maladaptation, also by Theron Randolph (see **brain allergy (12)**).

Changes in Sexuality at Various Levels of Reaction

++++ Performance commonly impossible
+++ Excessive desire: poorly co-ordinated performance
++ Hypersexuality in both desire and performance
+ Normal to slightly heightened sexuality
0 Normal
− Normal to slightly reduced sexuality
−− Debility and diminished desire and performance
−−− Female frigidity and male impotence occur
−−−− Frigidity and impotence the rule

Also see **target organs (104)**

99. Sick Building Syndrome

Few working people today are unaware that certain buildings have serious problems that affect the health of the occupants. Almost invariably these are modern offices and public buildings, incorporating the 'latest advances' in design and technology. Yet something is often seriously wrong and illness and absenteeism among staff working in affected premises sometimes reaches such major proportions that the cost to industry becomes a major concern.

Origins of this 'sick building syndrome' may be classified into different physical factors affecting the modern workplace, or according to the symptomatology produced. Taking the physical factors first, a number of possibilities have been suggested:

● chemicals
● electro-magnetism
● lighting
● humidity
● air flow
● carbon dioxide levels
● biological sources (mould, bacteria, etc.)

Several of these in turn are a function of other factors, such as temperature, the quality of air exchange and the structural materials present.

Classification according to symptomatology is less revealing. As with any environmental illness, potential manifestations are almost as legion as the individuals concerned. However, there seem to be important sub-groups, such as:

● headache and lethargy
● dry eyes and throat
● rhinitis (runny and/or blocked nose)
● type I **hypersensitivity (53)** reactions ('true' allergy)

PHYSICAL FACTORS

Chemicals

Clinical ecologists are well aware that minute ambient levels of toxic chemicals can make people ill. It may be supposed that this affects only a very small minority of people, but the number of sufferers will increase as the concentration of chemicals goes up or if the exposure continues for a long period of time.

Visitors to a building with a high chemical burden in its atmosphere may notice little more than an unpleasant smell and maybe an inconvenient attack of runny nose or itchy eyes. But if the exposure is continued for weeks, then months, as with an employee, then it is fairly certain that the phenomenon of sensitization will take place; that is, more and more people will become especially intolerant of the chemicals present. In fact this is exactly what seems to happen; serial studies have shown that the problem gets worse as a function of time.

Where do these ambient chemicals come from? Actually very many sources. New carpets, laminates, plastics, fabric treatments, polyurethane surfaces (desk tops, etc.), photocopiers and cleaning fluids all add their share of chemicals. Many of these are volatile organic substances, such as toluene and xylene, which have a high affinity for human (animal) tissue and readily get into the body and are taken up by the brain, being very fat-soluble.

From the moment it is built the actual fabric of a building begins to deteriorate. Bacteria and mould accelerate this process. Whatever humans can devise, usually there is some micro-organism or other that has the knack of breaking it down chemically. This is part of the very essence of Nature's process, decomposing, recycling and re-building. There are thousands of fungi that attack work-surfaces, walls, drapes, etc. and some of them are regular little laboratories that would be the envy of Du Pont. Polyurethane (foams in upholstery and varnishes on wooden surfaces) is made from cyanates and certain organisms attack it with facility, yielding back toxic cyanates in so doing. Urea-formaldehyde, it is well known, gives off highly irritant formaldehyde gas. Urea-formaldehyde foam is used in cavity-wall insulation. Not all buildings have it (it is banned in the US). But phenol-formaldehyde and melamine-formaldehyde also break down in the same way, and these are present in almost all modern buildings.

Electro-magnetism

Most offices have a great deal of electrical and electronic equipment. These give off significant electro-magnetic fields and also **microwaves (71)**. Some people are more susceptible than others and could be affected adversely by operating within these fields. Alternatively, the artificial fields may neutralize or overwhelm the body's familiar terrestrial magnetic field. We now know, from the unpleasant experiences of the early astronauts, that this field is essential to our well-being; we lose or disturb it at our peril.

Individuals who have a problem may need to ask for a less electrically 'polluted' workspace or to get unnecessary equipment switched off. Just re-siting the desk may help; the effect seems worse if the individual is located in an area surrounded by trans-mitting equipment. If it is all arranged to one side or the other, the impact seems to be less.

Lighting

Many people without medical training are aware that they feel unwell in the presence of fluorescent lighting, so typical of modern offices. No one is certain why. Various remedies have been advocated, from wearing something dark on the head to taking large doses of vitamin A.

Tests made with a field meter (see **electrical fields and allergies (32)**) show a distinct radiation field down to about shoulder level from fluorescent lights at average ceiling height. It can sometimes even be detected coming through the floor from the room below. The effects of electro-magnetic fields are probably far more serious than has been previously supposed, but this remains very much a research area at the moment.

Interesting experiments have suggested that it might be the frequency of the fluorescent light that is at the root of the problem. Fifty to sixty hertz is about the most biologically disagreeable frequency possible. Fluorescent lighting is more prone to flicker than the ordinary tungsten bulb and so the effect shows up more. Some workers claim that altering to a different frequency removes the unpleasantness of fluorescent tubes and that this is reflected in improvements in office health. Suitable frequencies seem to be about 500,000 hertz – tubes are available commercially with this in mind.

Humidity

We really mean *relative humidity*, expressed as a percentage of the total possible moisture content. That is what the human body perceives as 'damp' or 'dry' atmospheric conditions. The air on a dry, warm summer's day (50 per cent humidity) actually holds more moisture than on a wet, cold winter's day (100 per cent humidity). Relative humidity is a function of both the moisture content of the air and the temperature.

For any given moisture content, the humidity falls as the temperature rises (and vice versa). This is of crucial importance in our modern heated buildings. Air from outside is drawn in and then warms up. Unless extra moisture is added, the humidity inside will be less than that outside. The general view is that humidity needs to be between 40 and 75 per cent for comfort, but in fact most people would find 40 per cent unpleasant after any but the shortest exposure and 75 soon begins to feel 'clammy'; 45 to 60 per cent is a much better range. Thus air that is saturated at 5° outside may have a relative humidity of only 40 per cent at 20° inside; at 22° this may be an uncomfortable 35 per cent; remember this is the *same* moisture content.

The reverse of this is the way that water condenses when room air meets a wall or window and is suddenly cooled. The relative humidity rises sharply, until the saturation point (100 per cent) is reached and precipitation occurs. This is usually very obvious on the windows but less so on or in the walls. Yet in these damp conditions bacteria, mites and fungi can grow which have a great impact on health, especially for allergics. The resultant reactions can be dermal (skin-related) but are usually respiratory in type and can be sufficiently severe, when the individual is sensitized, to be a threat to life.

HUMIDIFIERS AND DEHUMIDIFIERS

Attempts to regulate the humidity of buildings may obviously involve adding moisture to air-conditioned atmospheres or removing water vapour in other circumstances. The equipment necessary is known as a humidifier or dehumidifier. The same principle can be applied, on a smaller scale, to the home.

The disadvantage of humidifiers is that the water they contain provides an ideal culture medium for micro-organisms – bacteria, mites and **moulds (75)** of all kinds. Once again, patients become sensitized to these and can experience serious reactions of the type 1 hypersensitivity kind which can be a serious threat to safety, as well as health.

Unfortunately, the same holds true of dehumidifiers, since the condensation surfaces become waterlogged (deliberately) and water accumulates in the collection chamber. Only constant maintenance can protect them (see **environmental allergies (34)**). Local air purifiers are better because they remove spores without changing the humidity level.

COOLING TOWERS

It isn't often appreciated that, even in cold and temperate climates, air-conditioning is largely concerned with keeping the atmosphere cool. A building full of human beings, each emanating heat energy at 65 watts, generates a considerable amount of heat which may not be satisfactorily dispersed in modern sealed-ventilation systems. Most air-conditioning systems therefore include cooling towers rather than heaters, an arrangement of baffles and plates that lower the air-temperature before recirculating the air. The expense of running these systems is actually a cooling cost rather than a heating cost. These too run permanently wet, due to the condensation process, and are equally subject to invasion and contamination by micro-organisms. Attention has especially been focused on this problem of water collection due to *Legionella* (Legionnaire's disease). Unfortunately, this infection carries around a 20 per cent fatality rate. The tendency now therefore is to run air-conditioning systems 'dry' and accept the loss in humidity. Up to a point this can be tolerated but there may be serious problems, as outlined below.

Air-flow Rate

People have now become keenly aware of smoking and other pollution in their place of work. The majority want adequate air-exchange to get rid of offensive odours and irritant pollutants. A satisfactory rate from the point of view of removing carbon dioxide exhaled and renewing oxygen levels would be about 1 litre per person per second. To clear the air of offensive odours, something nearer 5 litres is required and, in many UK boroughs, by-laws require this level of exchange. Recommendations may be higher, at 8 litres, and many engineering firms, erring on the side of efficiency, may supply 12 litres per person per second, levels which would be more suitable to public buildings and halls with a drinks bar and heavy smoking than a typical office.

Remember also that these are *fresh air* figures. Due to recirculation of a portion of existing air this 12 litres may be a part of a system handling 25 litres per second. A new factor then enters, which is wind-chill. Air moving at such a rate is necessarily perceived as cold. It needs to be warmed and, naturally, this lowers the humidity markedly. Moving dry air has very unpleasant dehydrating qualities and some people cannot tolerate it. The effects can be both pronounced and varied, producing sore eyes, dry, burning mouth and lips, dry skin and even eczema in susceptible individuals.

Ironically, this very low humidity tidal air is said by many experts to be the worst contributor to sick building syndrome. The best efforts to produce clean fresh air in quantity may make the problem paradoxically worse.

Carbon Dioxide (CO_2) Levels

It is widely supposed that the incentive to breathe is lack of oxygen. As the levels drop, the brain is stimulated to provoke more respiration and so rectify the situation. Actually, this isn't so. Nor is it logical: otherwise a brain knocked out by a deficit of oxygen couldn't rescue itself! In fact the drive to the respiratory centre is excess carbon dioxide. As it accumulates in the blood, the control centres recognize that breathing is too slow and speed up the rate. It works fine.

Except in some modern buildings, that is. Air subject to wet recirculation, such as that produced by cooling towers or humidifiers, is scrubbed of carbon dioxide. This may be made worse by alkaline solutions used for sterilizing purposes. The CO_2 content of office air can fall dramatically low.

This means that the respiratory centres lose their drive. Respiration rates will drop and this will produce an unwanted hypoxia (low blood oxygen). This is the *opposite* of **hyperventilation (54)**. The brain will be affected progressively, at first leading to mild dysfunction (yawning and lethargy) which gradually gets worse, with headache, serious malfunction and finally unconsciousness on the way down. Fortunately, office spaces rarely get down to zero carbon dioxide, so coma is not encountered, but lethargy and headache are very common in buildings of this type. In fact probably much more common than is supposed, since many people would be reluctant to report to their employer that they keep falling asleep at their desk.

Also see **chemical cleanup (19)** and **weather and health (111)**

100. Stress

It is common knowledge that stress makes allergies worse; it is a careless or lazy diagnosis, however, simply to dismiss a patient as neurotic because this is true. Worry or anxiety may make a rash worse, but if the rash is caused by a milk allergy, the real remedy is obvious.

There is the additional complication that many allergic reactions include a degree of **'brain allergy' (12)** that may result in the patient feeling anxious, tense, depressed or even out of touch with reality. This reinforces the idea that the patient has a psychosomatic illness. Doctors then switch off and won't even consider other possibilities. Many patients will testify that once any kind of psychiatric diagnosis is entered on their notes they can no longer obtain much sympathy or understanding for any other type of illness. Even tumours, bacterial invasions and gallstones may be written off as 'psychogenic' until the truth forces its way out despite the doctor's unwillingness to listen.

Even if there is a frankly psychogenic illness at work, it will be a lot easier to deal with when the patient is getting good nourishment and is free of environmental triggers.

STRESS AND THE IMMUNE SYSTEM

We are beginning to understand how emotions can affect the way our bodies react to disease. The term *psycho-immunology* has been coined to define the way in which mental attitude can influence functioning of the immune system. Many scientific papers have now emerged showing there is a direct relationship between mood or stress factors and cell performance; even the lymphocyte count can go down if the patient is depressed and negative. Some of this comes from work in studying AIDS cases, but it is also important in considering cancer, another disease of the immune system.

Patients with AIDS are now being taught to visualize their immune systems and create mental 'mock-ups' of white cells battling away against the virus. Remarkable though it may seem this can actually lead to a betterment of the blood-cell profile. This has now even reached the state where there are computer simulations in some hospitals, rather like electronic arcade games, depicting the body's immune cells at work 'zapping' the invader. This helps at a subconscious level to get the immune system moving, as if by creating a belief in 'self'.

Though we don't know the exact mechanism, it is possible to speculate that some sort of humoral (chemical) control exists via the hypothalamus, that very important regulatory centre at the base of the brain. It is already known to be widely implicated in the cross-over between our feelings and state of mind and the body's physiology. We may be talking of some kind of hormone; research is continuing and it is too early to say for sure.

The fact is, it does happen and can be observed and measured. The lesson to be learned for allergics therefore is quite straightforward and very important: think positive!

By the nature of their illness allergics have to avoid certain substances that are common in our environment. There is, therefore, a constant pressure to remain isolated and alone. This is wrong, no matter how tempting, because such individuals can become highly introverted and so plunge even more deeply into an obsession with their condition, which makes the problem far worse.

You must make a positive effort (and it may be an effort) to contact others and share in a normal life with friends and family. Be willing to take a few rebuffs; you will surely get some. But without being overoptimistic it is possible to state that most people have now heard of someone or other who is allergic and has to follow unusual lifestyle restrictions. See yourself, if you wish, as a pioneer from whom others can learn. It all comes under thinking positively!

STRESS FACTORS

Remember, not all stress is mental. Other factors can include fatigue, undernutrition, chemical toxins, drugs, hidden infections, hormone dysregulation and exhaustion.

These factors can all make allergies worse by lowering the body's resistance. Allergies themselves are stressful, which is rather a vicious circle in some cases and explains why sometimes a patient gets ill due, say, to a viral condition and then never really gets over it: the allergies themselves maintain the stress and recovery is not possible until the allergies are detected and defused.

Hans Selye's theory about stress is a good one (see **general adaptation syndrome (44)**) in that it explains the observed facts and enables us to make certain predictions. For example, if stress goes on too long there will come a time when no adverse effects can be observed, yet this will inevitably lead to a serious deterioration unless the stress is removed. The actual period of time this takes will vary according to the individual and the type of stress.

A lot of people ask for trouble by pushing themselves too far. It's a hectic society we live in and often relentless pressure assails the individual who wants to do a little more than just get by. Success comes at a price and often the price is too high. It isn't really worth striving for material goals if by the time you achieve what you want bad health prevents you from enjoying your triumph. The neurotic rich are a study in hang-ups and pathology. It is worth while stopping to consider whether you really want to join them.

Remember, the body begins to recover as soon as you remove stress. It may take a long time, but as soon as you control the adverse factors things will begin to look up. The fact is it's never too late to change. There are many worthwhile goals in life apart from a bigger house or more prestigious car. It may be time to set yourself some spiritual goals; perhaps more time with the kids, that special holiday you've always promised yourself. Remember, the harder it is for you to contemplate this sort of thing, the more in the grip of the rat race you are. People who can take time off at the drop of a hat and go for a few days' walking tour in Scotland are not really under much pressure. It is people who 'can't get away' who are the ones who must do so, for their own sakes.

Perhaps you are not doing what you most want to do in life. This can be built up into an unbearable stress and is a cause of a great deal of bitterness and frustration. A reappraisal of your career may be in order. The truth is, many people have switched tracks successfully later in life and been glad they did. Neither is being sacked the end of the world if the struggle to hold down a job is an unequal one. For some any change would be an improvement and lead to a more worthwhile and contented way of life.

Also see **body load (11)** and **hyper-ventilation (54)**

101. Sudden Infant Death Syndrome (SIDS)

Two fifths of all infant deaths (under the age of 12 months) are sudden and inexplicable. Having ruled out infections, suffocation, parental violence, congenital abnormalities and other detectable possible causes of death, 1,500 infant fatalities per year (over 2 per 1,000 births) happen without prior warning and in mysterious circumstances (these are the figures for England and Wales combined).

In the absence of any real explanation, this distressing phenomenon was labelled Sudden Infant Death Syndrome (SIDS), or 'cot death'. Its incidence began to rise alarmingly in the 1960s. In 1970 it became reportable (to the Registrar of Births, Deaths and Marriages). It is included in this book because there has been much discussion that SIDS might be an environmental or allergy problem.

Conventional medicine sticks within its own parameters. Was it a virus? Many SIDS victims were found to have upper respiratory tract infections but it is difficult to see, based on post-mortem findings, how this could prove fatal. In any case, these infections may have been secondary to some underlying killer pathology.

Hypothermia has also been suggested as a cause, since the incidence is much higher in the colder months. However, Australia and New Zealand have an extraordinarily high incidence of cot death, over a hundred times that in the UK. It is difficult to see how anyone could get hypothermia in the scorching Outback.

The first model was Professor Robin Coombs' work in Cambridge with infant guinea pigs. He showed that if they were challenged with an intra-tracheal dose of cow's milk after being sensitized they were liable to sudden anaphylaxis and death. Well aware that cow's milk allergy is common in children, this seemed a possible explanation. To my knowledge challenge feeding tests never prove fatal, but here was a model which was saying they might be, given the right circumstances. Post-mortem examination, however, does not usually reveal allergic airways disease, or milk in the bronchi.

In the mid-1980s clinical ecologists began to get interested in electro-magnetism as a phenomenon (see **electrical fields and allergies (32)**). Among the many diseases that were considered by researchers, SIDS was one. Roger Coghill, a research biologist specializing in electrical 'pollution' found that a number of the affected children slept in close proximity to electrical or electronic devices, close enough for him to expect physiological effects. In some instances the field strength was many times what it should be.

The National Radiological Protection Board are reviewing his findings as this is being written. However, I think there is a more probable theory.

GOSIO'S DISEASE REVISITED

The real answer, I believe, follows a brilliant trail of detective work done by Barry Richardson of Penarth Research International in Guernsey. He is a building scientist concerned with environmental and health problems in relation to places of work, etc.

Richardson has made a connection between SIDS and a once-common fatal condition known as *Gosio's disease*. Gosio was an Italian chemist and in 1893 he published a paper detailing his discovery that many mysterious deaths were due to arsenic poisoning – not the deliberately administered kind popular in Victorian melodramas but passed on innocently by a busy micro-organism. The villain was a fungus now known as *Scopulariopsis brevicaulis*. It lives wherever there are damp favourable conditions, and Gosio's discovery centred around the fact that certain green pigments used in making wallpaper were salts of arsenic (Paris Green and Scheele's Green). *S. brevicaulis* was splitting these salts chemically and giving off arsine gas. In the suffocating enclosed rooms popular at that time, enough of this gas was accumulating to cause fatal poisoning. Arsine gas is still sometimes known as 'Gosio's arsenic'.

The last reported case of Gosio's disease in the UK was in 1932. However, the fungus is still around today. It is common in meats, milk, cheese, wool and leather. You may recognize it, growing on damp old leather boots or other organic matter. Richardson's sensational discovery is that *every* baby's cot he has tested to date contains significant amounts of *S. brevicaulis*. Conditions within a mattress are ideal for it. A well-wrapped baby will perspire and create a damp patch around its body; organic matter is present in fabric, skin and possibly urine; even warmth is supplied by the child's body heat.

Where does the toxin come from? Since the late 1950s traditional cotton mattress coverings have been replaced by PVC. Conventional wisdom decreed that it would be best to add fire-retardants and these come in the form of antimony and phosphorous compounds. The jig-saw puzzle suddenly starts to make a discernible picture:

The baby lies enclosed in a microcosm of wrappings, sharing it with a fungus encouraged to grow by heat and damp. The fungus attacks the chemicals in the mattress and releases stibene and phosphene, which are heavier than air. The child breathes them in excess quantities. These gases are anti-cholinesterases, which cause progressive heart failure and vasodilatation, as well as being nerve toxins. The cardiac effect may explain the observation that the child sometimes goes limp and dies at the moment of being picked up. Lack of blood to the brain would do this.

Everything fits, especially the time sequence. SIDS did not really become a major health concern until the advent of modern chemicals and their application as treatments to mattresses. It even explains why the SIDS incidence is higher in winter, since the child tends to be more closely wrapped and ventilation is poorer (windows are closed because of low outdoor temperatures).

Unexpected support for this comes from the Antipodes. The incidence of SIDS is very high in parts of Australia and New Zealand. According to Richardson, mat—tresses in farming areas are usually covered with lambs' skins. The soil is rich in arsenic and antimony in certain localities and in these districts the sheep are accumulating it in their wool (much as arsenic passes into the hair of its victims). These mattresses are then particularly dangerous, and when attacked by *S. brevicaulis* would certainly give off large amounts of arsine and stibene.

ACTION

Until the debate is settled, the advice is:

- Use a fresh mattress with each child.
- Keep the mattress dry with a waterproof layer under the sheet.
- Do not over-wrap the child. Avoid putting the child in a prone position.

Also see **moulds (75)** and **mycotoxins (76)**

102. Sugar

A lot of patients ask about sugar. It would be silly and impractical to ask patients to avoid it altogether, unless a clear-cut reaction exists.

Patients with allergies need to be mindful of the source of origin of the sugar, as well as its physical form. Thus sugar from beet is different to cane sugar and it is possible to be allergic to one but not the other. In the UK, the British Sugar Corporation (*Silver Spoon*) used beet sugar exclusively and Tate and Lyle were traditionally only cane sugar manufacturers. Now either will buy whichever is cheaper in the marketplace. Companies in the US use a lot of corn sugar. Corn sugar is used as corn syrup in the UK but is not called 'sugar'. Demerara and Muscovado are, of course, cane sugars. Thus you can get brown cane sugar but there is no equivalent beet sugar (except a synthetic cheat, as described below).

If you are buying brown sugar it is important to get a natural product. The only way to be sure is to look on the packet and see 'Country of origin: Guyana' or some such wording. Billington's are reputable UK suppliers and a name to look for.

You must be on your guard against synthetic substitutes. These are usually white sugars dyed brown, flavoured and coloured with artificial caramel (more dyes and chemicals). Various names are used, such as 'soft brown sugar', etc. Usually the packet says 'manufactured in . . .some English town' (where true brown sugar could never originate).

'Fruit sugar' is also a deception. Certain suppliers market a product that is purportedly fruit sugar. The justification for this is that it is fructose, a glucose-type ingredient that occurs naturally in fruits. Years ago I found out that they faked it, starting with ordinary white sugar and degrading this chemically to fructose: it does *not* necessarily come from fruit. Other products are similarly suspect.

Glucose, a naturally occurring compound, is sold only as a synthetic product. The usual starting point is corn, so those with corn allergy may need to avoid it.

Many products are sweetened with corn syrup. Manufacturers avoid calling it sugar, thereby deceiving the innocent buyer.

Also see **bread (13)**, **food additives (41)**, **hypoglycaemia (55)** and **milk (73)**

103. Symptoms Table

Probably no recent development in the study of allergy has caused more confusion than the recognition of the multiplicity of symptoms it can produce. No doubt this has hampered progress, since the traditional medical view of patients with many and variable symptoms has always been that they were somehow neurotic and 'putting it all on.'

This dismissive tendency is made worse if the patient suffers psychological disturbances, yet few doctors have ever thought to question whether such personality changes could also be caused by an allergy. Even if they were not, if you had a chronic disease or symptoms that came and went in a baffling way – headache one week, sore throat the next, diarrhoea the next, and so on – wouldn't you expect to feel bad mentally? Some doctors now like to use the term 'pseudo-food allergy syndrome', which does not help patients at all. One of the sacred texts of this disagreeable trend appeared in the *Lancet* in an article by D. J. Pearson, K. J. B. Rix and S. J. Bentley entitled 'Food Allergy: How Much is in the Mind?' (*Lancet* i: 1259–61, 1983).

The trouble is, these researchers made no allowance for the fact that their tests might be at fault and assumed, because they got no reaction, that the patient was deluded (their tests were the equivalent of evincing the effect of eating a beef steak by allowing the patient only two capsules of beef). This is not to say that there are no neurotic individuals whose symptoms are an attempt to win sympathy from a world they find too hostile; merely that such people are in a small minority.

How do such changeable and mysterious symptoms come about? The modern allergist thinks in terms of **target** or shock **organs (104)**. The concept is really very simple: an allergic reaction is, of course, a manifestation of the whole person, but some part of the body, or a particular organ (for reasons which are not clear) receives more of the trauma than the rest. Symptoms will depend largely on the function of this organ.

FIVE KEY SYMPTOMS

The range of potential symptoms caused by an allergy is vast. Nevertheless, Dr Richard Mackarness gives five key symptoms that point the way to allergic illness and that have special importance. He believes that without one of the following symptoms diagnosis is unlikely:

1. Over- or underweight or fluctuating weight
2. Persistent fatigue that isn't helped by rest
3. Occasional swellings around the eyes, hands, abdomen, ankles, etc.

4. Palpitations or speeded heart rate, particularly after meals
5. Excessive sweating, not related to exercise

It needs mentioning that there should be no other explanation for these symptoms.

Table 103.1 lists symptoms commonly encountered with allergies and maladaptation syndrome. The list is far from complete.

It is important to say that most of the symptoms could be caused by some other illness, although several – such as sneezing attacks – are peculiar to allergies. What really matters is the spread of symptoms – the more of these you have, the more likely it is that your illness is allergic in origin.

Some are quite obvious; those denoting digestive disturbance would point particularly to a food allergy in the absence of any other pathology. Those affecting the brain show up clearly as mood changes, altered feelings, etc.

Abrupt changes from being well to unwell (well one minute, sick a few hours later) are also pretty characteristic of allergic reactions.

What often surprises people are those symptoms of feeling bad first thing in the morning. This is so common most people can't accept that it is even a disorder, never mind an allergy. It's almost considered normal to feel that way! The key is food addiction. By the time a person wakes up in the morning, he or she has often been off food for 12 to 14 hours: that's enough to start up withdrawal symptoms. He or she then has breakfast, which acts like a 'fix' and symptoms start to clear. Certainly these feelings are common, but that's only because masked food allergies are very common.

Another surprise is the 'four-day flu', which isn't really flu at all – it's a food allergy. Dr Arthur Coca, a pioneer of allergy detection and treatment, said, 'You don't catch colds, you eat them.' He had a point: a person eats a food, symptoms are centred on the nose and muscles so he or she experiences headache, runny nose, aches and pains, maybe even a temperature, but a few days later, when the food leaves the bowel, the symptoms disappear. That's too quick for the natural course of a viral disease.

Symptoms that May Be Attributable to Allergies and Maladaptation[1]

Eyes
redness, itching
blurred vision
'sandy' or gritty feeling in the eyes
seeing spots
heavy eyes
seeing flashing lights
dark rings under the eyes
double vision (comes and goes)
unnatural 'sparkle' to the eyes
watering

Ears
ringing in the ears
hearing loss
itching and redness of pinna (outer ear)
recurring infections (especially if the sufferer is a child)
earache

Cardiovascular System
rapid or irregular pulse
chest pain
palpitations, especially after eating
tight chest
pain on exercise (angina)
raised blood-pressure

Lungs
tightness in chest
wheezing
hyperventilation (over-breathing)
coughing
poor respiratory function

Nose, Throat and Mouth
metallic taste
post-nasal drip
mouth ulcers
stuffed up nose
frequent sore throats
sinusitis
stiffness of throat or tongue
sneezing

Gastrointestinal System
nausea

[1] (With acknowledgements to Theron Randolph, Richard Mackarness, Vicky Rippere and Marshall Mandell)

diarrhoea
dyspepsia
constipation
variability of bowel function
abdominal bloating
flatulence
hunger pangs
acidity
pain in the stomach
abdominal distress

Skin

eczema
urticaria (hives)
rash that isn't eczema
excessive sweating
itching
blotches
chilblains

Musculo-Skeletal System

swollen, painful joints
aching muscles
muscular spasm
shaking (especially on waking)
cramps
fibrositis
pseudo-paralysis

Genito-Urinary System

PMT
menstrual difficulties
frequency of urination
genital itch
bedwetting
urgency
burning urination

Head

mild or moderate headache
migraine
sick headaches
solid feeling
pressure
throbbing
stiff neck
stabbing

Nervous System

inability to think clearly
memory loss
'dopey' feeling
stammering (attacks)
terrible thoughts on waking
insomnia

maths and spelling errors
blankness
delusion
crabby on waking
hallucination
difficulty waking up
desire to injure self
convulsions
light-headedness
twitching

Mental State

STIMULATED, OVERACTIVE

silliness
anxiety
intoxication
panic attacks
hyperactivity
irritability
uncontrollable rage
tenseness
restlessness
smashing-up attacks
fidgeting
general speeding up
restless legs

DEPRESSED, UNDERACTIVE

'brain fag'
depression
feeling withdrawn
lack of confidence
melancholy
low mood
unreal or depersonalized feeling
confused
tearful

Other Revealing Symptoms

sudden tiredness after eating
sudden chills after eating
over- or underweight, history of fluctuating
weight
vertigo
abrupt changes from feeling well to unwell
feeling unwell all over
occasional swellings of face, hands, ankles
feeling totally drained and exhausted
persistent fatigue not helped by rest

Also see **allergy: a definition (5), diseases caused by allergies (28) and hidden allergy (49)**

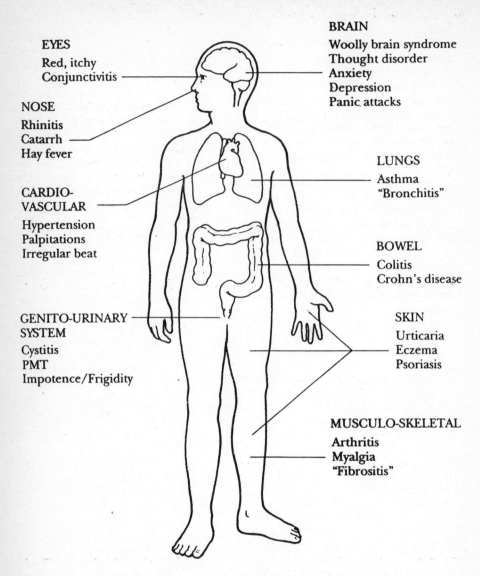

EYES
Red, itchy
Conjunctivitis

NOSE
Rhinitis
Catarrh
Hay fever

**CARDIO-
VASCULAR**
Hypertension
Palpitations
Irregular beat

**GENITO-URINARY
SYSTEM**
Cystitis
PMT
Impotence/Frigidity

BRAIN
Woolly brain syndrome
Thought disorder
Anxiety
Depression
Panic attacks

LUNGS
Asthma
"Bronchitis"

BOWEL
Colitis
Crohn's disease

SKIN
Urticaria
Eczema
Psoriasis

MUSCULO-SKELETAL
Arthritis
Myalgia
"Fibrositis"

Figure 104.1: Target organs: Some examples of symptoms and the relevant organs

104. Target Organs

The allergy-aware doctor today thinks in terms of target or 'shock' organs. The concept is really very simple: some part of the body, or a particular organ (for reasons which are not clear) receives more of an allergic reaction than the rest.

Whatever the environmental stressor, whether it is a food, a chemical, a hidden infection or some other insult to the tissues, the symptoms appear at the weak point and are 'referred' to this organ, regardless of the actual trigger. Thus you may also hear the term 'end-organ failure'. The symptoms experienced will depend largely on the function of this organ and whether it is excited (stirred up) or depressed (slowed down).

Thus, an allergy or intolerance attacking the lungs will cause asthma; one that attacks the bowel will produce abdominal pain, bloating and maybe diarrhoea or vomiting; one that attacks the joints will produce aching and stiffness; one that attacks the head will produce headaches, and so on. Incidentally, this tells us why sometimes even just one hand or just one joint is affected.

Undoubtedly the most sensitive organ in the body is the brain. It is the seat of our highest functions; our thoughts can easily become disordered by allergy. The resultant disturbance can be as mild as forgetfulness or as frightening as full-blown dementia. Probably the most common symptom of all is 'woolly brain syndrome', which is surprisingly common; so much so that many people consider it 'normal'. It is only when they try an exclusion diet or a similar unburdening step that they realize it was a pathological condition, because it clears.

No part of the body is spared. Allergies can and do mimic many diverse conditions, such as cystitis, colitis, hormone disorders, schizophrenia, hypertension, peptic ulcer, etc. The list is a long one and the reader is referred to other sections for a full discussion: **body load (11), diseases caused by allergies (28), general adaptation syndrome (44)** and **symptoms table (103)**.

Remember, this effect can also be modified by other important principles in clinical ecology, for example, biological variation and adaptation, in which the body fights constantly to adapt to each new stressor. This can cause the target organ to change. Thus a typical allergic history would include a number of manifestations: perhaps eczema in infancy, hay fever in childhood, migraine in the teenage years and arthritis in later life. Doctors might make the mistake of thinking the patient is suffering from different illnesses, but really these are simply changing reactions to the same disease, which is focussing on a new target organ. The good allergy doctor sees the underlying allergic individual, no matter what the varying manifestations might be.

105. Terpenes

There are a number of biological compounds, produced by plants and based on simple organic molecules of the aliphatic and aromatic series, that give rise to characteristic odours, taste, attractiveness (or otherwise) to insects and so on. We call these compounds *terpenes* and the potential number of them is probably almost infinite; certainly there are more of them than of any other plant or animal product.

For those interested in their chemistry they are based mainly on a simple carbon-5 isoprenoid unit. Monoterpenes have two 'units'; there may be multiple chains of 'units' (see Figure 105.1).

isoprene unit

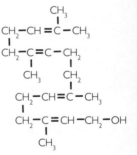

phytol, a terpene

Figure 105.1: Derivation of phytol, found in green plants

Terpenes are characteristically plant products and are well-known as components of many essential oils. Camphor, rubber and carotene are terpenes. But monoterpenes have also been found in animals. Cholesterol is probably the best-known terpene.

Citronellol has been isolated from the scent glands of alligators. Some insects produce monoterpenes as part of their defence secretions. Some of these compounds are endocrine precursors in animals. A lot of fascinating biochemistry lies before us and research is continuing.

TERPENES AND ALLERGIES

Resins and special oils in plants, especially coniferous trees, are terpenous. These can be severe allergens to certain individuals. The production of leaf terpene is greatest up to and just before the time of flowering. It then drops off rapidly. Here, then, is another seasonal allergen (see **environmental allergies (34)**). Conifers, of course, are with us all year round so, even when growth is at a minimum, there is some exposure. It is believed that the typical blue haze over pine-covered mountains is due to the atmospheric terpenes they secrete.

It is worth reminding the reader that petrochemical products, which can be so troublesome to the allergically sensitive individual, all come ultimately from coniferous plants laid down some 200 million years ago. So there is little wonder that a reaction to 'pine' is quite common.

DESENSITIZATION

Some doctors report successful results neutralizing patients to terpenes using the Miller serial dilution technique. Flowers, leaves and other vegetable products are gathered and soaked with saline solution or Coca's solution to extract the active chemicals. The resulting *supernatant* (liquid overlying the materials deposited by settling, precipitation or centrifuge) is filtered, diluted and injected for testing in the usual way (see **Miller's method (74)**). It can also be used sublingually (under the tongue).

'Pine terpene', a mixture of conifers, is important because it is so common an allergen. 'Grass' terpene is also significant. Most allergy doctors are aware that patients often react to grass that has been cut, without pollens being present. Dr Harry Morrow-Brown finally proved this scientifically to everyone's satisfaction. Therefore, relying only on pollen extract testing may miss the true cause of the patient's reaction.

Terpene solutions to be used in testing can be made from all growing plants. A mixture of tree leaves is called 'tree terpene.' Weeds can be made up separately or put together as a group. Flowering plants are used in their entirety; that is, leaves, petals, stamen and pistil. In fact, everything that grows in an area can be a 'terpene' solution for that locality. English doctors are now having to use 'rape terpene', as rape is a relatively new but powerful irritant in the UK.

Also see **phenolic testing (86)** and **plant toxins (87)**

106. Thermal Chamber Depuration

The use of repeated saunas to increase sweating and thereby 'washing away' xenobiotic (foreign) chemicals is an idea that is attributed to the late, eccentric American philosopher, L. Ron Hubbard. Clinical ecologists have taken over his idea for removing body toxins and refined it, but the approach described here is still known as the Hubbard method.

He himself called it the Purification Rundown and gave it spiritual overtones; it is sometimes also known as the **detoxification (26)** programme. However, the term detoxification is not strictly correct. In medical parlance it really means to render a chemical less toxic by altering its structure. Depuration is a better word – that is, getting rid of impurities.

The term 'sauna' might also cause misunderstanding. Concern exists within the medical profession that traditional Finnish high-temperature saunas, i.e. those kept at between 175 and 195°F/80 and 90°C, could be dangerous if used for more than very short periods of time. Hubbard's method relies on the sweating process being continued for many hours and so a lower temperature is used, in the region of 120 to 150°F/50 to 65°C. Hence the adoption of the term *thermal (heat) chamber*. In practice, an ordinary sauna is used but at the lower temperature settings.

Hence we have the term thermal chamber depuration.

LSD TRIPS

Hubbard originally developed his method to help remove traces of street drugs in the system. I was medical adviser to Hubbard's programme in its early years and observed some remarkable results. It was not rare for someone using the method to experience a 'flash-back' or 'trip', even if it had been 10 years or more since he or she had last taken the drug. LSD is stored in body fat; the Hubbard programme mobilized the drug in sufficient quantities to cause a new hallucinogenic experience.

We know from basic pharmacology that many volatile, organic compounds are fat-soluble and remain in adipose tissue this way. Remember, too, that the brain has a high percentage of fat, which is why some drugs, such as anaesthetics, have a strong affinity for brain tissue. This is how they achieve their particular effects. There is special concern that many of our toxic effluent chemicals – **pesticides (85)**, etc. – will find their way selectively into the brain, where they have maximum impact.

Once in this fat tissue 'dustbin', chemicals simply stay there. Until the heat depuration technique there was no way to get rid of them. Fortunately, it didn't take Hubbard long to realize that all these other toxic waste chemicals as well as the hallucinogenics were being cleared in the sweating-excretory process. Since then careful estimations of volatile and halogenated organics on subjects before and after the programme have confirmed his claims.

METHOD

There are several steps to the Hubbard procedure:

1. A daily period of aerobic exercise to promote circulation and to initiate sweating. Running, jogging, cycling and swimming are recommended.
2. This is followed by increasing exposures to heat in a thermal chamber, with occasional cool-off periods, until the individual is able to tolerate up to five hours per day. This level is then maintained for a number of weeks.
3. Ever-increasing doses of multivitamins are taken, with particular emphasis on reaching Niacin (vitamin $_3$) levels of 3 g or more a day.
4. Polyunsaturated oils are taken.
5. Calcium and magnesium supplements are taken in an acid medium (cider vinegar).
6. Other nutritional supplementation is administered.

Large doses of Niacin (as opposed to Niacinamide, which does not have this effect) cause unpleasant flushes of the skin not unlike sunburn. Hubbard claimed that the purification programme was in fact 'running out' radiation, though this could hardly be said to be more than conjecture. Nevertheless, I have an interesting observation to report: my wife did this programme in 1980 and, during the course of the Rundown, developed 'sunburn' patches on the skin outlining exactly a swimming costume she had worn some *15 years previously*, when she had been quite badly burnt. The shape was quite distinctive and could not have been confused with the outline of any other garment.

Generally, the Rundown is concluded when the individual feels subjectively it has achieved its effect. Most people describe feeling 'clean' and 'purified', or whatever subjective term seems appropriate.

Those who wish to may carry out the Rundown for themselves. One word of warning: it is very strenuous, particularly in the latter stages, and should only be undertaken under the supervision of your doctor.

Normal warnings on sauna usage should be followed. If at any stage you feel dizzy or weak you must remove yourself from the heat at once and take a cold shower. If this happens twice on the same day you should consider terminating the routine for that day. Drink plenty; loss of fluid can be quite considerable.

Salt and potassium supplements are not mandatory but are necessary if the symptoms of salt deficiency (heat exhaustion) occur. These include clammy skin, tiredness, weakness, cramps, nausea, dizziness and, sometimes, fainting.

Nutritional Supplements

The Hubbard method will not work in the presence of nutritional deficiencies. A comprehensive supplement programme is therefore essential. It should include (as a minimum) vitamins A, B complex, B_1, C, D, E; a multi-mineral with zinc, iron, magnesium, calcium, manganese, copper, potassium and iodine; and a daily calcium-magnesium liquid formula consisting of:

one level tablespoonful of calcium gluconate,

half a teaspoonful of magnesium carbonate,

one tablespoonful of cider vinegar,

stirred well and brought to a full glass with boiling water, stirring until all solids are dissolved. After cooling the liquid can be drunk. The solution is good for two days.

NIACIN (VITAMIN B₃)

Niacin (nicotinic acid) is one of the most important B complex vitamins. Its actions are subtle and far-reaching; we are only just beginning to understand some of them. Niacin seems to be involved in one or more metabolic detoxification pathways. One study showed that it protected rats from the effects of paraquat. Without question, it is the *key* supplement for the whole depuration procedure; the Rundown would be ineffective without it.

The starting dose is 100 mg a day. Even this low level is usually sufficient to cause the unpleasant 'sunburn' flushing, but after a few days the individual adapts and the effect disappears. The dose levels are then steadily increased. The flushing will reappear until adaptation to the new levels occurs, then amounts are increased again, and so on. It is important that as the niacin dose gradually rises, other vitamin doses are increased to keep pace with it.

The aim is to get up to 3,000 to 5,000 mg daily. Care is needed, as overdosing will produce unpleasant symptoms: a flu-like state, diarrhoea, nausea, muscle aches and pains and frightening or even terrifying hallucinations and nightmares. If this happens, the dose should be levelled off until tolerated once again. It was one of Hubbard's sayings that 'What turns it on will turn it off,' meaning that if any of these alarming manifestations appears, just keep going (without increasing the dose) and eventually the effect will vanish.

Do not be tempted to substitute niacinamide (nicotinic acid amide) for niacin. This product is sold commercially because it avoids the flush, but this defeats the whole object of the programme and as such is worthless.

Twinning

There is no doubt, as already stated, that niacin mobilizes xenobiotic chemicals stored in the body. Those with a history of drug-taking may experience some kind of hallucinogenic crisis, do something crazy and hurt themselves or others. It is therefore advisable for such individuals to do this programme with a 'buddy' – this is known as 'twinning'. The 'twin' also carries out the programme, including the exercise and saunas. Obviously, this buddy system would not be necessary in a properly supervised clinic or in-patient facility.

ENDING OFF

The programme can be ended when it is 'flat'; in other words, when no new manifestations occur over a period of several days and a sense of really zestful well-being supervenes. Typically this takes three to four weeks.

It is recommended that the nutritional supplements are not suddenly discontinued but are staged down gradually in the seven to ten days subsequent to the conclusion of the programme. This gearing-down procedure could rightly be considered part of the programme itself.

107. Universal Reactors

Universal reactors suffer from what has sometimes been called 'total allergy syndrome'. While this did give some insight into the origin of the problem it was grossly overstated and was the cause of much confusion and misinformation about real allergies.

There *are* persons who have a very tough time from a wide variety of foods and environmental excitants, and they find it difficult to share our ordinary way of life. Sometimes the sheer number of triggers can seem endless and baffling. Even clinical ecologists have tended to use the term *universal reactors* for such people, without stopping to think what this means. Nobody can be sensitive to everything, so the term has no meaning.

What is actually being described is a condition in which most of the immediate substances in view seem to cause symptoms. In other words, allergics trying to find a safe diet and encountering only foods that cause symptoms may well in despair get the idea that they are allergic to 'everything'.

Others are alarmed about chemicals in the environment: they wear masks, panic at the sight of a ball-point pen, claim they react to yesterday's aftershave on visitors and would rather starve than eat food that *might* have been sprayed with pesticides. There is something irrational about the beliefs of patients who reach this level of anxiety about chemicals. Many such 'chemical victims' have lost sight of, or are unaware of the irony that the foods they allow themselves to eat contain high levels of some of the toxic chemicals they claim to react badly to. Many foods are highly toxic in nature, especially when eaten raw (see **plant toxins (87)**).

ISOLATIONISM

There could be, in the environmental view of disease, the germ of fanaticism; the foundation of the (erroneous) notion that all one has to do to enjoy good health is to isolate oneself from the outside world. It is a tempting notion on the surface and I have seen many examples of people trying to cope with their problems in this way. But their 'victory' has come at such a cost.

Health in its fullest sense means well-being of body, mind and spirit. This cannot really be achieved by severing all practical contact with other human beings. I am

talking about holistic medicine and that means the *whole* self. To fixate on the body at the expense of the mind and spirit is a sad slight to the totality of our humanity.

If this isn't reason enough, there is a very sound technical reason why extreme avoidance is wrong. It means the patient will unmask large numbers of food and chemical allergies simultaneously. It can then become extremely difficult to find a way back without having to pass through many reactions while readapting to the environment. This can actually fuel the impression that you react to everything.

THE WAY OUT

Urgent reduction of **body load (11)** is needed. This applies also to psychological burdens: counselling may be called for.

All means of reducing body load are legitimate. A holiday, however fearful to contemplate, can be soul-saving in the event. Sometimes just such a simple measure can break what has hitherto been a vicious circle. Exotic foods are better than starvation. Malnutrition will only add to the body's problems.

Some kind of desensitization is essential. The best general programme I know lies with a **rotation diet (95)** and neutralizing drops, in accordance with **Miller's method (74)**, or the phenolics system (see **phenolic testing (86)**). Unfortunately, those who are very sick benefit least from Miller's method. **Enzyme potentiated desensitization (36)** (EPD) may be a workable alternative, but there are those so overloaded that even this is doomed to fail. EPD has, on occasion, made such patients worse.

The **environmental control unit (35)** approach may be the answer, where available.

Also see **chemical cleanup (19)** and **general adaptation syndrome (44)**

108. Urine Therapy

Drinking one's own urine as a medication is a very old idea, its beginnings lost in antiquity. Naturally, it has been dismissed as folklore, unworthy of serious study by modern medicine. Yet it is a curiously persistent notion – a fact that of itself bears some consideration.

Many investigators have independently and unequivocally demonstrated the presence of physiologically significant quantities of competent antibodies in normal human urine. In fact it could be a unique therapeutic agent since only that patient's urine could possibly contain the exact correct antibodies to his or her allergens. Certainly it has strong theoretical plus points.

BACKGROUND

The earliest scientific report, dating back to 1863, is in the *Physiological Memoirs* of Surgeon-General Hammond of the US Army. But the paper that seems to have generated most interest among fellow doctors was an account in 1947 by Dr Jonas Plesch, who was, incidentally, personal physician to Albert Einstein. He left Germany at the time of the Nazi takeover and set up a fashionable practice in London. Dr Carl Eckhardt of Riverside, California read his paper while serving in Europe during the Second World War and put it to the test when he returned home.

He tried it out first on a member of his family with severe incapacitating eczema: the condition cleared up completely. From that time until his death in 1976 he carried out approximately 70,000 treatments on 9,000 cases with remarkable success and relatively few side-effects.

Dr William Fife, from Sacramento, California, next took up the mantle. Fife himself was an allergy sufferer and had been forced to retire due to ill-health. By chance he heard of auto-immune urine therapy (AIU) and, after a course of treatment, his health and vigour were restored. He has since claimed that several clinical trials have shown that over 80 per cent of patients have experienced various degrees of clinical improvement, lasting up to many years without further treatment.

However he does caution that it is wrong to talk of a cure. AIU lowers the individual's sensitivity and allows more contact with previous offending allergens, but sensitivity

is only reduced, not abolished, so frequent injudicious antigen exposure will still cause trouble.

FIFE'S TECHNIQUE

The patient is given a sterile plastic urine container and a medicated swab with instructions on how to collect a sterile specimen of mid-stream urine. This is tested before use in the normal way for specific gravity, pH, glucose, proteins, etc.

The patient then lies face-down on the examination table and the urine is injected slowly over several minutes into the subcutaneous fat of the upper outer quadrant of the buttock (the dose depends on the patient's body weight). Two ml of 2 per cent Carbocaine (or Lignocaine in the UK) can be added to the injection solution for anaesthetic purposes, unless the patient is sensitive to such a drug.

Treatments are generally given once a week but it is not detrimental if one or more is omitted. The intervals need not be exactly one week, but usually this is convenient from the point of view of scheduling appointments.

Observation shows that improvement is frequently manifest in two stages:

1. Almost immediate relief of symptoms, indicating an immune blocking effect
2. A build up of tolerance after several months, suggesting an antibody mobilization, similar to that of immunization.

Advantages

There are a number of possible advantages for auto-immune urine therapy:

1. Extensive allergy testing for all possible antigens is not essential to treatment, as the body makes its own antibodies to all the antigens it is reacting to.
2. The medication is cheap and, being fresh, no preservatives are required.
3. There are no toxic chemicals or drugs required which hypersensitive patients might react to.
4. It has a high safety factor. Urine is naturally sterile. Since it is autogenous,

unaltered and the antigens have been attenuated by passage through the body, the most sensitive patient is spared the danger of anaphylactic shock. Fife claimed to have given over 100,000 treatments without a single serious reaction.

Side-effects are relatively minor, though some researchers have reported a severe though short-lasting depression. More common is a flaring up of previously experienced allergic symptoms or the premonitory feeling of coming down with a cold. There may indeed be mental stimulation and a sense of well-being or euphoria. This stimulation is appreciated by the tired and depressed but can be temporarily disturbing to some tense schizophrenics, so they should be under adequate supervision. These symptoms may last for a few days after a treatment.

Rarely, a local inflammatory reaction at the site of the needle penetration occurs; this may subside voluntarily or with the aid of an antibiotic injection. There is a notable lack of any local tissue destruction caused by the urine.

Increasing the Chances of Success

Since the success of this treatment, theoretically at least, depends on the presence of effective antibodies in the urine, it is sensible to try to boost these just before treatment. Thus the patient is told to expose him- or herself to moderate amounts of known or likely antigens the evening before reporting to the clinic. This may mean eating several suspect foods or spending some time breathing in the air in suspicious locations. Foods expected to produce a severe reaction are not eaten until arrival at the clinic (the AIU injection will then probably switch off the symptoms quickly).

The best time of all to collect urine is when the patient is at the height of a symptom attack. It may not be possible to identify any known or possible allergens for the patient but if, at the time of collecting the sample, the patient is reacting then it seems logical that at that time the urine will be loaded with antibodies. The patient may thus

be told to report at once to the clinic if a reaction starts up.

As with all treatments, there is little hope of success if the patient doesn't also carry out at least some corrective procedures in his or her environment and diet. Thus it is necessary to advise the patient to avoid addictions, such as to drugs, tobacco, alcohol, coffee, cola, wheat, sugar, milk, junk food, etc., as appropriate. Chemical fumes must also be avoided and dust or mould may need to be radically reduced in the home, depending on the nature of the problem.

Objections

Opponents of AIU say it may be dangerous. Fife points out that no one has been able to produce any disease by injecting normal, unaltered urine and that when one ureter is severed and opened into the peritoneum no serious or fatal effects result.

Probably one of the main objections is aesthetic: in our culture people cannot easily accept that urine can be beneficial.

Also see **enzyme potentiated desensitization (36)** and **Miller's method (74)**

109. Vega Machine

In Germany in 1952, the acupuncturist and doctor Voll came up with the first device for measuring the electrical resistance of acupuncture points. His system involved over 700 readings on the body, a process that was demanding for both patient and doctor. Many electro-acupuncture techniques have been developed since.

One of these is the Vega machine, developed by Schimmel and now increasingly in use world-wide. Research into so-called *bio-energetic regulatory* systems (BER for short) continues apace and BER is rapidly developing into one of the most exciting advances in medical skills.

The Vega machine (known in the US as the Dermatron) is basically a wheatstone bridge – meaning it checks comparative resistances. The patient holds one electrode in his or her hand while the practitioner uses the other electrode as a probe to touch one of several convenient acupuncture points,

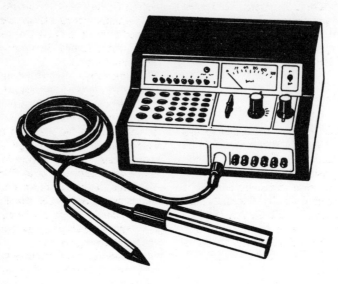

Figure 109.1: The Vega testing machine

usually on the foot. The electrical response results in a *read* (a swing of the needle, which may be accompanied by an audible signal if desired). The circuit includes a metallic honeycomb into which phials of different solutions are placed for testing.

The machine is first calibrated by putting poison, such as a phial of paraquat, into the honeycomb. This produces a 'disorder read' (a drop in register). The pathogenic potential of any test substance that gives the same read as paraquat should then be obvious.

The Vega machine is said to be useful in detecting many conditions including stressed organs, early cancer, imbalances and even too much electro-magnetic radiation from living close to high-tension electric cables. Cross-filtering of test phials may enable the 'stressed' organ to be identified and a nidus of infection – early tumour, etc. – shown as the cause. The machine's therapeutic potential lies in the fact that medicines can be tested to see if they eliminate the disorder read *before* they are administered to the patient. The

possibilities are fascinating.

From the point of view of this text, the important capability of the Vega machine is that it can be used for allergy testing. Obviously, if milk, pork, egg and tomato give the same reading as paraquat, the patient should not eat them!

Such testing can be swift and effective and consequently cheaper than many more formal techniques. This means testing is made more accessible to those of limited financial means. Accuracy may not be as high as with some methods, but it is easy to re-check and missed allergens may turn up on subsequent testing. It is even possible to use a Vega machine to evolve 'neutralizing drops', as with **Miller's method (74)**. The correct dose will be the one that eliminates the disorder read.

The main drawback is that the machine can prove difficult to use. Basically, the Vega machine seems to be a form of sophisticated electronic dowsing: some people have the ability, others haven't. Users of the machine emphasize that practice will eventually enable the majority of would-be practitioners to master it. Here we enter the world of mysterious 'energies' and even accomplished practitioners find they cannot perform when tired or stressed.

Also see **applied kinesiology (9)** and **phenolic testing (86)**

110. Water

Modern-day tap water in Western cities has become something of a health hazard in its own right. What comes out of the tap is often so toxic that sensitive individuals react to it. Moreover, there are an increasing number of reports of accidental toxicity: unusually high loads of chemicals have been dumped into the water supply, often by mistake, and members of the public made ill as a consequence. These accidents serve to highlight the nature of the problem.

If you want convincing about the amount of chemicals in tap water, simply boil some away in a pan and you will see you are left with a white powdery residue: these are the chemicals and toxins left behind.

The problem of tap water pollution is twofold. There are the chemicals added deliberately by the water board, for hygiene and cosmetic purposes. These include chlorine, alum (used to remove cloudiness) and sulphur dioxide. But the largest number of pollutants, however, come from contamination of ground water and river supplies. One survey identified over 128 chemicals including **pesticides (85)**, fertilizers, weed-killers, dyes, degreasers, PCBs and trihalomethanes. **Nitrates (78)** are also a major problem in some areas, usually from slurry and run-off from agricultural land.

It is important to remember that although repeated surveys may show contamination levels are within normal limits, there can be times, however transitory, during which safety margins are exceeded many times over. It is unlikely that the water companies will report these to the public; they will only be discovered by accident.

Few people are aware that many water processing plants recycle sewage water. Whereas this water may be hygienic and free of pathogenic bacteria (although this is not always the case), the problem is that chemicals are not removed – all those disinfectants, detergents and toxins that are washed down the toilet or sink reappear back in the water supply, in steadily increasing concentrations.

Traditionally, allergy patients resort to bottled spring water. It tastes better and is free of chlorine and other deliberate contaminants. Unfortunately there are major questions about the purity of most bottled waters, since they undergo few quality control tests. A better answer in the light of up-to-date knowledge is to filter incoming tap water to remove the majority of contaminants. This is safe, simple to do and has the added advantage of being less trouble and expense than carrying home weighty bottles of spring water.

The simplest type of water filter is a jug with activated carbon cartridges. These are inexpensive in the short term, though the true cost over several years is surprisingly high. They do not remove nitrates but dramatically reduce organics (chlorinated hydrocarbons, pesticides, PCBs and phenols), heavy metals and chlorine.

Plumbed-in units are better and more convenient. Some contain silver impregnation to avoid the build-up of bacteria once the chlorine has been removed; the presence of this silver may be troublesome to some allergics.

An alternative water treatment is that of reverse osmosis. This process also removes nitrate and fluoride left behind by the carbon filters. Enthusiastic salespeople usually fail to make it plain, however, that reverse osmosis filtering is very inefficient and wasteful, needing up to 10 gallons of tap water to produce 1 gallon of filtered water. It may take all day long doing it as well, and so requires a holder tank; this in turn leads to hygiene problems.

The only sure, reliable way to purify water is distillation. A number of distilling plants are available on the market. However, these may not be the best answer because in the process of distillation everything is removed including friendly substances such as carbonates, calcium and magnesium – important minerals needed for health.

Certainly it would be most unwise to rely exclusively on distilled drinking water, though it may be possible to use a combination of distilled and other water to reduce your contamination load without altogether eliminating natural chemical substances.

Also see **atmospheric pollution (10)** and **chemical cleanup (19)**

III. Weather and Health

METEOROLOGICAL STRESS

It is beyond doubt that weather conditions act as a stressor to some people, though it may be anything but easy to see why. Most doctors pay scant attention to patients who say they are worse during certain types of weather. Their 'training' and textbooks tell them boldly this cannot be so; therefore the patient is assumed to be a humbug or hypochondriac. This is a great pity.

Weather effects can include a wide range of psychological and somatic changes such as migraine, headache, mood swings, tension, increased accident-proneness and even heart attacks. Tests have shown that sodium is lost from the tissues and glucocorticoid hormones are released from the adrenals to cope with this kind of stress. There may be other physiological changes.

There are several well-known examples of atmospheric conditions making people ill. Hot, dry winds seem to be the chief offenders, possibly due to static build up. Positively-charged ions, most inimical to well-being, are generated in the upper atmosphere by the sun's radiation. They tend to reside there but can be brought down by certain freak pressure combinations, causing downwinds with devastating effects. Examples include the *sharav* of Israel, the *sirocco* of southern Europe and the North African *khamsin*.

Northern Europe and North America do not suffer such climatic extremes. Nevertheless, minor disturbances occur from positive ions coming down to fill low-pressure areas. This probably accounts for the widespread tendency for people to find overcast days 'heavy' and 'oppressive'.

It is common knowledge among homoeopaths – who take careful case histories – that some people are adversely affected by the lead-up to thunder storms. Once again, static build-up is the key. Electrical fields before a storm can reach up to 50,000 V/m (see **electrical fields and allergies (32)**).

Sometimes the cause isn't quite as obvious as it looks. Some patients experience unpleasant symptoms prior to the onset of cloudy and rainy weather. This may give an important clue to **mould (75)** sensitivity. Moulds spore in advance of the damp conditions and patients may begin to react at this time. Those who claim they can tell when it will rain because their nose twitches may be speaking from experience based in scientific fact, not folk nonsense.

Humidity

We use the term 'humidity' loosely to refer to the 'damp' feeling in the atmosphere. Strictly speaking, humidity means only the moisture content of the air (MC); what we usually mean in this context is *relative humidity*. This is defined as the ratio of MC to the theoretical maximum (saturation) at a given temperature. Thus air that is fully loaded with moisture is said to have 100 per cent relative humidity. It is saturated, that is, any more moisture would simply precipitate out (as rain, dew or condensation).

Absolutely dry air (which can't be obtained in practice) would be said to have zero (0 per cent) relative humidity. Thus air that contains half the possible loading of moisture would be said to have a relative humidity of 50 per cent. Over 70 per cent relative humidity feels rather damp and oppressive ('muggy'); under 40 per cent would feel very dry.

Extremes of humidity are more often met with indoors. As outdoor air enters a building and is warmed up its humidity drops. It can become unpleasantly dry and this is undoubtedly one of the contributors to so-called **sick building syndrome (99)**.

'Outdoor' humidity, which of course affects non-air-conditioned buildings, is most likely to lead to symptoms when it is too high for comfort.

Smog

The term smog is derived from the words smoke and fog; it was coined in around 1950, when atmospheric pollution reached its peak in the Western world.

Actually, atmospheric pollution has been around a long time. In London in the thirteenth century laws were enacted to control smoke emissions from domestic fires. With the coming of the Industrial Revolution the problem of smoke, grime and chemical pollution began to manifest themselves in a serious way. But it was only with certain combinations of pollution and atmospheric conditions that smog occurred. Typically, these took place in winter, when temperature inversions in the atmosphere meant that a band of cold air would become trapped under a warmer zone. The cold air, being heavier, would not disperse. Smoke and industrial fumes were trapped in this lower layer, which could remain stable for days.

The greatest smog ever was in London in 1952. It contributed to the deaths of around 4,000 people, most of them elderly or already infirm with heart disease and bronchitis. This tragic event resulted in the Clean Air Act in Britain and since that time we have had no repeat episodes, at least not of such severe proportions. Many other countries have since followed the UK's lead.

Domestic fires were the main cause of pollution before the Clean Air Act came into being. Today industry is the main pollutor. Every year 25 million tons of sulphur dioxide, emanating from factory combustion processes involving fossil fuels, fall on Europe alone. Major areas such as Scandinavia and the Black Forest face ecological disaster, as their trees are affected.

The internal combustion engine follows as the second largest pollutor; it causes a different kind of smog.

Types of Smog

We are now able to recognize two types of smog:

1. 'Reducing smog', much as described above, with oxides of sulphur, carbon and nitrogen plus debris and a mixture of hydrocarbons. It results from incomplete combustion sources and the strange atmospheric conditions described above.
2. 'Oxidant smog' resulting from petrochemical pollution. This also requires a meteorological ingredient, in this case sunlight acting on vehicle exhaust gases, ionizing them and producing dangerous ozone. Nitrogen dioxide – itself an active oxidant – is the main culprit but hydrocarbons are needed to act as catalysts.

The reaction is a merry-go-round, starting and ending with nitrous oxide (NO_2).

Ultraviolet (sun-) light + NO_2 = NO + O
O_2 + O = O_3 (ozone)
O_3 + NO = NO_2 + O_2

Once again, atmospheric temperature inversions cause build-ups. The Los Angeles basin is notorious, but most travellers know that approaching any city by plane reveals a pall of murky pollution overhead in all but the most exceptional meteorological circumstances.

During warm weather, ozone levels in a city may reach startling proportions. It can cause damage to plants and affects humans suffering from asthma at levels of 50 parts per billion (ppb). The permitted level in factories is 80 ppb. Yet in many cities, levels can at times exceed 100 ppb. In July 1976, during an unusual hot spell in Britain, levels reached 260 ppb and stayed there for a week.

The dangers of oxidation to the tissues is a major new ecological issue (see **antioxidants (8)**).

Also see **chemical cleanup (19)** and **ionizers (60)**

112. Zinc

Zinc plays many roles in nutrition and metabolism. Lack of it has been found to be associated with stunted growth, infertility, behavioural disturbances, poor wound healing, hair loss, lowered immunity and skin conditions such as eczema, among others. Zinc is required as a co-factor to at least 80 human enzymes.

Yet our diets are notoriously lacking in zinc. Studies show that an average diet does not meet the recommended requirements (15 mg daily). Partly it is removed in the processing of food, especially in refining grains. Phytate inhibition further reduces the bio-availability of zinc. To make matters worse, crops grown in Europe and the US may be short of zinc because the soil has become exhausted.

Signs of a lack of zinc are said to be white flecks in the finger nails and an impaired sense of taste. Professor Bryce-Smith's zinc status test rests on the fact that zinc-deficient individuals cannot taste the metal in solution as zinc sulphate. After adequate supplementation, taste appears to return.

Zinc works in concert with other vitamins and co-enzymes. For example, vitamin A metabolism needs zinc. B_6, so helpful in many conditions, is far more effective in the presence of zinc (and **magnesium (66)**). Zinc appears to counteract copper and an imbalance of the ratio of these two metals is associated with an increased tendency to allergies.

Zinc is necessary in the metabolism of **essential fatty acids (38)** and their conversion to **prostaglandins (92)**. Thus zinc deficiency will produce the same symptoms as EFA deficiency.

Zinc supplements reduce the average duration of the common cold. Other clues suggest the importance of zinc in immunity. Allergics would do well to ensure they are not zinc-deficient. However, although zinc is clearly needed for competent T-cell mediated immunity, it has the opposite effect on neutrophils and macrophages, causing a reduction in their motility and ability to ingest invaders. Thus, supplementation of zinc in immune-deficient or allergic patients needs careful monitoring.

SUPPLEMENTS

Zinc is available in a large number of proprietary preparations such as in the gluconate or orotate form. Doses of around 15 mg are required, but beware: quoted weights usually include the whole formula. A tablet with 100 mg of zinc as gluconate may have only 2 mg of elemental zinc!

Experiments suggest that the citrate form is best absorbed. For cheapness and convenience I often give zinc sulphate as a powder, 7 g dissolved in a pint of water. The patient takes a teaspoon per day of this liquid, providing about 15 mg daily.

Also see **nutrition and allergies (81)**

Appendix A
Food Families

This appendix gives a list of food families and also foods without commonly-eaten relatives. Use this as a guide in making up your own **rotation diet (95)**.

There is a great deal of cross-reacting between different members of a food family. However, this does not mean that if you are allergic to one food all other members of that same family need be condemned. For example, it is possible to be violently allergic to potato but OK with tomato. This *does* mean, however, that you should be more suspicious of related foods.

Note that ham and bacon belong with pork, dairy produce with beef, and eggs with chicken. Once again, though, it doesn't follow automatically that you will be allergic to all products from a certain animal. It is possible to be very allergic to milk and dairy produce and yet (reasonably) safe with beef.

Study the table carefully; it will repay your effort.

THE PLANT KINGDOM

Apple family: apple, pear, quince, medlar
Avocado family: avocado, cinnamon, sassafras
Banana family: banana, arrowroot, plantain
Beechnut family: beechnut, chestnut
Black pepper
Blueberry family: blueberry (various names), cranberry, wintergreen
Buckwheat family: buckwheat, rhubarb
Carrot family: carrot, celery, parsnip, parsley, dill, fennel, anise, caraway, cumin, coriander
Cashew family: cashew, pistachio, mango
Chicle
Chinese artichoke
Citrus family: orange, grapefruit, lemon, lime, tangerine, citron, kumquat, clementine, ugli
Coffee

Cola family: chocolate, cola, gum karaya
Composite family: lettuce, endive, chicory, globe artichoke, jerusalem artichoke, sunflower, dandelion, chamomile, goldenrod, safflower
Crucifer family: cabbage, brussels sprouts, broccoli, cauliflower, kale, collards, kohlrabi, mustard, turnip, rutabaga, swede, rape, horseradish, chinese leaves, cress
Elderberry
Ginger family: ginger, turmeric
Ginseng
Gooseberry family (saxifrages): gooseberry, blackcurrant, red currant
Grape family: grape, muscatel, raisins, sultanas (note: 'currants' are dried grapes)
Grass family: bamboo, barley, wheat, rye, oats, rice, millet, sugar cane, sorghum, corn
Guava family: guava, allspice, clove
Gum acacia
Lily family: garlic, onion, shallot, leek, chives, asparagus
Lychee nut
Macadamia nut
Maple sugar
Mint family: peppermint, spearmint, horse mint, water mint, basil, lavender oil, rosemary, marjoram, sage, horehound, savory, thyme
Mulberry family: mulberry, figs, breadfruit
Mushrooms, fungi
Nightshade family: tomato, potato, eggplant, tobacco, green and red peppers, capsicum
Nutmeg family: nutmeg, mace
Okra family: okra (bindi), cottonseed
Palm family: coconut, sago, date, Taro, poi
Papaya
Persimmon

Pineapple
Plum family: plum, prune, peach, apricot, almond, cherry, greengage
Pulses (legumes) *family*: peanut, pea, beans, lentils, licorice, gum tragancanth
Quinoa
Sarsaparilla
Spinach family: spinach, chard, beetroot, sugar beet
Squashes family: melon, watermelon, pumpkin, squash, cucumber, courgette, marrow
Strawberry family: strawberry, raspberry, blackberry
Sweet potato
Tapioca
Tea
Vanilla
Walnut family: walnut, pecan, hickory
Water chestnuts

THE ANIMAL KINGDOM

Sea Food

Anchovy
Bass, mullet, grouper
Butterfish
Carp
Catfish
Cetaceae; whale, dolphin (these are, of course, mammals)
Cod, haddock, hake, coley, whiting
Conger eel
Crustacea: shrimp, lobster, crayfish, crab,
Eel
Fish (there are many families here, which make a confusing array. Only the main fishes and groups are included):
Sturgeons
Flounder, turbot, halibut, plaice, dab, sole
Grunt
Herring, pilchards, sprats, shad
Mackerel, tuna, bonito

Molluscs: (Pelecypods) clam, oyster, mussel, scallop; (Gastropods) snail, conch, abalone; (Cephalopods) squid, octopus
Pike
Puffer
Red snapper
Salmon, trout
Yellow perch, walleye pike

Amphibia

Frog

Reptiles

Turtle, snake, alligator

Birds

Duck family: duck, goose
Eggs: all pretty similar, but experiment. Egg white is usually the most allergenic
Grouse family: grouse, turkey, guineafowl
Pheasant family: chicken, pheasant, quail, partridge, prairie chicken, peafowl
Pigeon
Snipe, woodcock

Mammals

Cattle: cow, sheep, lamb, mutton, goat, buffalo
Deer: venison, elk, moose, caribou, reindeer
Horse
Lion, tiger
Pig: pork, ham, bacon, gammon
Rabbit family: rabbit, hare
Rodents: domestic guinea pig
Seal

Appendix B
Food Contacts Lists

Patients often find it helpful to have lists of all the possible foods and drinks in which banned (allergenic) substances might be found. Here is a starter list, but I do encourage patients to use their resourcefulness, as there are bound to be omissions. The doctor cannot always be present to watch what is being eaten, it is the patient who needs to have control and a full understanding of all the data available.

Keep in mind that food manufacturing techniques change, ingredients are altered as market forces come into play and items differ from one country or ethnic group to another.

Use these lists as a guide until you get the hang of what to look for.

Remember: not all types of food listed *always* contain a specified ingredient. Often items are listed that simply *may* do so. If there is any real doubt, contact the manufacturers and ask.

Individuals vary. It is sometimes possible to eat a food in some forms but not in others. Thus a certain amount of experimentation is called for.

Where non-food contacts are interesting, I have supplied hints concerning these also.

WHEAT CONTACTS

Beverages: beer, gin, whiskies, (in fact any drink containing neutral spirits, see **alcohol (2)**), malted milk, *Ovaltine*, *Postum*

Breads: white bread, wholewheat bread, rye bread, hot breads, multi-flour breads (such as German cornbread), rusk, biscuits, muffins, popovers, pretzels, rolls and any foods made with batter (such as waffles, griddle cakes and crackers)

Cereals: bran flakes, corn flakes (often), *Weetabix*, *Grape Nuts*, *Puffed Wheat*, *Krumbles*, *Crackles*, *Pettijohns*, *Rice Crispies*, *Shredded Wheat* and other malted cereals (such as barley malt), farina, wheat germ

Flours: corn flour, gluten-free flour, rice flour, rye flour, white flour, wholewheat flour. One should not overlook mixtures with wheat flour in them

Meat, Eggs or Cheese: casseroles, croquettes, timbales, meat loaf, patties, hamburgers that include bread, flour or breadcrumbs as ingredients, sausage, wieners, cold cuts, soufflés, meat and fish rolled in flour (Swiss steak)

Pastries and Desserts: cakes, biscuits, doughnuts, pies, pastries, puddings, ice-cream cones, ice-cream (thickening), bread pudding

Potatoes or Substitute/Pastas: scalloped floured potatoes, packet creamed potatoes, macaroni, noodles, vermicelli, spaghetti, any pasta, dumplings, soufflés and any casseroles or puddings that include flour, bread or breadcrumbs as ingredients

Soups: bouillon cubes, all cream soups thickened with flour, any canned cream soups

Sweets: candy bars, chocolate drink – all chocolate (except bitter cocoa and bitter chocolate)

Vegetables: scalloped tomato, fried vegetables (if floured or breaded), vegetable soufflés, casseroles or puddings including flour, bread or breadcrumbs as ingredients

Miscellaneous: breaded foods, mixtures containing breadcrumbs, flour or bread, mayonnaise (check the label), malted products, gravies, sauces, any fat used for frying food with wheat in it, foods rolled in flour or breadcrumbs and pancake mixtures

CORN CONTACTS

Note: Maize is the same as corn

Baking: corn flour, corn starch, non-specified flours, stock cubes, tinned and packet soups, batters, baking mixes, doughs, baking powder, gravy mixes, corn oil, any non-specified vegetable oil, confectioner's sugar, jellies, glucose syrup, grits, monosodium glutamate

Beverages: beers, ales, lager, spirits, colas, squashes, lemonade, *Lucozade*, most carbonated soft drinks (they use corn syrup as a sweetener), instant coffee, instant tea

Breads: bread, cornbread, polenta, pizza, pasta, tortilla

Cereals: cornflakes, sugared corn flakes, e.g. *Frosties*

Confectionery: cakes, biscuits, muffins, waffles

Dairy: instant desserts, *Delight*, custard powder, blancmange, branded yoghurts, ice-cream, margarine, dairy-free margarine, processed cheeses, soya milk

Drugs and Medicines: aspirin, paracetamol and all white pills and *most* other tablets, syrups, liquid medicines, suppositories, lozenges, capsules, some vitamin pills

Jams, etc.: jam, peanut butter, sandwich spreads, potted meat

Meats: sausage, ham, bacon, wurst, variety meats, bolognas, frankfurters; some meats are injected with dextrose to 'sweeten' them

Sauces: ketchup, *OK*, mayonnaise, French dressing, gravy mixes, vinegar, pickles

Sweets: popcorn, chocolate, chocolate 'flavour', chewing gum, sherbet, glucose tablets, any dextrose-containing food, candy, chocolate bars, other

Miscellaneous: paper cups, cartons for fruit juice, milk, etc., envelope gum, stamp gum in some countries, sticky labels, talcum powder, toothpaste and dentifrices, clothing starch, plastic food wrappers (may be coated with corn starch), some wines (may appear on labels as 'modified starch'), etc.

Tip: On a corn-free diet you should avoid all manufactured foods, then it's easy!

YEASTS, MOULDS AND FERMENTS CONTACTS

Definition: any substance derived from, cross-reactive with or containing either substantial or trace amount of yeasts (sometimes called leavening), moulds (also called fungi), ferments (process of souring, fermentation, fermentation hydrolysis)

All Cheeses: including fermented dairy products, cottage cheese, natural, blended and pasteurized cheeses and sour cream

All Fermented Beverages: beer, wine, champagne, whiskies, rum, brandies, tequila, root beer, ginger ales, as well as all substances that contain alcohol: extracts, tinctures, cough syrups and other medications

All Malted Products: milk drinks that have been malted, cereals and sweets that have been malted, malted breakfast cereals

All Raised Doughs: breads, buns, rolls, prepared 'icebox' or frozen breads, some biscuits and crispbreads

All Vinegars: apple, distilled, wine, grape, pear, etc. This includes all foods containing any vinegar, e.g. salad dressings, mayonnaise substitutes, pickles, catsup, sauerkraut, olives, most condiments, sauces (barbecue, tomato, chili, green pepper), mince pie preparations and many others

Antibiotics: penicillin, Amoxycillin, and many other '-illins'. 'Mycin' drugs and related compounds such as Erythromycin, Streptomycin, Chloramphenicol. Tetracyclines and related derivatives: all the cephalosporin derivatives and all others derived from moulds and mould cultures

Cereals: those fortified with added vitamins such as thiamin, niacin, riboflavin, etc.

Dried Fruits: prunes, raisins, dates, figs, apricots, etc. Again, some batches may be mould-free but others will have commercially acceptable amounts of mould on the fruit while drying

Ferments and Moulds: soya sauce, pickles etc., truffles, mushrooms

Flours: those that have been 'enriched' (i.e. most flours).

Juices: fruit juices – canned or frozen. (In commercial preparation the *whole* fruit is used, some of which may be mouldy but not sufficiently so to be considered spoiled): fresh, home-squeezed should be yeast-free

Milks: if enriched or fortified with vitamins

Vitamins: B, B complex and multiple vitamins containing B complex. Products containing B_6, B_{12}, irradiated ergosterol (vitamin D); all products containing brewer's yeast or derivatives

MILK CONTACTS

Beverages: milk, cream, chocolate or cocoa drink mixes, cocoa made with milk

Breads: any bread made with milk, milk solids, butter, oleo-margarines (check labels)

Cereals: any cooked cereal or gruel prepared with milk or cream

Desserts: puddings made with milk, whipped cream toppings, ice-cream and sherbet, cake, biscuits, prepared flour mixes, pudding mixes, custard

Fats: butter, oleo-margarine churned in milk

Meat, Eggs or Cheese: scrambled egg made with milk or prepared in butter or oleo; any meat or fish seared or fried in butter or oleo; all cheeses (au gratin); cold cuts; packaged mixed dishes

Potatoes or Substitute: creamed or scalloped potatoes, gravy, any vegetable seasoned with butter, oleo, milk, cream, cheese (au gratin)

Soups: cream soups made with milk, cream, butter, oleo; all canned cream soups

Sweets: all sweets except plain sugar candy

Vegetables: creamed vegetables, any vegetable seasoned with butter, oleo, milk, cream, cheese

Miscellaneous: creamed foods, boiled salad dressing, white sauces. Read labels on all prepared foods

SOYA CONTACTS

Bakery Goods: soybean flour containing only 1 per cent oil is now used by many bakers in dough mixtures for breads, rolls, cakes and pastries. This keeps them moist and saleable several days longer. Roasted soya nuts are also sometimes used in place of peanuts

Cereals: soy flakes, soya bran

Cheese Substitutes: Tofu, vegetarian cheeses (some), miso

Low-fat Spreads and Butter Substitutes: oleo-margarines, *Granose*, shortening

Meats: sausages, wurst, bologna, saveloy, luncheon meat

Milk Substitutes: soya milk, *Wysoy* (Wyeth), soya ice-cream. Some bakeries use soy milk instead of cow's milk

Nuts: soya beans may be roasted and salted and used instead of peanuts

Pastas: soybean noodles, macaroni, spaghetti

Salad Dressings: many of the salad dressings and mayonnaises contain soy oil but only state on the label that they contain vegetable oil. Present conditions have necessitated the use of soy oil in many brands of oil previously free of soybean

Sauces: ketchup, *OK* sauce (brown sauce), soya sauce, *Lea & Perrins*, Worcester sauce (any)

Sweets: soya flour is used in hard candies, nut candies, and caramels. Lecithin is invariably derived from soybean and is used in candies to prevent drying out and to emulsify the fats

Miscellaneous: varnish, paints, enamels, printing ink, candles, celluloid, cloth, massage creams, linoleum, paper sizing, adhesives, fertilizer, nitroglycerine, paper finishes, blankets, soap, fish food, custards, fodder, glycerine, textile dressings, lubricating oil, illuminating oil

Appendix C
Chemical Pollutants in the Home

To follow a comprehensive low-chemical lifestyle, you will need to eliminate as many as possible of the following contacts from your home and immediate environment. The list isn't comprehensive but no list is a substitute for common sense. Think it through. Note that it is not necessary to get *zero load* to get zero symptoms.

HEATING

Odours from hot radiators, grills, heating bars.

Stoves, cookers, furnaces and fires fired by:

    kerosene (paraffin)
    coal
    oil
    gas
    wood

Ducted warm air heating

Free-standing butane or propane stoves are particularly bad and heavily pollute the indoor environment with oxides of carbon, nitrogen and sulphur, plus hydrocarbons – *avoid*.

CLEANSERS

(With or without additional scents)
Lysol
Phenol (carbolic)
Bleaches
Soaps
Detergents
Ammonia
Polishes
Lavatory cleaners
Oven cleaners
Degreasers

COSMETICS

Talc

Toilet water
Perfumes
Creams
Cleansers
Powder
Nail polish, nail polish remover
Aftershave
Deodorants

FABRICS

Synthetic upholstery, curtains, rugs
Printed fabrics
Clothes conditioners
Permanent pressing
Drycleaning fluid
Clothes should be aerated in the sun after being sent to dry cleaners.

FLOOR COVERINGS

Waxes
Linoleum
Rubberized tiles
Foam-backed carpet
Treated (stain-resistant) carpets

SOLVENTS

Newsprint
Paint strippers
Carbon tetrachloride
Chloroform
Trichloroethylene
Dry-cleaning fluid
Shoe polish
Metal polish
Newspapers and magazines should be opened and read by someone else first. Baking them in an oven speeds up removal of chemicals.

AEROSOLS (FLUORINATED HYDROCARBON PROPELLANT)

Insecticides
Deodorants
Air fresheners
Hair sprays
Degreasers
Furniture polish
Easing oil
Beware: so-called 'ozone friendly' sprays usually contain butane, which is certainly not human friendly and a serious fire hazard.

MEDICINES

Ointments
Impregnated bandages and dressings
Sticking plaster
Surgical spirit
Medicines
Patent 'remedies'
Rubbing alcohols
Toothpaste
Dentrifices

PAINTS AND VARNISHES

Polyurethane paints
Textured paint
Turpentine and substitute (white spirit)
Paint stripper
Varnish
Oil paints

MOTOR CARS

Petrol
Oil
Plastic cockpit fittings
Upholstery
Cellulose paints

FOAM RUBBER

Pillows
Cushions
Mattresses
Lounge chairs and sofas
Carpet backing

LEAKAGES

Refrigerator
Heating boilers (flue)
Petrol/oil (garage)

ADHESIVES

Thixotropic adhesives
Glues
Cement
Shellac
Fungicides in wallpaper paste

PEST CONTROL

Insecticides
Fungicides
Weedkiller
Moss treatment
Mothballs
Rug shampoo can contain DDT.
Note: Pest exterminators use dieldrin, chlordane, pentachloraphenol.

MISCELLANEOUS

Evaporating oil from any motor.
Air filters of glass wool or fibreglass usually have oiled filters, but one can get them without.
Pine Christmas trees
Pine in wood burning fireplaces
Creosote
Odours from prolonged use of TV sets
Plastic wrappings (cellophane is best)
Coloured paper
Several of my patients have had trouble with chemical pollution coming from the house next door. Be alert to this possibility. But do not get into fights or litigation: it's stressful and nobody wins except lawyers.

Appendix D
Top Ten Allergens

I am often asked which are the most common allergens. This table lists the top ten according to three different sources. The first was a study carried out on adults by Vicky Rippere, a clinical psychologist at the London Institute of Psychiatry. The second was taken from a migraine trial at Great Ormond Street Hospital conducted by Professor Soothill and others. The third study was carried out by Dr Joseph Egger in Munich, who was studying hyperactive children – all of whom completely recovered when put on a diet that excluded the allergenic foods listed.

	Rippere	Soothill	Egger
1	wheat and wheat products	cow's milk	chocolate
2	dairy produce	egg	colourings
3	food additives	chocolate	cow's milk and chemicals
4	coffee, alcohol	orange	egg
5	chocolate	wheat	citrus
6	citrus	additives	wheat
7	corn	tomatoes	beet sugar
8	egg, cane sugar	rye	nuts
9	tea	fish	cheese
10	oat	pork	pork

My own experience would simply reiterate that, in adults at least, wheat is the most common allergen, dairy produce the second and instant coffee, third. If one were simply able to persuade the entire population to give up just these three foods, the change in the health of the nation would be dramatic.

Appendix E
Seven-day Stone Age Diet Menu Plan

Many people, I know from experience, would like to try the Stone Age diet but find it daunting. It *is* something of a revolution. Here are some suggestions for those of you who want to know how to go about it. My nurse Marion Whiting went to the trouble of working out a 7-day menu plan, complete with recipes where relevant.

This is not a strict regime, merely a guide. You can vary it as you wish, once you have grasped the idea. Variety is the key note. Make sure you don't eat the same few foods over and over. This risks developing new allergies. It is safer to eat *new* foods.

Vegetarian dishes are included.

DRINKS

Keep your fluid intake up in whatever way you like. Herb teas are an acquired taste. Try them very weak to start with. Hot water on its own can seem delicious after a few days.

Dilute fruit juices with carbonated spring water and make filtered water ice-cubes; add a slice of apple, a sprig of mint and you have a delicious drink.

SOUPS

Soup daily will fill the gap. Soups can be made in advance and frozen in portions if necessary. They make a good start for lunch and the evening meal, and are handy to have ready prepared to eat after a busy day before you start to cook for the evening or bath the baby! Prepare recipes beforehand.

PUDDINGS

As such these do not exist on the diet, but by making fruit salads that vary their base daily and using the day's juice you can make a surprising number of different tastes. Add chopped nuts and dried whole fruits (that you have soaked per instructions).

SPECIAL NOTE FOR CHILDREN

We usually allow rice cakes and Tomor margarine (wheat- and dairy-free). If your child is uncooperative and refuses to eat for the first 48 hours, don't worry: hunger will soon be on your side. He or she may be sulking and may indeed be suffering from withdrawal symptoms. Encourage drinks, dilute some of the fruit juice and don't worry about cravings for sweets and 'good things'. By day 3 he or she will be feeling happier.

Once the child realizes there is no alternative, he or she will eat what is prepared. Offer some kind of tangible reward. Children are very good at playing the game when they know the rules.

Purée foods for a small baby, adding a calcium supplement – *not* soya milk (most baby formulas contain sugar and corn) and he or she will do fine.

DAY I

Breakfast
SPECIAL SAUSAGE

Fresh minced beef, pork or lamb
Fresh herbs, i.e. sage or mint, chopped
Sea salt and black pepper to taste
Potato flour as needed
Mix first meat, herbs and seasoning together, press into spoon-sized shapes and roll in potato flour. Alternatively, ask your butcher to make these. He will if you ask for 5 lb at a time, and then they will be in sausage skins. Freeze individually and use as required. To cook, fry in hot fat.

BUBBLE AND SQUEAK

Cooked mashed potato (can use leftover jacket potatoes)
Cooked green-leaf vegetables, chopped
Salt and pepper to taste

Potato flour as needed

Mix vegetables and seasoning together and either make small portions by rolling in potato flour or put whole lot in frying pan and keep turning until brown and crisp. Small portions freeze well.

Soup
FRENCH ONION

1 lb/455 g onions, sliced
1 pint/570 ml/2½ cups stock (without thickener)
2 tbsp sunflower oil
Salt to taste
Fry onions in oil until browning. Add stock and simmer for half an hour.

Main Meal
ROAST TURKEY AND VEGETABLES

Roast as much turkey as you like and eat with any vegetables you fancy. Cook extra potatoes to use for day 2. Use the turkey's giblets to make gravy and stock for days 2 and 7.

Vegetarian Main Meal
SAVOURY CHESTNUT BAKE

1 onion, peeled and sliced
1 stick of celery
2 tbsp oil
2 oz/55 g chestnuts, chopped
2 cloves of garlic, peeled
4 oz/115 g walnuts
4 oz/115 g cashews
2 fl oz/60 ml/¼ cup apple juice (more if needed)
6 oz/170 g dried chestnuts, soaked overnight. Drain and simmer with enough water for 2 – 3 hours. Keep water for stock.
Salt and pepper to taste
Set oven at 375°F/195°C/Gas Mark 5. Line a loaf tin with greaseproof paper and brush with oil. Fry onion and celery in oil for 10 minutes. Remove from heat and add to other ingredients and blend in a food processor. Add seasoning, and pile into the baking tin. Cover and bake for 45 minutes. Uncover and bake for another 15 minutes.

DAY 2

Breakfast

Use potato from the night before, slice thinly and sprinkle with sea salt. Quickly fry in a small amount of oil until crisp.

Banana slices make a good alternative to mushrooms, but don't overcook them.

Soup
COURGETTE SOUP

1 lb/455 g courgettes, chopped
1½ pints/850 ml/3¾ cups turkey stock (from giblets of yesterday's turkey)
Salt and pepper to taste
1 tsp oil
Lightly fry courgettes in oil and add stock, salt and pepper. Simmer for half an hour, until the skins are soft. Liquidize. Make double quantities and freeze for next week.

Main Meal
STIR FRY

1 tbsp oil
Selection of at least 5 vegetables, chopped
Meat of choice (turkey leftovers?)
Salt and pepper to taste
Sweet potato (for side dish)
If possible, pre-set your oven and leave a sweet potato to cook in its jacket – if you can arrange this, this will be a quick meal.

Pour oil into a heavy-lidded pan or wok. Add vegetables and cover for 3 minutes, shaking while cooking. Add cooked meat, salt and pepper. Cook for 2–3 minutes. Serve immediately with sweet potato.

Vegetarian Alternative
BEAN LAYER PIE

6 oz/170 g black-eyed peas
Water as needed
1 large onion, chopped
2 tbsp safflower oil
3 medium tomatoes, skinned and chopped
2 sticks of celery, chopped
1 small pepper, seeded and chopped
1 tsp parsley
Salt and pepper
Mashed potatoes
Green vegetables, boiled

Cook beans in double their volume of water for 30 minutes. Drain. Fry the onion in oil and then add tomato, celery and pepper and cook for about 5 minutes.

Place layers of beans and vegetables in a greased pie dish, adding parsley and seasoning to taste. Cover with mashed potatoes and bake in moderate oven – 275°F/170°C/Gas Mark 3 – for 30 minutes. Serve with green vegetables.

NB: Cook double the quantity of potatoes for tomorrow's fish cakes. Put lentils to soak for tomorrow's soup.

DAY 3

Breakfast
FISH CAKES

Fish of your choice, cooked
Mashed potato
Salt and pepper to taste
Potato flour as needed
2 tbsp oil
Tomatoes, cooked
Mix together fish, mashed potato and seasoning. Roll mixture in portions in potato flour. Fry in hot oil until brown. Serve with cooked tomato. You can use soft tomatoes to make homemade ketchup by blending them in a liquidizer.

Soup
LEEK AND LENTIL SOUP

4 oz/115 g red lentils, soaked overnight
6 oz/170 g chopped leeks
3 tbsp oil
1 pint/570 ml/2½ cups vegetable stock
Sea salt
Fresh herbs of your choice
Boil lentils for at least 1 hour. Fry leeks in a heavy pan in the oil for 10 minutes. Drain lentils, then liquidize along with the leeks. Add to vegetable stock and season. Bring to the boil then simmer for 2 minutes. Garnish with chopped herbs.

Main Meal
ROAST DINNER

Use lard for roasting vegetables and basting meat. Keep fat for the next roast and use the meat juices for stock or gravy.

Vegetarian Alternative
STUFFED AUBERGINES (FOR 1)

1 aubergine
Oil as needed
1 onion, chopped
2 tomatoes, chopped
¼ lb/340 g mushrooms, chopped
2 oz/55 g pine kernels
Salt to taste
Halve the aubergine, scoop out the flesh and chop. Heat the oil and fry the onion until soft. Add tomatoes and mushrooms and cook until soft, but not mushy – about 5 minutes.

Place the aubergine shells in a greased dish, fill with vegetable mixture, sprinkle on pine kernels and bake in moderate oven for 30 minutes, or longer, if necessary, at a lower heat. Good with a green salad.

NB: For tomorrow, prepare breakfast by making bacon-mushroom mix and pre-setting the oven for the potato.

DAY 4

Breakfast
JACKET POTATO WITH FILLING

4 rashers of streaky bacon, chopped
4 mushrooms, chopped
Lightly fry bacon, add mushroom, turn off heat and shake in frying pan. (Reheat mixture if you made it last night.) Use this mixture to fill potato, stirring the mix in with the potato. Pop under the grill until crisp.

Soup
LIGHT VEGETABLE SOUP

1 tbsp sunflower oil
1 small onion, peeled and finely chopped
6 oz/170 g carrot, cut into 'match sticks'
3 sticks celery, sliced
1½ pints/850 ml/3¾ cups vegetable stock
Celery leaves
2 tbsp chopped parsley
Black pepper, pinch of salt
Heat oil and fry onion without browning, about 5 minutes. Add carrot and celery and cook until oil is absorbed. Add stock, bring to the boil and then simmer for 20 minutes until the vegetable is tender, but not soggy. Add parsley and seasoning. Can be frozen.

Main Meal
RATATOUILLE

1 tbsp oil
1 large onion, peeled and chopped
1 large aubergine, cut into 1-inch cubes
3 small courgettes, sliced
1 green pepper, seeded and diced
1 red pepper, seeded and diced
10 oz/285 g tomatoes, skinned (dropped into
  boiling water for 2 minutes) and chopped
1 tbsp fresh basil
Salt and pepper to taste
Fry the onion for 10 minutes and then add all the other ingredients. Cook, covered, for 15 minutes stirring frequently. Can be frozen.

Vegetarian Alternative
HAZEL NUT SAUCE (SERVES 4)

Jacket potato (side dish)
1 tbsp oil
1 onion, peeled and chopped
1 tbsp hazelnut butter
4 oz/115 g chopped roast hazelnuts (roast
  under grill)
½ lb/225 g tomatoes, chopped and skinned
  (see above)
Salt and pepper to taste
Cauliflower, broken into florets and steamed
  till tender
Have jacket potato baking in oven for at least 1 hour.

Fry onion, then add all other ingredients except for the cauliflower. Season and pour mixture over cauliflower. Serve piping hot with jacket potato.

DAY 5

Soup
LEEK AND POTATO SOUP

1 tbsp sunflower oil
1 small onion, peeled and sliced
1 large (8 oz/225 g) leek, washed and sliced
12 oz/340 g potatoes, peeled and cut into
  ¼-inch cubes
1½ pints/850 ml/3¾ cups homemade
  vegetable stock
Bay leaf
Salt and pepper

Heat oil and fry onion for 3–4 minutes. Add the leek and potatoes and stir well. Leave on a low heat for a few minutes, covered, until oil is absorbed. Add stock, bay leaf and plenty of black pepper. Cover, bring to the boil and then simmer for 15 minutes. Remove bay leaf and serve piping hot.

Main Meal
BEEF BURGERS

2 medium onions, finely chopped
1 lb minced beef
Salt and pepper
Potato flour
Sunflower oil
Put onions, beef and seasoning into the food processor on a low setting. Make ¼-lb (115-g) portions of meat mixture for each burger, roll in potato flour and flatten. Cook in hot oil for 5 minutes each side, making sure each burger is well cooked through.

Vegetarian Alternative
MILLET AND COURGETTE RISOTTO

2 tbsp oil
2 onions, peeled and chopped
1 red pepper, chopped and seeded
1 lb/455 g courgettes, sliced
2 cloves of garlic, finely chopped
8 oz/225 g millet
1 pint/570 ml/2½ cups water
Salt and pepper
Fry onions, red pepper, courgettes and garlic in a saucepan for 10 minutes. Add millet and water and bring to the boil. Cover and turn down the heat; cook for 20 minutes, until the millet is cooked and fluffy. Season. Serve with crispy lettuce.

NB: For tomorrow, put the lentils to soak. Make the gazpacho if you have time and leave it in the fridge.

DAY 6

Soup
GAZPACHO

1 medium onion, skinned and chopped
2 tbsp oil
1 small green pepper, chopped and seeded
½ pint/285 ml/1⅓ cups tomato purée
  (blended, skinned tomatoes)

1 clove garlic, crushed (optional)
Small quantity other vegetables to hand, e.g. courgettes
Seasoning
Watercress
5 oz/140 g cucumber, chopped

Sauté onion in oil for 5 minutes. Add other ingredients except seasoning, watercress and cucumber. Simmer for 15–20 minutes, season and chill. Serve garnished with watercress and with chopped cucumber on the side to use as croutons.

Main Meal/Vegetarian Alternative
ITALIAN LENTIL CASSEROLE

12 oz/340 g green lentils (soaked overnight)
2 pints/1.14 1/5 cups water
2 tbsp oil
1 onion, skinned and chopped
6 oz/170 g mushrooms, chopped
1 lb/455 g tomatoes, chopped
Clove of garlic, crushed
1 tsp fresh marjoram or basil (but any other herb will do)
Salt and pepper

Boil lentils in water for 35–40 minutes. Drain. Heat oil and fry onion, then the other vegetables; cook for 5 minutes. Grease casserole, add lentils to the vegetable mixture, add herbs and seasoning to taste and bake for half an hour at 325°F/180°C/Gas Mark 4.

Keep 2 tablespoons of tomato purée for tomorrow's paella.

DAY 7

Soup
CARROT SOUP

2 pints/1.14 1/5 cups turkey stock
1 lb/455 g carrots, chopped
3 large leeks (or 1 large onion), chopped
Parsley, chopped

Put all ingredients except parsley into a pan and simmer until the vegetables are soft. Liquidize and return to heat. Serve garnished with parsley. If you want to, you can leave vegetables in whole pieces for a luncheon-type soup.

Main Meal

Joint of ham
Water to cover
½ pint/285 ml/1⅓ cups pineapple juice
Jacket potatoes
Carrots, chopped
Salt and pepper to taste

Soak ham joint for 2 hours (shoulder is an inexpensive cut). Put the joint in a pan and bring to the boil, then tip away the water and cut off the rind. Put the joint into a roasting tin or oven-proof dish. Baste with pineapple juice and roast at 325°F/180°C/Gas Mark 4 for 30 minutes, or until fat is brown. Bake jacket potatoes in the oven. Use skewers through each to shorten cooking time. Carrots can be put in a lidded casserole with some water and seasoning and cooked with potatoes in a low oven for 2 hours, a hotter oven for 1 to 1½ hours.

NB: For tomorrow, cook enough ham to have cold. Plus extra potato for bubble and squeak (back to Day 1).

Vegetarian Alternative
PAELLA

Sunflower oil for frying
3 oz/85 g mushrooms, sliced
5 oz/140 g brown rice, uncooked
½ pint/285 ml/1⅓ cups pineapple juice
½ pint/285 ml/1⅓ cups water
2 tbsp tomato purée
2 oz/55 g sultanas
½ small green pepper, chopped
2 oz/55 g nuts
Pineapple rings to garnish

Sauté the sliced mushrooms in a large pan. Add the rice and cook for a few minutes. Add juice, water and tomato purée. Simmer for about 25–30 minutes until the liquid is absorbed and rice is tender. Add sultanas, green pepper and coarsely chopped or grated nuts. Heat through and serve with pineapple rings.

Recommended Reading

Bread

Dr Amy McGrath, *One Man's Poison: The 'Glucose' Factor* (Tower House Publications, 1990).
You can get a copy by writing to Tower House Publications, 23 Primrose Hill, Tower, County Cork, Eire. Tel: 021 385720.

Chemical Cleanup

Richard Mackarness, *Chemical Allergies* (formerly *Chemical Victims*) (Pan, 1980).

Detoxification

J. A. Timbrell, *Introduction to Toxicology* (Taylor and Francis, 1989).
Dr Sherry Rogers, *Tired or Toxic?* (Prestige Publishing, 1990) Prestige Publishing, Box 3161, Syracuse, New York 13220, USA.

Electrical Fields and Allergies

Harold Saxton Burr, *Blueprint for Immortality: The Electric Patterns of Life* (C. W. Daniel Company Ltd, 1972).
Cyril Smith and Simon Best, *Electromagnetic Man: Health and Hazard in the Electrical Environment* (J M Dent and Sons, 1989).
Michael Shallis, *The Electric Shock Book* (Souvenir Press, 1988).

Food Additives

Caroline Walker and Geoffrey Cannon, *The Food Scandal* (Century, 1984).

General Adaptation Syndrome

Hans Selye, *The Stress of Life* (McGraw-Hill, 1976).

Geopathic Stress

Kathe Bachler, *Earth Radiation: The Startling Discoveries of a Dowser* (Wordmasters Ltd, 1989).
(This is available by post from 23 Edge Lane, Manchester M21 1JH.)
Gustav Freiherr von Pohl, *Earth Currents: Causative Factor of Cancer and other Diseases* (Stuttgart: Frech-Verlag, 1987: English edition distributed by Ilse Pope, 1 Gary Close, Romford, Essex, RM1 4EA).

Hair Analysis for Minerals

Jeffrey Bland, *Hair Tissue Mineral Analysis* (Thorsons, 1983; Pan, 1987).
Dr Stephen Davies and Dr Alan Stewart, *Nutritional Medicine: The Drug-free Guide to Better Family Health* (Pan, 1987).

The Hay System

Doris Grant and Jean Joice, *Food Combining for Health* (Thorsons, 1984).

Irradiation of Foods

Tony Webb and Dr Tim Lang, *Food Irradiation: The Facts* (Thorsons, 1987).

Microwaves and the Electromagnetic Spectrum

Roger Coghill, *Electro-pollution: How to Protect Yourself Against It* (Thorsons, 1990).

Migraine and Headaches

Dr John Mansfield, *The Migraine Revolution* (Thorsons, 1989.)

Pesticides and Health

Robert van den Bosch, *The Pesticide Conspiracy* (Doubleday and Co, 1978).

Preconceptual Health

Dr Ellen Grant, *The Bitter Pill* (Corgi, 1985).

Belinda Barnes and S. G. Bradley, *Planning for a Healthy Baby* (Vermilion, 1992)

Premenstrual Tension (PMT)

A. Nazzaro and D. Lombard with D. Horrobin, *The PMT Solution* (Adamantine Press, 1985).

Bibliography

(Published in the UK unless otherwise indicated)

Of course this list is far from complete but the many references contained in each of these works should lead you on to much more of interest. Some of the books are now out of print, but you may be able to find them at the public library.

GENERAL

S. Faelten, *The Allergy Self-help Book* (Aurum Press, 1987).

N. Golos and F. Golos Golbitz, *Coping with Your Allergies* (New York: Simon and Schuster, 1979).

D. Pearson, *The Natural House Book* (Conran Octopus, 1989).

Sir G. Stapledon, *Human Ecology* (The Soil Association, 1964).

CANDIDA

W. G. Crook, *The Yeast Connection* (Jackson, TN: Professional Books, 1984).

O. Truss, *The Missing Diagnosis* (P.O. Box 26508 Birmingham, AL: 1983).

CHEMICAL ALLERGIES

R. Mackarness, *Chemical Allergies* (formerly *Chemical Victims*) (Pan, 1980).

P. Mansfield and J. Monro, *Chemical Children* (Century Hutchinson, 1987).

T.G. Randolph, *Human Ecology and Susceptibility to the Chemical Environment* (Springfield, IL: Charles C. Thomas, 1962).

T.G. Randolph and R. W. Moss, *Allergies: Your Hidden Enemy* (Thorsons, 1981).

P. Saifer and M. Zellerbach, *Detox* (New York: Ballantine Books, 1984).

CHILDREN AND ALLERGIES

W. G. Crook, *Tracking Down Hidden Food Allergies* (Jackson, TN: Professional Books).

B. F. Feingold, *Why Your Child is Hyperactive* (New York: Random House, 1974).

D. J. Rapp, *Allergies and the Hyperactive Child* (Thorsons, 1988).

——, *Allergies and Your Family* (New York: Sterling Publishing, 1980).

FOOD ALLERGIES

J. B. Brostoff and L. Gamlin, *Food Allergy and Intolerance* (Bloomsbury, 1989).

H.J. Campbell, *The Food Watch Alternative Cookbook* (Ashgrove Press, 1988).

A. McGrath, *One Man's Poison: The 'Glucose' Factor* (Tower, Eire: Tower Hill Publications, 1990).

R. Mackarness, *Not All in the Mind* (Pan, 1985).

J.B. Miller, *Relief at Last* (Springfield, IL: Charles C. Thomas, 1987).

K. Mumby, *The Food Allergy Plan* (Allen & Unwin, 1985).

E. Workham, V. Alun Jones and J. O. Hunter, *The Allergy Diet* (Martin Dunitz, 1985).

FOOD INDUSTRY

A. Gear, *The New Organic Food Guide* (J M Dent and Sons, 1987).

M. Hanssen, *E for Additives: Supermarket Shopping Guide* (Thorsons, 1986).

T. Lobstein, *Children's Food* (Unwin Hyman, 1988).

T. Webb and T. Lang, *Food Irradiation: The Facts* (Thorsons, 1987).

GEOPATHIC STRESS

Kathe Bachler, *Earth Radiation: The Startling Discoveries of a Dowser* (Wordmasters Ltd, 1989).

S. Skinner, *The Living Earth Manual of Feng-Shui* (Arkana, 1989).

G. F. von Pohl, *Earth Currents: Causative Factor of Cancer and other Diseases* (Stuttgart: Frech-Verlag, 1987: English edition distributed by Ilse Pope, 1 Gary Close, Romford, Essex, RM1 4EA).

HORMONES

E. Grant, *The Bitter Pill* (Corgi, 1985).

A. Nazzaro and D. Lombard with D. Horrobin, *The PMT Solution* (Adamantine Press, 1985).

NUTRITION

S. Boyd Eaton, M. Shostak and M. Conner, *The Paleolithic Prescription* (New York: Harper and Row, 1988).

S. Davies and A. Stewart, *Nutritional Medicine: The Drug-free Guide to Better Family Health* (Pan, 1987).

M. Lesser, *Nutrition and Vitamin Therapy* (Thorsons, 1985).

H. L. Newbold, *Meganutrients for Your Nerves* (New York: Berkeley Publishing Corporation, 1975).

C.C. Pfeiffer, *Zinc and Other Micronutrients* (Connecticut: Keats, 1978).

——, *Mental Illness and Schizophrenia* (Thorsons, 1987).

F. Pottenger, *Pottenger's Cats* (La Mesa, CA: Price-Pottenger Nutrition Foundation, 1983).

J.V. Wright, *Dr Wright's Book of Nutritional Therapy* (Pennsylvania: Rodale Press, 1979).

PHYSICAL FACTORS

P. Bunyard, *Health Guide for the Nuclear Age* (Papermac, 1988).

R. Carson, *Silent Spring* (Penguin Books, 1962).

R. Coghill, *Electro-pollution: How to Protect Yourself Against It* (Thorsons, 1990).

H. Moolenburgh, *Fluoride: The Freedom Fight* (Mainstream Publishing Co, 1987).

M. Shallis, *The Electric Shock Book* (Souvenir Press, 1988).

B. Small, *The Susceptibility Report* (Longueuil, Canada: Deco Books, 1982).

FOR THE DOCTOR

J. C. Breneman, *Basics of Food Allergy* (Springfield, IL: Charles C. Thomas, 1987).

J. Brostoff and S. J. Challacombe, *Food Allergy and Intolerance* (Bailliere Tindall, 1987).

L. D. Dickey (ed.), *Clinical Ecology* (Springfield, IL: Charles C. Thomas, 1976).

J. W. Gerrard (ed.), *Food Allergy: New Perspectives* (1980).

J. B. Miller, *Food Allergies: Provocative Testing and Injection Therapy* (Springfield, IL: Charles C. Thomas, 1972).

W. H. Philpott and D. K. Kalita, *Brain Allergies: The Psychonutrient Connection* (Connecticut: Keats, 1980).

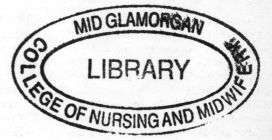

List of Useful Names and Addresses

Several groups and organizations are mentioned in the text. Contact addresses are given below. Others are included as groups of environmental interest.

GROUPS

Action Against Allergy
23–24 High Street,
Hampton Hill,
Middlesex TW1 1PD

National Society for Research into Allergy
PO Box 45,
Hinckley,
Leicestershire

British Nutrition Foundation
15 Belgrave Square,
London SW1X 8PG
Tel: 071–235 4904/9

The McCarrison Society
Honorary Secretary: Miss Pauline Atkin,
23 Stanley Court,
Worcester Road,
Sutton,
Surrey

Medic-alert Foundation
12, Bridge Wharf,
156, Caledonian Road,
London N1 9UI
Tel: 071–833 3034

Complementary Therapies

British Holistic Medical Association
23 Harley House,
Marylebone Road,
London NW1 5HE
Tel: 071–487 4227

British Touch for Health Association
[Kinesiology]
29 Bushey Close,
High Wycombe,
Bucks
Tel: 0494 37409

Institute for Complementary Medicine
PO Box 194,
London SE16 1QZ
Tel: 071–237 5165

Society for Environmental Therapy
Secretary: Mrs Davidson,
521 Foxhill Road,
Ipswich IP3 8LW

Environmentalists

British Ecological Society
Burlington House,
Piccadilly,
London W1V OLQ
Tel: 071–434 2641

Friends of the Earth
26–28 Underwood Street,
London N1 7JQ
Tel: 071–490 1555

Greenpeace Ltd
Canonbury Villas,
London N1 2PN
Tel: 071–354 5100

Disease Support

Arthritis Care
18 Stephenson Way,
London NW1 2HD
Tel: 071–916 1500

British Dyslexia Association
98 London Road,
Reading,
Berks RG1 5AU.
Tel: 0734 668271

British Migraine Association
178a, High Road,
Byfleet,
West Byfleet,
Surrey KT14 7ED
Tel: 0932 352468

Coeliac Society of the United Kingdom
PO Box 220,
High Wycombe,
Bucks HP11 2HY
Tel: 0494 437278

Hyperactive Children's Support Group
Secretary: Sally Bunday,
71, Whyke Lane,
Chichester,
West Sussex PO19 2LD

ME Action Campaign
PO Box 1126,
London W3 0RY

ME Association
P.O. Box 8,
Stanford-Le-Hope,
Essex SS17 8EL

MENCAP (Royal Society for Mentally
Handicapped Children and Adults),
Mencap National Centre,
123 Golden Lane,
London EC1Y 0RT

Multiple Sclerosis Society of Great Britain
and Northern Ireland
25 Effie Road,
Fulham,
London SW6 1EE
Tel: 071–736 6267

National Association for Colitis and Crohn's
Disease
98a London Road,
St Albans,
Herts

National Asthma Campaign
Providence House,
Providence Place,
London N1 0NT
Tel: 071–226 2260
(Formerly Asthma Research Council and
Asthma Society, now combined).

National Eczema Society
4 Tavistock Place,
London WC1H 9RA
Tel: 071–388 4097

Schizophrenia Association of Great Britain
Bryn Hyfryd,
The Crescent,
Bangor,
Gwynedd
LL57 2AG

Seasonal Affective Disorder Association
51 Bracewell Road,
London W10 6AF

Women's Nutritional Advisory Service
(Incorporating the PMT Advisory Service),
Box 268,
Hove,
East Sussex
Tel: 0273 771366

Preconceptual Health

Foresight Association
28 The Paddock,
Godalming,
Surrey GU7 1XD
Tel: 0428 684500

SUPPLIERS

Organic Growers

British Organic Farmers
35a, High Street, Potters Bar,
Herts EN6 5AJ
Tel: 0707 56644

Henry Doubleday Research Association
The National Centre for Organic Gardening,
Ryton-on-Dunsmore,
Coventry CV8 3LG
Tel: 0203 303517

Organic Growers Association
Aeron Park,
Llangeitho,
Tregaron,
Dyfed
Wales
Tel: 0974 23272

Organic Wine Company
PO Box 81,
High Wycombe,
Bucks HP11 1LJ

The Pure Meat Co.
1, The Square,
Moreton Hampstead,
Devon
Tel: 0647 40321

Soil Association
86 Colston Street,
Bristol BS1 5BB
Tel: 0272 29066

ECOLOGICAL PRODUCTS

The Allergy Shop
2 Mount Place,
Lewes,
East Sussex BN7 1YH

Chemico – The Country Chemical
Company Ltd,
553 Stratford Road,
Shirley,
Solihull,
W Midlands B90 4LB
Tel: 0217 442294

Faith Products
52–56 Albion Road,
Edinburgh EH7 5QZ
Tel: 031–661 0900

The Healthy House
Cold Harbour,
Ruscombe,
Stroud GL6 4DA
Superb mail order catalogue.

Little Green Shop
16 Gardner Street,
Brighton,
E Sussex BN1 1UP
Tel: 0273 689011

Natural Therapeutics
25 New Spalding Road,
Lincs PE11 1DJ

Safe House
Ecover, Full Moon Distributions,
Charlton Court Farm,
Mousse Lane,
Steyning,
Sussex BN4 3DG
Tel: 0903 851614

Wholistic Research Company
Bright Haven,
Robin's Lane,
Looworth,
Cambridge CB3 8HH

World of Difference
21 Endell St,
London WC2H 9BJ
Tel: 071–379 8208
Non-toxic paints and SAD lighting

Air Purifiers

National Safety Associates
Basic Elements
Back Sload Farm,
Balkram Edge,
Wainstalls,
Halifax,
N Yorks HX2 0UB

Chelating Multi-vitamins and Minerals

Lambert's
PO Box 1
Tunbridge Wells
Kent

Environmental Control Units

Airedale Allergy Centre
Elmsley Street,
Steeton,
Keighley,
West Yorkshire

Full-spectrum Lighting

Full Spectrum Lighting Ltd,
25 Hanworth Road,
Sunbury-on-Thames,
Middlesex TW16 5DA
Tel: 0932 789700

Truelite SML
Unit 4,
Wye Trading Estate,
London Road,
High Wycombe,
Bucks HP11 1LH

Geopathic Stress

Ecological Design Association
20, High Street,
Stroud GL5 1AS
Tel: 0453 752928

Gaia Environments Ltd,
Managing Director David Pearson,
Umbrella Studios
12, Trundle Street
London SE1 1QT

Geophil Mat
Sanoway International
Boecklinstrasse 90
A-1020 Vienna
Austria

R. Wiggenhauser GmbH
Multipolaris
Lachenweg 15
D7760, Radolphzell
Germany

Greenscreen Charcoal Filter Masks

Greenscreen International Ltd
40 Woodstock Road,
London NW11 8ER
Tel: 071-372 1487

Testing for Parasites

The London Clinic
20 Devonshire Place
London W1N 2DH
Tel: 071-723 6581

Vacuum Cleaning Products

Taylormaid Products Ltd (Medivac)
18a, Water Lane,
Wilmslow,
Cheshire SK9 5AA

GOVERNMENT AGENCIES

Department of the Environment
2 Marsham Street,
London SW1P 3EB
Tel: 071-212 3434

Employment Medical Advisory Service
1 Chepstow Place,
Westbourne Grove,
London W2 4TF
Tel: 071-299 3456

Health and Safety Executive
Regina House,
259 Marylebone Road,
London W1 5RR
Tel: 071-723 1262

FOR HEALTH PROFESSIONALS

British Society for Allergy and
Environmental Medicine
c/o The Burghwood Clinic,
34 Brighton Road,
Banstead,
Surrey SM17 1BS

British Society for Nutritional Medicine
PO Box 3AP,
London W1A 3AP
Tel: 071-436 8532

The Nutrition Society
Chandos House,
2 Queen Anne Street,
London W1N 9LE

USA

Kinesiology
Touch for Health
1174 N. Lake Avenue,
Pasadena, CA 91104

231

Nutrition

Price-Pottenger Nutrition Foundation
PO Box 2614,
La Mesa, CA 92041

Suppliers of Ecological Products

GREENSCREEN CHARCOAL FILTER MASKS

Greenscreen USA
981 1st Ave
New York, New York 10022
Tel: (212) 675–7157

TESTING FOR RADON GAS

Tech/Ops Landauer Inc.
2, Science Road
Glenwood, Illinois 60425–1586
Tel: (312) 755–7911)

Government Agencies

National Institute for Safety and Health
Parklawn Building
5600 Fishers Lane,
Rockville, MD 20857
Tel: (301) 443–2140

Occupational Health and Administration
US Department of Labour,
200 Constitution Avenue, NW
Washington, DC 20210
Tel: (202) 523–8148

For Health Professionals

American Academy of Environmental
Medicine
PO Box 16106,
Denver, CO 80216